An Existential Approach to Interpersonal Trauma

An Existential Approach to Interpersonal Trauma provides a new existential framework for understanding the experiences of interpersonal trauma building on reflections from Marc Boaz's own personal history, clinical insight and research.

The book suggests that psychology, psychotherapy and existentialism do not recognise the significance of the existential movements that occur in traumatic confrontations with reality. By considering what people find at the limits and boundaries of human experiencing, Boaz describes the ways in which they can disillusion and re-illusion themselves, and how this becomes incorporated into their modes of existing in the world and in relation to others. In incorporating the experience of trauma into the way people live – all the existential horror, terror and liberation contained within it – Boaz invites them to embrace an expansive ethic of (re)(dis)covery. This ethic recognises the ambiguity and spectrality of interpersonal trauma, and expands the horizons of our human relationships.

The book provides an important basis for professionals wanting to work existentially with interpersonal trauma and for people wanting to deepen their understanding of the trauma they have experienced.

Marc Boaz is an existential psychotherapist and visiting professor in public mental health at the University of Northampton. He is a founding member of, and policy adviser to, the UK Trauma Council, hosted by the Anna Freud Centre for Children and Families. Marc also serves on the Disability Advisory Committee of the Equality and Human Rights Commission. He focuses on the relationships between philosophy, social policy, practice and lived experience in the fields of disability, mental health, long-term conditions and youth.

An Existential Approach to Interpersonal Trauma

Modes of Existing and Confrontations with Reality

Marc Boaz

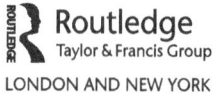

Routledge
Taylor & Francis Group

LONDON AND NEW YORK

Cover image: © Ian Hodgson, 'Marionette', graphite on paper

First published 2022
by Routledge
4 Park Square, Milton Park, Abingdon, Oxon OX14 4RN

and by Routledge
605 Third Avenue, New York, NY 10158

Routledge is an imprint of the Taylor & Francis Group, an informa business

British Library Cataloguing-in-Publication Data
A catalogue record for this book is available from the British Library

Library of Congress Cataloging-in-Publication Data
A catalog record has been requested for this book

ISBN: 978-1-032-02063-1 (hbk)
ISBN: 978-1-032-02060-0 (pbk)
ISBN: 978-1-003-18167-5 (ebk)

DOI: 10.4324/9781003181675

Typeset in Baskerville
by Newgen Publishing UK

Contents

Acknowledgements

My deep appreciation goes to Charlie – for the love, the movement, the wisdom, the joy, the expansion, the journeying and the unknowing. No doubt you will see echoes of the long conversations, moments of discovery and our shared realisations and explorations rippling through the ideas contained in these pages. Without you this book would not be possible. We have lived half our lives growing together, explored the world together, confronted reality apart and together. Each day I am grateful that we continue to find a path alongside one another and create new ways of exploring our connection, love, joy and playfulness.

My deep gratitude goes to my current and previous therapists (Tim, Sabine and Roberta) who have encouraged me in this project of unknowing and growth over the years, and helped me confront and make sense of my own traumatic experiencing. Thanks especially to Sabine for her support and with whom I have explored the themes in this book in depth, and latterly to Tim for continuing to expand my horizons and modal movements as I finished rewriting and editing the manuscript.

I am extremely grateful to all my supervisors (especially Martin Adams, Dani Hecht and Jonathan Rosen) and peers who have supported my clinical practice over the years. My thanks also go to my former supervisor Chloe Paidoussis-Mitchell who provided invaluable reflections on my earlier thinking and articulation of the ideas contained within this book.

The insights and reflections of my clients and colleagues have been a vital source of wisdom and challenge to me as I have developed this manuscript. My heartfelt thanks go to them for the explorations we have shared, movements we have experimented with and realities we have confronted together.

This book remains a tentative contribution to existentialism and psychotraumatology, not least because in many respects, rather than the written word, the ideas and expressions contained within these pages might be better articulated through embodied movement. My thanks go to my movement leaders and teachers for their guidance and holding of growthful and expansive spaces over the years (especially Bodie, Alex, Kate and Emi); and to Kai, Eric, Daan and all the queer spirits who made their way to Berlin, for opening up beautiful, spiritual and magical worlds of intimacy in my life. Further thanks to the AndroTechne artists collective, and Homos and Houmous, for kindly providing the space and opportunities to engage in private and public experimental movement performances – the experimental endeavours have deepened my understandings of modal movement and appreciation of expansive horizons of experiencing.

A special thanks to all my friends and family who have explored the themes in this book with me, discussed and sometimes debated the emerging ideas and provided ongoing encouragement. Thanks especially to Phoebus for the years of close friendship, hours of conversation, tears and laughter, and in memory of the three of us cycling through the empty locked-down streets of London and for the kindness and grace you have always offered.

Finally, my thanks to Daradi Patar, Joanne Forshaw, Sunantha Ramamoorthy and the team at Routledge for all their support and for making this project possible. And especially to my copy editor Leigh Westerfield, and earlier in the process to Kelly Derrick.

Permissions

Portions of Chapter 3 were adapted from *Addressing Adversity* (ISBN 978-1-5272-1946-5), which was co-authored and edited by the author: Bush [Boaz], M. (2018) 'Childhood Adversity and Trauma', in M. Bush [Boaz] (ed.) *Addressing Adversity: Prioritising Adversity and Trauma-Informed Care for Children and Young People in England*. London: YoungMinds/Health Education England, pp. 26–55.

The sections exploring adverse childhood experiences (ACEs) in Chapter 3 build on a seminar presentation given at the Social Science Research Unit (SSRU) of the Institute of Education (UCL) in May 2019. The description of the operations of the triune brain in Chapter 4 is derived from a synthesis compiled in dialogue with clinicians for Bush [Boaz], M. (2017) *Beyond Adversity: Addressing the Mental Health Needs of Young People Who Face Complexity and Adversity in Their Lives*. London: YoungMinds.

Chapters 6 and 8 include partial content redrafted from two recent articles by the author: 'Refractions in Time: A Minkowskian Understanding of Being Dislocated in Time' (2020) and 'Paradox, Polarity and the Pandemic: Making Sense of the Existential Impacts of COVID-19 on People's Lives' (2020), both published in volume 31, issues 1 and 2, of the Society for Existential Analysis (SEA) journal, *Existential Analysis*.

The author thanks the Society for Existential Analysis and YoungMinds for the permission to include redrafted portions of these works in this book.

Introduction

This book is about interpersonal trauma and what it tells us about our human existence. In thinking about interpersonal trauma, it can be difficult to know where to begin. Seemingly, we live in a world where every other situation or life event is labelled 'traumatic' and negative emotions are frequently described as forms of psychological trauma. In the media, academia, online and in everyday conversations, we hear narratives and accounts of psychological trauma and the impacts it can have on people's sense of self and relationships with others. Whole industries have grown up around the identification of psychological trauma, its causes, how to treat it and how to become 'trauma-informed' in our response to it. Increasingly, contemporary discourse makes it harder to discern what the specific features of interpersonal trauma might be; the ways that people respond, adapt and make sense of these adverse experiences; and how their responses might obscure the reality of what people have confronted in their lives. In this book, I invite the reader to pause for a moment, to consider, in more depth, what lived experiences of interpersonal trauma can disclose about the foundations of our human existence.

I originally trained as a sociologist and ethnographer. I researched intensely in and among the everyday worlds of people situated in the environments in which they lived and worked. Over the years I have had the benefit of speaking to many people about their experiences of interpersonal trauma, and how they have made sense of it. These encounters have taught me the importance of engaging with personal philosophy and the ways we attempt to make meaning for ourselves, in relation to others and the world around us. Additionally, I have journeyed through structuralism, postmodernism, interactionism and various forms of realism in my life as an academic, social policy negotiator, advocate and researcher. Inevitably the residue of these explorations is present throughout this book.

The creation of this book is, in itself, a process of making sense of my own traumatic experiences. It is part of cultivating a *new mode of existing*; a way of relating to others that extends beyond my own traumatic experiencing. It constitutes part of what the psychiatrists Judith Herman (2015 [1992]) and Irvin Yalom (1980) might describe as a form of personal activism. By personal activism, they mean a life project that helps us find meaning, purpose, *movement* and healing in the world. I hope that the explorations and reflections in these pages provide insight

DOI: 10.4324/9781003181675-1

for others who have experienced interpersonal trauma, and more broadly contribute to continued debate in the fields of existentialism and psychotraumatology about the fundamental structure of human existence.

So where do I begin this work? At this early stage of the book, Martin Adams, the personable and ever-pragmatic existential psychotherapist, might kindly suggest: 'You could start anywhere and we will find our way to a beginning'. In supervisions with Martin, he encourages me to be open to all the different ways a beginning can present itself. At times, he has suggested that 'we are never really caught in a circular thought; each rotation is like a spiral, a new path. And with each and every turn we take, we get new understandings and perspectives'. He tells me that we can start at any point of the spiral, and as we continue to delve backwards, or surge forwards, we will see what has gone before, where we are now and sense what might emerge in the future.

So, by way of introduction, I will start with a description of a brief encounter I had along my path for greater understanding, a quest for deeper knowledge about the nature of interpersonal trauma, and the way it impacts our lives. From there we will find our way to the other reasons I am writing this work, and what I found in my inquiries.

What do you mean by 'trauma'?

I found myself sitting nervously in the waiting room of a sexual health clinic, waiting to be seen by a psychosexual psychotherapist. I had recently finished having therapy for over three years with a tender and insightful integrative psychotherapist. As much as I would have loved to continue working with her, she was heavily pregnant, and we continued towards what was a good ending. Sitting in this cold, clinical and yet friendly waiting room was a world away from the soft furnishings, scent of incense and warm lighting I had grown accustomed to as a therapeutic environment.

I sought psychosexual psychotherapy as I felt I had made significant progress in understanding my experiences of sexual trauma and wanted to take brave steps towards making a greater commitment to human connection, joy and ease in my life. The mists of my dissociation were finally clearing, and I could see on the horizon the beauty that closer and more intimate relationships could offer me. The world was feeling less like a continuous threat, and I was softening into it.

My name was called by a woman a little older than I. Let's call her *Keres*. She invited me into her office, introduced herself and took some preliminary, factual details about me and my circumstances. She informed me that her approach was based on 'her own unique version' of cognitive behavioural therapy (CBT), and that it would be very directive and confronting. I responded by telling her that I had had to confront so many things in my life already, so more confrontation with reality through our relationship would be very welcome.

Keres asked, 'So tell me about this sexual dysfunction'. She was right, she was very direct, though the way she pronounced and used the word 'dysfunction' took me aback. Keres continued, 'You didn't like that, did you?' Still a little stunned, and having hardly spoke until now, I cautiously replied that I didn't feel I was there to speak about a 'dysfunction'. For me it was more about finding a greater understanding about the impact that sexual trauma had had on my sexual relationships and forms of intimacy.

Keres looked quizzical and pointed to the screen behind her (we were in a room usually used for sexual health testing). She said, 'It says here your GP has referred you for a "sexual dysfunction"?' Again I stared at her and laughed nervously. She nodded and continued, 'Tell me about that'. I almost choked while trying to swallow her words. A little intimidated, I heard myself say more distantly, 'I'm not experiencing a dysfunction. I need to talk to you about my sexual trauma and the impact it's having on my sexuality, the way I relate to people'. Evidently changing tack, Keres asked, 'What sexual trauma?' I went on to briefly describe enduring harmful sexual behaviour and rape from a male peer in my childhood. I stopped, moved in my seat, looked at Keres, studied her face and waited for her response.

After about 20 seconds, though what seemed like an eternity to me, Keres retorted, 'So where is the sexual trauma in what you've said?' I was astounded, unable to speak. I stared at her blankly, feeling myself dissociate. The walls around me become animated in movement and I thought I was going to faint. Keres coolly continued, 'It's normal for boys to experiment, so that isn't trauma'. I was so out of my body, it was hard to concentrate on her. Only her lips seemed to be in dialogue with me; it was like her presence had left her body too. 'It's normal ... that isn't trauma' repeated over and over again in my mind. I had spent most of my childhood and adult life dissociated from the world around me, at great cost. I had spent years in therapy slowly and carefully making sense of these experiences. It had taken me years to recognise what constituted interpersonal violence and rape, and here I was being negated. What I had come to know of my world and what I had experienced was being totally invalidated by Keres's 'It's normal'.

I brought to mind my previous therapist, the hours she had spent holding me as I had made sense of the experience of violence, the impact it had on my sense of my body, the distance I created between myself and others, the projects of survival I had engaged in. I summoned all the strength and courage I had and mustered a reply: 'My understanding is that if it isn't consensual and it involved significant coercion, public humiliation and ...' Keres interrupted with, 'How do you know it wasn't consensual?' I stared at her. It was a serious question. From that moment on, I was gone; I nodded my head politely, she delivered vague psycho-educative messages, I agreed when she scheduled the next meeting, and smiled when she shook my hand.

I walked out of her room, down the stairs and out onto the bustling street. I breathed deeply, touched my face, shook my head, my body trembling with rage and shock, and never returned. With the chorus of 'It's normal ... that isn't trauma', ringing in my ears, I was spurred on to find another psychotherapist, this time an existential psychotherapist.

Purpose of this book

What I mean by trauma is a fundamental focus of this book. The psychological and philosophical investigation I set out in these pages is grounded in the many years I have spent working in mental health, before and since sitting in that room with Keres. It draws on my personal experience, my academic work and insights from the people I have talked to about their lived experiences of interpersonal trauma. I have had the benefit of speaking with so many different people while working professionally in research, policy and practice change across the fields of disability, youth, health and mental health.

The forms of interpersonal trauma I have spoken to people about vary significantly: from familial and institutional neglect and abuse; to hate crime and harassment; to domestic and partner violence; to rape and sexual violence; to bullying, victimisation and gang membership; to torturous, inhuman and degrading treatment. While all very different and distinct in their nature, experience and response, I have discerned commonalities across them, which seem to illuminate fundamental features of human relating. In this book, I will seek to describe an existential framework for understanding experiences of interpersonal trauma, and the impacts on ourselves, our relationships with others and the world around us. Specifically, I will focus on the commonalities in experiences of these various forms of interpersonal trauma.

To do this, I will describe the dominant and contemporary psychological and psychotherapeutic understandings of trauma. Some of the terms used do not always translate well to existentialist frames (i.e. dissociation, somatisation, defences etc.). For the purposes of conceptual coherence, I retain the terms and formulations used by the literature base I am drawing upon throughout this work. Latterly, I will introduce, and then apply, my own terms or those I am reinterpreting or reconceptualising from wider existentialist thought.

Using the psychological and psychotherapeutic literature as a basis of common understanding, I will turn to the existential and phenomenological contributions to explore conceptions of trauma within the existing literature base. Emerging from this exploration, I will propose a new existential framework for understanding what I will term *traumatic experiencing*. Having established the existential features of traumatic experiencing, I will more fully delve into the phenomenon and consider it from a number of existential and thematic perspectives, to build a more descriptive, multidimensional understanding of the proposed model.

Meanings of trauma

Definitions of trauma have varied significantly over time, cultures and societies. Broadly, the word 'trauma' (τραῦμα) was used by the ancient Greeks to refer to a *wound*. This is primarily meant to be a physical wound and was routed in the word to 'pierce' (τιτροσχω). Most notably, the founding father of psychoanalysis, Sigmund Freud, used the term 'trauma' to describe the piercing of a traumatic situation (such as war, sexual violence or an accident) into the psychic world of a person. Joseph Breuer and Sigmund Freud (1982 [1908]) noted a number of ways that this 'trauma' creates psychic wounds in the perceptions, memories, relationships and dreams of their patients. The rapid growth of contemporary psychiatry and psychology saw the popularisation of definitions of trauma, which put an emphasis on enduring and complex physic wounds.

Many Western academics, clinicians, professionals and laypeople continue to use this definition of psychic wounding as a common consensus. That said, there remains a substantive use of the word 'trauma' in everyday parlance, to refer to the actual situation, event or enactment someone has faced, rather than its psychological or emotional impact upon them. This dualistic external/internal locale of trauma is frequently *bridged* by a recognition of the dialogic nature between the traumatic situation and traumatic psychological wounds. In that, it is the person who has the wound, who has been wounded – *or in the case of intergenerational trauma has been proximate to those wounding and/or wounded.*

This bridge is further articulated in the various post-traumatic phenomena that are described within *psychotraumatology*. These could include medically unexplainable somatic pain, sexual dysfunction, maladaptive daydreaming and significant aversion or nausea when exposed to specific textures, smells, sounds or tastes. In exploring the ways that people exhibit the consequences of their 'psychic trauma', psychotraumatologists recognise the dialogue between the traumatic experiences – the psychic wounds – and the impact of the interactions between these on people's experiences of themselves, their emotional worlds and the world of others.

For me, the notion of 'trauma' defined fundamentally as a psychic wound feels problematic – even if we use contemporary bridges to transcend a dualistic notion of external/internal wounding. Existentially, I feel there is a simultaneous binding up of the situation and person(s) within trauma, which is more fundamental, complex and ambiguous than just a physic or emotional consequence, or the physical manifestations. In the case of interpersonal trauma, the people involved are inextricably entangled within the encounter. Their entanglement will be a theme within my exploration in this book, and I will consider what it means for our existential understanding of the experience(s) of trauma.

Likewise, the idea that there is an ahistoric universality in the events, actions or encounters that constitute a traumatic situation is problematic for me. Having a background in sociology, human rights and childhood studies, it would be remiss of me not to explicitly note the moment in time that I am writing this work. This moment in time contains specific conceptions of the interpersonal actions that constitute a traumatic situation. Being located within the United Kingdom means that the inquiry is written from a primarily Western and European perspective of what a traumatic situation is composed of. While I draw on studies from around the world, and various cultural standpoints, these are nevertheless being rendered through a European philosophical tradition and mobilised within the operations of these systems of thought. It will be for the reader to note this and make their own judgement as to whether this becomes a limitation or point of contrast for them in the examination that will ensue.

Let us consider what 'traumatic situations' might describe from the moment in time in which I am writing. Having spent much of my professional career in social policy advocating for institutional reform, I remain despairing that a wide variety of state and independent organisations harboured and buried the realities of intentional and systemic physical, sexual and emotional abuse of children, when they were meant to be a place of safety for them (Independent Inquiry into Child Sexual Abuse, 2018). That it took until 2004 for the UK government to remove the defence of 'reasonable chastisement' from parents who corporally punished their children astounds me (s. 58 Children Act [2004]; following ECHR [1997] *A. v. UK*). The fact that smacking remains legal in England at the time of writing, seems to me a dismissal of children's human value and personhood.

For me, it is somewhat horrifying to realise that it is only within *recent* history that rape within marriage was deemed an illegal and criminal act in the United Kingdom (*R v R* [1991] UKHL 12; *R v R* [1991] 3 WLR 767; Sexual Offences Act 2003), and that it remains permissible in many societies around the world. It feels like progress to me that (at the time of writing) the extension of the definition of, and protections against, 'domestic abuse' is currently being considered by the UK Parliament, and especially that it gives additional prominence to the economic, psychological, emotional forms and to the existence of controlling or coercive behaviour (Domestic Abuse Bill 2020). However, it has been concerning to read of the rise in reporting of domestic violence (ONS, 2020) and child sexual abuse (NSPCC, 2020) cases resulting from the lockdowns and social isolation due to the 2020 COVID-19 pandemic.

We need only look back a generation to see that in Britain's recent past we pathologised and criminalised communities, and allowed for the permittance of state-sanctioned torture and inhuman and degrading treatment (Drescher, 2009). I am personally filled with disgust when I recall the ways in which psychiatrists and psychologists were instrumental in the sanctioned chemical castration of gay men (Hodges, 2014 [1983]). Further, I am rageful that despite progress (Anton, 2010; NHS England et al., 2015; Policing and Crime Act [2017]), sadly today a small minority of misguided therapists and faith-based healers continue to advocate for humiliating and torturous so-called conversion treatments.

The harrowing treatment just described is not an exhaustive list of all contextual changes in our recent understanding of what constitutes an interpersonal, traumatic situation. Rather, the examples here are included by way of illustration. I am highlighting that these ways of being and acting towards one another are, and were, permissible to lesser and greater degrees in the near past. Many of the listed ways of relating to each other are still seen as normative and fully permissible in other countries and cultures today; this is despite the plethora of international conventions from the United Nations and World Health Organisation monitoring, prohibiting and sanctioning the offending States.

You may be wondering by this point, what I mean by the term 'interpersonal trauma'. By 'interpersonal' I mean the direct relationships, (inter)actions and encounters between two or more people, which are experienced as traumatic (consciously or non-consciously) by at least one of the people involved. The use of 'direct' here denotes an actual contact or connection between these persons, whether or not they are 'known' to each other. This definition would include acts, actions and relations that we describe as neglect of a child or adult; child, peer and domestic abuse (including emotional, psychological, physical, sexual forms, controlling, humiliating and coercive behaviour, grooming, gang membership); physical or sexual violence (including rape, assault, attacks, people trafficking); torture, inhuman and degrading treatment (including some culturally specific practices such as female genital mutilation). This is in contrast to trauma resulting from environmental or natural disasters, acts of war or terrorism, major emergencies or crises, or indeed global pandemics like COVID-19.

The interpersonal forms of trauma can occur within the family, online communities, relationships and institutions by state sanctioning or opportunistically within a given context. The majority of my discussion in this work is primarily focused on child neglect; child, peer and domestic abuse; and physical, emotional or sexual violence. That said, in places I do draw upon other forms of interpersonal trauma. With some reticence I have included traumatic bereavement within elements of the discussion. This was on the encouragement of other clinicians and professionals whom I shared earlier drafts of this work with. They suggested that the themes and conceptual concerns I develop in the coming pages could apply to traumatic bereavement, although I continue to believe that a more substantive treatment of this is warranted as a stand-alone work. *Ultimately, for me, the existential features I present are equally applicable across all forms of interpersonal trauma.*

Finally, this work is not a stance on the morality of traumatic interpersonal actions, nor is it a treaty on the origins of threats and enactments of violence towards other people. The relevance of mentioning this definition of interpersonal trauma, and framing it within recent social categorisations and reforms, is to draw readers' attention to the changing notions within a given society of what interpersonal trauma means over time. This goes to demonstrate both the ever-changing ideas about what a traumatic situation is, and its significant variance across different societies, cultures and systems. The socio-historical constructions of interpersonal trauma have important legal, ethical and personal meanings for people and the systems they live within. They help us individually and collectively understand what is permissible within any given society, and what is deemed to be intentional harm-inducing behaviour.

This book is not a sociolegal critique of these constructions, nor does it advocate for the removal or reform of categories of illegality or harm. Rather, I am delving within the categories to understand the complexities and nuances of what we can say of interpersonal trauma in philosophical, psychological and experiential terms. Further, as I cannot escape the historical moment in which I am writing this text, my intention is to tease out an existential understanding of interpersonal trauma, which enables us to see what these experiences disclose about the foundations our human existence.

Confrontations with reality

In this book I will argue that what we call 'trauma' would more usefully be thought of, and described, in terms of a movement, that is, a movement towards a confrontation with both the reality of a traumatic situation and the basis of our human existence. Further, trauma defined in this way is not just a movement towards and within the confrontation, but also the movement beyond and in the wake of the confrontation. I will go on to describe this movement as the modes of existence that we embrace in an attempt to respond to our confrontations with reality. It is significant here to note that in the case of interpersonal trauma, the confrontation is not necessarily chosen nor does it necessarily arise from spontaneity or opportunity. This gives the modes of movement – the forms of confrontation – specific qualities, and these qualities are also the subject of inquiry in this book.

With this emerging definition in mind, you may be considering how this sense of confrontation with reality resonates with me, as the author of this work and someone who has himself experienced interpersonal trauma. Rollo May reminds us of the important relationship between lived experience and the generation of new philosophical investigations, explorations and elaborations. He writes: 'There is not authentic experience without a concept, and there is not vital concept without experience. The concept gives form to the experience; but the experience had to be present to give content and vitality to the concept' (May, 1972: 77). With this in mind, I turn briefly to my own experience.

I was born into a family still making sense of intergenerational and cultural trauma (the Holocaust), and in the close wake of a significant familial bereavement and distress. My early years included being surrounded by attachment figures navigating significant traumatic loss and grief. In my mid-childhood I experienced harmful sexual behaviour and rape by a male peer. These experiences endured over time, with an increasing level of control and coercion used to ensure compliance and maintain silence. Later on (in early adolescence), these experiences included acts of public inhuman, degrading treatment and humiliation. This period was defined by enduring and significant feelings of threat, fright, horror, terror, stress, disorientation and shame. All of these feelings were deepened by my emerging sexual identity: witnessing the death, illness and the survival of my lesbian, gay, bisexual, transgender and queer or questioning (LGBTQ) community during the AIDS crisis; experiencing the state-sponsored stigmatisation and criminalisation of homosexuality in the United Kingdom; and the resulting threats of harm that I was confronted with by my peers at school and in the communities in London in which I lived. While there have been other challenging experiences in subsequent years, the echoes of these ones, and the ways in which I responded to them over time, have had a foundational impact on my life, my relationship with myself and with others.

Understandably, from childhood I began to develop a sense of unreality. The lines between the 'real' and 'unreal' became blurred for me. Clinically defined as forms of dissociation, I experienced a world and a self filled with derealised phenomena. I lived in a material world that was in animated contact with me, which only heightened my sense of terror and stress. In later childhood and adolescence, I constructed complex ways of convening with, entering into dialogue with and mitigating the forces (mainly water elements) of the animating spirits I was perceiving. The significant ideation around self-injury (more prominent) and suicidality led to a number of expressions and enactments during childhood, and a brief moment of hospitalisation when I was 19.

I also experienced flashbacks, maladaptive daydreams, panic attacks and night terrors. Associated with this was significant somatisation, including shaking, numbness in certain parts of my body, (later) psychogenic seizures and anhedonia (especially in relation to sexual contact). The chronic experience of stress triggered a greater expression of an underlying genetic condition that continues to impact my peripheral nerves to this day.

Through studying and working in disability, health, mental health, social policy and justice causes, I found meaning, purpose and a way of making sense of my own traumatic experiences. That said, this continued to perpetuate my mode of surviving in complex and challenging environments. Entering individual psychotherapy, and with the loving understanding and support of my partner, I better understood the impact that these experiences had on my life and acquired new ways of relating to myself, other people and the world around me. Establishing, and committing to, movement practices (initially judo, then yoga, dance and improvised movement) enabled creative exploration of my traumatic embodiment, and facilitated new ways of experiencing pleasure, joy and creativity through the movement through space and time.

Finding new movements within the confrontation of reality, and in existing in the wake of it, have inspired me to find my way back to myself, others and the world around me. Movement is a fundamental mode of our existence; it is part of our animation, experience of time and space and relationality with our world. For this reason, movement has become a core lens through which I have come to understand and make sense of interpersonal trauma and its existential dimensions. As an existentialist, I believe we remain in a state of perpetual becoming, and as such my movements are far from over. It is not that I have *recovered* from my experience of trauma; rather, it is more the case that my movements now incorporate my experiences and I am able to explore more expansive modes of existing.

Ontological status of trauma

Before the substantive inquiry begins, it feels important to situate this book within a broader philosophical concern, one that perhaps goes to the heart of Keres's dismissive comment that 'it's normal … that isn't trauma', and to the dentition of what 'trauma' could be.

Within existentialism, there is an ongoing debate about what trauma is, and the extent to which it relates to the fundamental basis of our human existence. Alice Holzhey-Kunz (2016) advocates for the differentiation between two forms of trauma.[1] As a Daseinsanalyst, she draws on the work of the existential philosopher Martin Heidegger to describe 'ontic' and 'ontological' forms of trauma.

By ontic, she means traumas that are contingent on the 'concrete possibilities and limitations' of our lived experiences and circumstances (ibid.: 17). In contrast, ontological trauma is seen as an 'unshielded exposure to [...] the human condition in its pure facticity' (ibid.: 18). What she wants to draw our attention to, is that one (ontic trauma) derives from 'a horrible' (to put it lightly) experience, and another arises from a 'special sensitivity for the ontological truth' (ibid.: 21).

Holzhey-Kunz's formulation is understandable. She is concerned that 'trauma' is increasingly being seen in clinical and philosophical terms as relating purely to a tangible, known or knowable threat, or catastrophic event, which causes the person significant (and possibly enduring) psychological distress. This is reflected in her formulation of a 'concreteness' to the ontic experience of interpersonal trauma (ibid.: 18) – *an assertion that I will seek to problematise within this book.* Her paper attempts to bring our awareness to the possibility that there is another group of people who experience trauma. These are people who have *not* experienced a traumatic event or situation but have been confronted with the realities of the human condition, and they could find this confrontation itself traumatising at an ontological level.

For me, there is something unsound and unsettling about her attempt to differentiate between ontic and ontological forms of trauma. If we were to follow her line of argument, we would unnecessarily or unwittingly create a hierarchal dynamic in the study and understanding of trauma. Much of her argument draws on Kierkegaardian or Heideggerian notions of an existential 'angst' (as opposed to an ontic anxiety/fear), and that this results in an ontological traumatisation (ibid.: 19–22). In doing so, Holzhey-Kunz seemingly sets aside interpersonal and other forms of trauma as something lesser, not worthy of a substantive ontological analysis.

Her comparison between an ontic fear and ontological angst is misleading. As this book will explain, what we might think of as ontic fear, might actually be manifestations of existential horror and terror. This can involve a deep confrontation with what Holzhey-Kunz calls an ontological trauma in the confrontation of our existence. What she calls 'ontic fear', in the context of interpersonal trauma, is so much more than that. It is greater than a 'fear of something or someone perceived as dangerous' (ibid.: 19); it transcends the anticipation of a specific something or someone, and enters the realm of horrific and terrifying confrontations at an ontological level.

This is where Holzhey-Kunz's differentiation is philosophically, psychotherapeutically and practically unhelpful. Using her terms, it pits people who experience this 'special sensitivity' (angst resulting from non-trauma-based psychoses and neuroses) against those who have ('horrible' ontic) experiences. Further, it communicates the notion that this 'special sensitivity' to ontological questioning is a more authentic or pure form of confrontation with the foundations of our existence. The so-called specialness seems to ignore the encultured embodiment of our lives, and the many social, environmental and interpersonal factors that might cultivate or stifle this special sensitivity. Moreover, it does not account for the high probability that people who would otherwise have this 'special sensitivity' are also thrown into confrontation with this existential questioning because of the contingencies of their traumatic (ontic) lived experience.

There is an interesting parallel here of the experience of many victims of interpersonal trauma. There is a parallel here with the silencing and dismissiveness of psychological and social systems around the experiences of interpersonal trauma. Historically psychological and social disciplines created permissive cultures where the realities of actual traumatic experiences were dismissed, to give way to generalities of theoretical and practice elaboration. Perhaps the best-known example is Sigmund Freud's abandoning of the seduction thesis (c.f. Freud, 1909); a change of heart that resulted in the very real experiences of child sexual abuse and rape, of girls and young women, initially being written out of mainstream psychiatric, psychological and psychotherapeutic understandings and practices at the time.

Philosophically, psychologically and practically, would it not suffice to say that we all have the potential to be confronted with the realities of our existence? Further, would it be not more useful to hypothesise that there is something about the ontic/ontological nature of interpersonal trauma, which creates *specific kinds of movements towards and through the confrontation*? This will be the argument I will pursue. Somewhat confusingly, Holzhey-Kunz (2016: 26) almost recognises this herself, noting that even ontic trauma can simultaneously disclose something greater than the immediate and contingent experiences of trauma, namely an ontological traumatisation, although this is then subsumed back into her differentiation between the two forms. Subsuming interpersonal trauma into the generalities of human suffering, or diminishing it as 'purely ontic', fails to recognise what it discloses about *specific realities of our existence*.

Overview of this book

This book is a form of movement. It is an attempt to find new ways of describing what is found at the boundaries of human experiencing, and what this discloses about the structure of our existence. At times I weave between philosophical, psychotherapeutic, experiential and personal discussions. Professionally and academically I have always been queer – that is, existing-between-worlds – caught between the worlds of conceptual and applied philosophy, of structural policy reform and clinical practice change, of sociology and psychology, of insider and outsider research, of the system and a so-called maverick beyond it, of static writing and improvised movement, to name but a few. My discussion in this book follows the weaving between these worlds, attempting to use the orientations and disorientations to find new insights and glimpses at the nature of human experiencing. I hope the reader will join me on the meandering between these different worlds, to consider what I have found, and perhaps begin to formulate their own understandings.

I draw on insight from philosophy, sociology, psychology and psychotherapy in an attempt to understand a new existentialism of traumatic experiencing. The reader, depending on their own orientation or interest, will find my approach either irritating or liberating. Irritating because I am less concerned with philosophical coherence. I focus on moving across, in between and within different traditions to find ways of describing and making sense of experiences and the structure of our existence. Liberating because at heart I am transdisciplinary and pluralistic, allowing more fluid moments between knowing and unknowing than many traditions allow for.

Ultimately, I believe that the structure of our existence is unintelligible to the human mind; we lack the means (even with human-created augmentations) to fully comprehend it. As such, our individual and collective experience is our primary means of exploring our reality, through which we can infer structures of our human existence.[2] Turning away from Holzhey-Kunz's Heideggerian analysis in this book will allow us to see that there are specific ontological (existential) dimensions to (so-called) ontic trauma. These existential features reach beyond the familiar themes of finitude and nothingness and emerge from the specific confrontations disclosed in the realities of interpersonal trauma.

I begin by describing early and contemporary psychiatric, psychological and psychotherapeutic understandings of interpersonal trauma. This includes a consideration of the genesis of major Westernised ideas of psychological trauma from the twentieth century forwards. The intention is to ground the reader in the dominant frameworks and foundational texts, in order to identify the existential and paradoxical features contained within them. My analysis then turns to considering what existentialists have written about human suffering and more specifically interpersonal trauma. Having reviewed the major philosophical and psychological contributions, I set out a new existential framework describing the way in which traumatic experiences constitute confrontations with the reality of human existence. The framework of traumatic experiencing is considered in depth from different existential perspectives, including our embodiment, time, space, identity and relationships with others. This leads me to describe and explore the ambiguities of interpersonal trauma, and the spectral, liminal and queer movements and qualities that emerge from these features of our existence. Within this inquiry, I consider the existential horror emerging, and the terror arising out of, traumatic confrontations with reality. The work concludes with an application of my existential framework to working with interpersonal trauma psychotherapeutically. I distinguish between psychotherapeutic movements of (re)covery, (dis)covery, and (re)(dis)covery. In doing so, I advocate for the establishment of communication on the horizon, which allows for specific modes of inquiry into traumatic confrontations with reality. Further, I describe an existential attitude of courage that enables us to confront both the traumatic reality we have experienced and the existential movements we have made to incorporate the confrontation. Finally, I briefly turn to note the value of psychotherapeutic awe and wonderment, alongside curiosity, in opening up new horizons of experiencing and modes of existing.

In the drafting of this work I have been asked whether this is a theory or practice book. During the course of writing, my response has been that it is both a theory and practice book, and about theory and practice. The ambiguity of my answer remains even with the book complete. In one sense it is all about theory and practice and how we might find queer turns between and within contemporary fields of psychotraumatology. In another sense, this is the culmination of my own inquiries to date, and as an existentialist I believe we are always in a state of emergence and becoming. So, in another way, this is a longer articulation of my own paths to understanding and where I find myself on my own philosophical and personal journey at this moment in time.

As a reader, I would ask that you critically engage with what I have written in this book. As the title suggests, here I set out one approach to working existentially with interpersonal trauma. My account is purposefully non-Heideggerian, though inevitably his influence on the genesis of existentialism will be present and sensed by those who know his work. In developing a new approach, I hope to synthesise what has already been formulated existentially about interpersonal trauma and use this synthesis to provide an alternative way of working psychotherapeutically with clients. The reader will ultimately be the judge of the success of this intention.

When examining my own line of inquiry, descriptions and suggestions in this book, you might want to follow the existential aphorism of the philosopher and theologian Jon Macquarrie. Macquarrie (1972: 26) proposes that 'the test is to compare the description offered with our own first-hand understanding of existence […] and the phenomena themselves as we have access to them'. This is a tentative contribution to existentialism and psychotraumatology, and Macquarrie offers wise words indeed for any reader or practitioner engaging with this text.

Notes

1 Based on an important lecture, originally given to the World Congress for Existential Therapy in London in May 2015.
2 Having studied under Professor Margaret Archer, some might sense the spectral remnants of critical realism within this work (not least where I borrow some of Archer's terminology).

Part I

Early and contemporary psychotraumatology

1 Early psychiatric and psychoanalytic psychotraumatology

In this chapter, I set out for the reader some of the dominant earlier understandings of 'trauma' within the fields of psychiatry, neuroscience and clinical psychology. Rather than a full sociohistorical analysis of the genesis of knowledge and practice in these professions, I will give a description of some of the foundational constructions of psychological trauma. As we will come to see, within these disciplines, the term 'trauma' has been used in various ways to describe the lasting impacts that specific experiences have on people's psychological and emotional worlds.

I have gone back to some of what are considered to be the foundational ideas and texts within interpersonal psychotraumatology to explore their notions of what constitutes psychological trauma. I will focus primarily on the literature relating to developmental, childhood and sexual trauma, which are the areas I have researched in more depth previously. Where possible, I have left out substantive discussion of intra-psychic processes and mechanisms, as it can detract from the focus of our inquiry and create an unnecessary complexity that does not translate well across the different approaches presented.

This close reading of the original texts is not exhaustive, but provides sufficient grounding for my later discussion. Inevitably, having done my training and research in the United Kingdom, the majority of works are taken from European and British schools of psychiatry, psychology and psychotherapy, with wider contributions from international schools, where they are based on European or British traditions. Further, I have included the writers and texts that either I have been exposed to through my own training, supervision or teaching, or that I have sought out to help make sense of my own experiences or those of my clients in the therapy room.

The ideas presented in what follows will provide an initial orientation and context for the analysis and discussion in subsequent chapters that investigate a more existential approach. I hope those readers who are new to the world of psychotraumatology, or who are looking to refresh or deepen their knowledge, will find these pages a useful navigation and summary of what is a colossal literature base in the recent founding works on psychological trauma. Those readers who are well versed on these works may want to meander their way through the

DOI: 10.4324/9781003181675-3

following initial discussion and head towards the next chapter to explore what I see to be the emerging paradoxes that are disclosed across this canon.

Pierre Janet: emotional shock and the disaggregation of ideas

Let us begin with a near history of the partial genesis of 'trauma' within the fields of neurology, psychiatry and psychology.[1] Neurology was thriving in the late 1800s in Europe, with significant interest being given to the governance and disciplining of people's behaviours, minds and nervous systems (following Foucault, 2009 [1961]). By the start of the century, attention, within the growing field of neurology, turned to what were seen to be medically unexplainable symptoms. Neurology more specifically marked a rationalist search for medically unexplainable physical symptoms. Neurologists attempted to move away from explanations of witchcraft, spirit possession and mesmerism (Porter, 1985), towards understandings of an underlying neuropathology as the basis of the phenomenon of 'hysteria' (Tasca et al., 2012).

In France, social reform was spearheaded by Philippe Pinel (1806), who instigated a transformation in the models of care delivered at both the Bicêtre and La Salpêtrière Hospitals (then asylums) in Paris. Initially, it was Paul Briquet (1859) who undertook a decade-long detailed evaluation of 430 cases of hysteria at the Hôpital de la Charité in Paris. This important study shifted understandings of hysteria and relocated the origins of medically unexplainable symptoms (in women) from their wombs to their brains and neurological functioning.

The renowned French clinician Jean-Martin Charcot (1873; see also Micale, 1985) worked at La Salpêtrière, which was a teaching hospital in Paris. His clinical observations were instrumental in investigating unexplainable physical presentations of seizure, paralysis, fainting, shaking and other somatic phenomena. Charcot's inquiry eventually led him to the conclusion that these 'hysterical', unexplainable symptoms had their roots in people's emotional responses to traumatic experiences. In this, Charcot suggests that the way that his patients emotionally made sense of their experiences of traumatic events is at the heart of the unexplained symptoms.

The French psychiatrist Pierre Janet studied under Charcot at La Salpêtrière, initially following his own interest in hypnosis, catalepsy and altered states of consciousness. Like Charcot, Janet recognised the reality of traumatic life events in his patients' lives. He noted that 'the various symptoms of hysteria' that he and his contemporaries were describing were 'not spontaneous manifestations, idiopathic of the disease', but rather had a 'close connection with the provocative trauma' (Janet, 1901: 496). Building on the work of Charcot, Janet similarly suggests that it is the emotional consequences of traumatic experiences that render them traumatic. As such, he focuses on the emotional shock of these events, and its impact on people's ideas about themselves, others and their environment (ibid.: 320, 375).

Janet suggests that it is this emotional shock that affects people's memories of lived events and prevents them from being able to behaviourally adapt to stressful lived experiences, and their potential reoccurrence in the future (ibid.: 150, 203, 230, 249, 461). Importantly, Janet demonstrates how this emotional shock overwhelms the person and exposes them to intense feelings of 'sad[ness], despai[r]; continual weariness, disgust of life, fear, terrors, extreme despair [...] [and] bursts of wild cheeriness [that] are merely accidents' (ibid.: 213).

Reflecting on his patients' emotional states of 'monotonous sadness', Janet suggests that they have 'lost a will and sentiment, and they are disgusted with their miserable existence' (ibid.: 213–214). This formulation begins to give us a sense of Janet's understanding that the emotional consequences of a traumatic event have a substantive impact on the person's attitude towards themselves and commitment to action in their lives. The emotional shock, he writes, can lead to 'mental accidents', which include the 'accidental phenomena [...] of impulsions and fixed ideas' (ibid.: 198–199).

Heim and Bühler (2006: 113) explain that for Janet, 'ideas' are not 'abstract thought', but rather 'a given psychological experience that includes [...] memories [...] emotions as well as various responses to persistent emotional influences'. They contend that for Janet, thoughts and experiences are part of a reflexive structure, which enables us to consciously synthesise the internalised experiences of our world, and results in more complex emotional and behavioural responses (ibid.). The 'special element' that is affected by the emotional shock of traumatic events, is the ability to create and retain new ideas (Janet, 1901: 199–200).

Janet suggests that the synthesis of new ideas into existing or older ones is disrupted in many ways, including through the use of an *exaggeration*. An exaggeration is an 'immense development', where an old idea remembered, or a new idea formed, loses its original context and becomes dreamlike and/or substantively abstracts from reality (ibid.: 200–201). Putnam (1989) suggests that Janet's identification of exaggerations is an early development of dissociation being on a continuum of normative and psychopathological responses to everyday life and traumatic experiencing.

Janet (1901: 202) continues that abstracted new ideas, or remembered old ideas, can 'pass before us like the colours of a kaleidoscope', and while seemingly incoherent, they have a 'certain vague unity about them'. This 'vague unity' suggests for Janet that the patients do not incorporate and synthesise the memories or new ideas. Rather, people gloss over these ideas, or relate them back to a circular or 'monotonous story' about themselves, others or their lives (ibid.). van der Kolk and van der Hart (1989: 1533) note Janet's astute identification of this phenomenon in his patients, and the ways in which this kept them attached to the emotional shock of the traumatic event.

Rather than connecting to the present moment, these patients 'no longer know how to adapt the present to the future, and in their lack of forethought, they, so to speak, confine human existence to the present moment' (Janet, 1901: 203). For Janet, there are two core conditions that result in so-called mental accidents resulting from a traumatic event. The first is the localisation of psychological and somatic phenomena 'according to the laws of emotion', which in this case is the emotional shock of the traumatic event (Janet, 1911: 636, my translation). The second is an 'original or acquired mental predisposition to decrease synthesis and disaggregation of the mind' (ibid.). Both the disaggregation of ideas *and* the manifested phenomena (psychological, somatic or otherwise) around the emotional shock are prerequisites to what Janet and others called traumatic hysteria (see also Ellenberger, 1970: 331–417). Of the two conditions, Janet (1901: 453) sees the abstraction of old and new ideas as existing at the 'bottom of all hysterical symptoms'.

The abstraction of new, and old (or seemingly forgotten), ideas is described by Janet as a 'disaggregation of consciousness' (ibid.: 149, 220) and latterly the disaggregation of the mind or spirit (Janet, 1911: 189, 443, 634–636).[2] This description indicates that the 'psychological disaggregation' is a 'subconscious phenomenon', which is developed 'outside of the will and personal perception of the patient' (ibid.: 197, 278–280).[3] This makes disaggregated ideas an automatic abstraction from *the synthesis of conscious thought* (ibid.: 264, 278; see also van der Hart & Horst, 1989).[4]

When ideas disaggregate (*désagrégate*), or disassociate (*dissocier*), and become systematised, they are 'transformed' into what Janet calls 'fixed ideas' (1901: 278–356). Heim and Bühler (2006: 112) usefully summarise fixed ideas as a 'kind of distorted experience, memory, imagination, or appraisal of the traumatic event'. Fixed ideas orientate around the emotional shock resulting from the traumatic event(s); however, they are not fully synthesised into conscious thoughts, and disrupt the subsequent acquisition and synthesis of new ideas (Janet, 1901: 280). In my reading of Janet, it is not that the ideas are fixed per se, as this would run contra to his more dynamic model of the human psyche. Therefore, it is through the dynamic process of not being synthesised into conscious thought, that ideas become fixed-like, in that the person returns to them in seemingly repetitive and obsessive fashion. Echoing this, Janet suggests that the fixing of ideas becomes a 'crisis of terror', where the person re-experiences the 'repetition of an emotion' related to the original traumatic event or accident (ibid.: 284). As Janet reflects, it is the relationship between the event and the idea of the event that 'may be more or less direct, but it exists always' (ibid.: 496).

So-called hysterical responses are marked out as different from the responses of the other psychiatric patients Janet treated, by the fixed idea that seemingly eludes them, and that they struggle to remember, express or articulate (ibid.: 279–282). The elusion can be to the extent that people seem to forget the traumatic events and lose the origin of the fixed idea (ibid.: 230, 290, see also 147 for the case of Bertha). The emotional shock, and the fixation of ideas, become manifest in people's feelings, sensations and bodily states, many of which they cannot themselves explain nor make sense of (ibid.: 230, 290–291). These seemingly unexplainable bodily states disclose the forgotten emotional shock of the traumatic experiences people have had, and/or the fixed ideas they have formed in relation to it (Janet, 1911: 662).

Fixed ideas, through a lack of synthesis of new ideas, result in a repetitious circularity of the associated emotions and somatic manifestations. The person's inability to incorporate new ideas into their thinking and action is seen by Janet to constitute a 'weakness of mental synthesis', and it is this weakness that maintains and sustains the fixed ideas (ibid.: 634–637). This results in a 'persistency of an idea or dream' that continually eludes the person (Janet, 1901: 496, see also 354).

Together these features of 'mental accidents' prevent the person from being able to adapt to new situations. In each new situation, the emotionality of disintegrated or dissociated fixed ideas is restimulated or arises from the subconscious. Being unable to respond with newly synthesised ideas, people respond with maladaptive and/or non-adaptive fixed ideas (see van der Kolk, Brown & van der Hart, 1989; van der Kolk & van der Hart, 1989). The inability to adapt to new stressful situations results in hysterical and unconscious phenomena, manifesting in the person's actions, words, dreams and unexplained somatic responses (Janet, 1901: 280–281; 1911: 634; van der Kolk et al., 1989; van der Kolk & van der Hart, 1989).

Sigmund Freud: memory and experience in the traumatic neuroses

Meanwhile, in Vienna, the neurologist Joseph Breuer had been working with a patient called Bertha Pappenheim who had developed a hysterical cough, and other unexplainable symptoms, while caring for her father, who had tuberculosis and subsequently died from the illness. The case of Bertha Pappenheim (who was given the pseudonym Anna O.), would become foundational in the creation of psychoanalysis. Around this time, a young Sigmund Freud returned from his studies in Paris under the guidance of Charcot and joined Breuer in his clinical studies. Freud also saw Pappenheim as a patient. Through their experiences with Pappenheim, and other (predominantly female) cases of 'hysteria', they developed a 'talking cure' as the basis for treating medically unexplainable symptoms (Breuer & Freud, 1982 [1908]).

Building on these cases, Breuer and Freud (ibid.: 166) suggested that people's affect (emotional experiences and expressions) were being unconsciously converted into somatic symptoms as a form of symbolic communication. Freud suggests that conversion could occur 'as immediate effect' (ibid.: 124) of experiencing a trauma, or after a 'short period of working-out [or] "incubation"' (ibid.: 96; 131). Further, in Freud's initial description of the case of Frau Emmy von N., he notes that 'however these motor symptoms may have originated, they all have one thing in common [...] an original or long-standing connection with traumas' (ibid.: 95).

Breuer is the more explicit of the two in reflecting on the significance and prevalence of interpersonal trauma in the lives of the patients he worked with, and the wider society at the time of writing. In his misleadingly titled 'theoretical material', Breuer (ibid.: 185) writes of sexual violence against women:

> Marriage brings new sexual trauma. One wonders that the wedding night does not more frequently act pathogenically, for unfortunately it is more often rape than erotic seduction. To be sure, hysterias of young women, traceable to

this experience, are not rare. But also in the further course of many marriages sexual trauma occur.

Notwithstanding the outmoded views on female sexuality contained within his work, Breuer does draw our attention to the realities of sexual violence within the lives of his patients and how this results in a traumatic impact on both the emotional understandings of the women involved, and their experiences and presentations of their bodies. Freud similarly notes within his case presentation the reality of incestuous sexual advances by an uncle of a patient named Katharina, and the silence surrounding this within the family (ibid.: 129–133). Other leading neurologists at the time, including Briquet (1859) (see also Mai & Merskey, 1981), were also noting the significant experiences of trauma in the lives of the women in their care.

However, this line of inquiry came to be somewhat confused within Freud's writing when he seemingly abandoned the reality of people's experiences of trauma (the so-called seduction thesis) and emphasised alternative accounts of infantile sexuality and fantasy. As Freud (1909: 189) justified after the abandonment of the thesis:

> By chance my former rather meagre material furnished me with a great number of cases in which infantile histories, sexual seduction by grown-up persons or older children played the main role. I over-estimated the frequency of these (otherwise not to be doubted) occurrences [...] and [therefore placed an over-] emphasis [...] on the 'traumatic' element of the infantile sexual experience.

We can see the emerging tension within Freud's work about the reality of exposure to sexualised situations in his discussions of the *primal scene*. During his analyses of the traumatic neuroses, Freud initially writes of the reality that the early witnessing of parents, or other significant adults, having sex has on the development of the child (c.f. the case of Katharina in Breuer & Freud, 1982 [1908]: 127–130). After the abandonment of the seduction thesis, Freud displays confusion over the extent to which the memories of witnessing sexual acts between adults are unconscious phantasies. For example, in the revised discussion of the case of the 'Wolf Man', Freud suggests that it is unclear (*non liquet*) as to whether the witnessing of sexual intercourse between parents within cases of traumatic neurosis is real, or if it is a transferring of seeing sex between animals onto the parents, and/or a phantasy of the child (Freud, 1953 [1914/1918]: 36–38, 57–60, see also 79–80, 226).

In his later papers, Freud recognises the tensions he has created between traumatic and non-traumatic neuroses in his work. He suggests that he has a 'fair degree of certainty' about the development of neuroses resulting from the experiences of ego development in infancy, and that this cannot be said of the 'traumatic neuroses' (Freud, 1963 [1940]: 83). For him, the relationships between the infantile development and traumatic experience 'eluded investigation' (ibid.). He does go on to recognise that experiences of sexual abuse, incest or early exposure to sexual behaviours increase a 'child's susceptibility' to later neuroses. These real experiences, Freud sees as 'instructive' and of an initial 'attraction'; however, after a short couple of paragraphs he asserts that his interest (and ours) should 'be still more attracted' to the influence of the Oedipal situation, to which he believes all children are subject (ibid.: 87–89). Thus, he puts the ambiguity of the relationship between neuroses and traumatic situations to one side and renders the developmental drama as the 'traumatic experiences [...] [that] no human individual is spared [of, nor] escapes the repression to which they give rise to' (ibid.: 84, see also 89–99).

Writing much later in his career, Freud (1940) continues exploring the relationship between memory, emotion and early experiences. Freud says that what he considered to be the symptoms of 'neuroses' are the 'consequences of certain experiences and impressions [...] [that] belong to early childhood' (ibid.: 118–119). He suggests that the common characteristics of trauma are their origins in 'early childhood' before the age of five years, 'impressions' of a 'sexual and aggressive nature' and a seeming loss of memory (ibid.: 119–120).

Freud suggests that within neurosis we can see both positive and negative effects of trauma (ibid.: 122–123). The positive effects seek to 'remember the forgotten experience, or, better still, to make it real' (ibid.: 122). This can lead to a fixing of the traumatic experience or impression in one's mind and an active compulsion to repeat this within new relationships. In contrast, the negative effects are to defend against or avoid the memory or repetition of the traumatic experience or impression. Freud suggests that both these positive and negative effects are present within a person's response to trauma, and to varying degrees the reactions conflict with each other (ibid.: 123). Further, the responses can have such a compulsive hold over people's view of themselves and the world that they lose a rational sense of what is actually occurring in their external reality (ibid.: 123–124).

Let us now turn to understand what Freud meant by a fixation on traumatic experiences of impressions. Writing more specifically about the 'traumatic neuroses', Freud (2012 [1920]) earlier suggested that his patients became 'fixated' on a traumatic event from the past, and specifically childhood. He locates the grounding of the fixation in the 'moment of the "traumatic disaster"', be that war or a traffic accident, and describes how his patients seemingly 'regularly live over the traumatic situation' (ibid.: 232), such as sexual attacks in childhood, within their waking and dream worlds (see Freud, 1931[1899]: 88).

In a similar way to Janet, Freud suggests that fixation arises from people's 'inability to meet an overpowering emotional experience' of the traumatic situation (Freud, 2012 [1920]: 232–233). The fixation becomes a repetition, in which the person can become 'completely absorbed in their retrospections' and disconnected from the relationship with the present and future (ibid.: 233–234). Again, echoing the observations of Janet, Freud suggests that people lose the conscious connection between the traumatic experience and subsequent compulsive fixation. As such, it becomes an 'unconscious psychological process', where they are unable to grasp the motivation of their thinking or action in new situations (ibid.: 234–237). As such, people unconsciously 'transpose' the traumatic situation and its overwhelming emotions into a new situation, which can lead to the hysterical 'attacks' and other symptoms that Freud noted (ibid.: 232).

Continuing to explain the relationships between experiences, emotions and memories, Freud introduces the notion of *Nachträglichkeit*. Frustratingly, Freud never explicitly defined the term. It was initially translated by James Strachey (Freud, 1966 [1895]: 356) as 'deferred action', and this became the dominant form in English. Thomä and Cheshire (1991: 407), among others, have drawn attention to the inaccuracy of this translation as it misinterprets the German meaning. The authors offer English alternatives of 'retroconstruction', 'retrospective attribution', 'an after-effect' and 'postportation' (ibid.: 424). Elsewhere, Freud (1940: 109–110, 117, 125–125) refers more simply to an 'incubation period' and 'latency' between the traumatic incident and the presentation of symptoms; however, this framing loses some of the complexity contained within the term *Nachträglichkeit*.

However we choose to translate it, the phenomenon of *Nachträglichkeit* is best understood within Freud's own discussion of a patient's memory of a traumatic experience (Freud, 1966 [1895]: 353–356). In some ways, this will also enable us to understand his inclusion of both traumatic experiences and impressions in his case descriptions (Freud, 1940). Let us take, for example, the case of Emma.

Emma is unable to go into shops alone. In conversation with Freud, she recalls a first memory of being 12 years old, going into a shop, being laughed at by two shop assistants for what she is wearing and finding one of the two assistants sexually attractive (Freud, 1966 [1895]: 353–356). She then recalls a second, earlier memory, from when she was eight years old. She went into a sweet shop and the shopkeeper 'grabbed at her genitals through her clothes' (ibid.: 354). She returned to the sweet shop a second time and the shopkeeper repeated the attack. Emma disapproved of herself going back into the sweet shop a second time and sees this as provoking the attack. Freud notes that in both situations she enters the shop alone. She associates the 'laughing' of the shop assistants in the first memory with the 'grin' of the shopkeeper in the earlier memory (ibid.).

Freud writes that Emma's later experience of the two shop assistants gives new meaning to the earlier one with the shopkeeper. Between the two time periods, Emma has gone through puberty, and Freud suggests that she connects a 'sexual release' with the shop assistants, which is transformed into an anxiety. He proposes that this sexual release was not consciously present (or the adult significance/meaning was not present) at the time of the earlier attack. Having now experienced puberty, the situation with the two assistants, and made an association with the earlier memory of the shopkeeper (the laughing/grin, being alone and the presence of clothes), Emma experiences an anxiety. The anxiety is that the shop assistants might attack her sexually, in the way that the shopkeeper did. As a result, she runs away with an 'affect of fright' (ibid.: 353).

Freud concludes that it is the experience of puberty and the later situation with the two shop assistants that alters the memory and understanding of the first with the shopkeeper. Emma's traumatic feelings are 'intensified' as, according to

Freud, she has had a 'premature' beginning of a sexual release, and one she could not yet understand at the time (ibid.: 357, see also 270). In this way, he argues that the memory of earlier events becomes traumatic, through the emotional response we latterly have to it rather than the experience itself (ibid.: 356–357; see also the similar discussion on the case of the 'Wolf Man', Freud, 1953 [1914/ 1918]: 57–58).

Nachträglichkeit can therefore be understood as referring to both the delayed after-effect of an experience, when subsequently reconstructed through memory, by way of new meanings and experiences.[5] The temporal delay here adds to his formulation of possible underlying relationships between trauma, memory and presentations of traumatic hysteria and neuroses. The important contribution Freud makes here is that it is our memories, and the emotions associated with them over time, that influence the ways in which we understand experiences to be traumatic.

We can note that in the case of a 'little boy' from the 'petite bourgeoise', Freud suggests (1940: 126–129) that it is the *threat* of castration by his father, voiced by his mother, which results in a 'very strong traumatic effect'. This case is couched within the Oedipal complex and drama between mother and male child. He tracks both the immediate effects and the 'return of the repressed' memory following the period of latency and the later death of his father (ibid.: 129). As such, *Nachträglichkeit* can be understood to relate to both the actual and perceived experience of the child.

Freud's ideas about *Nachträglichkeit* were taken up particularly by French psychoanalysts following Jacques Lacan's (1991 [1975], 2001 [1966]) identification and reappraisal of the concept (translated as *après coup*) in Freud's writings (c.f. Laplanche, 1999). Following French psychoanalysis, some contemporary psychoanalysts have sought to expand Freud's formulation. They suggest that in addition to a retroactive (new) meaning being ascribed to an earlier traumatic event, *Nachträglichkeit* can also contribute to the construction of the meaning of an experience or situation for the first time (Faimberg, 2007; Stern, 2019).

The American relational psychoanalyst Donnel Stern draws attention to the difference between Freudian psychoanalysis and contemporary French and constructionist schools. Within these latter traditions our minds, and the meanings of self and other, are typically seen as being 'constructed and then reconstructed, over and over again', influenced by the experiences we draw into our unconscious (Stern, 2017: 511). The reconstruction happens at both an unconscious and conscious level. Stern (ibid.: 516–517) writes that the act of construction is in the present, and thus the person retroactively seeks to reinterpret past meanings, experiences and emotional responses through the present-reconstruction, as well as anticipating what this might mean for future experiences.

For Stern (2003, 2017, 2019), we all have 'unformulated experiences'. Unformulated experiences are previously unaccepted aspects of our life, through which we are confronted with unknowing, confusion, puzzlement and possibly 'intrigue' (Stern, 2003: 37). Our confusion and puzzlement is seen by Stern to be a global vague sense of uncertainty about what we have experienced previously, what its significance might be, why we are feeling an emotional charge and how it relates to what we are constructing of ourselves in the present. For Stern, the experience is 'unformulated', as we have not yet articulated it to ourselves or others. As such, unformulated experiences are 'raw materials of conscious [and] reflexive experience' (ibid.).

The present-constructive nature of our mind means that experience is experienced as emergent and spontaneous. It is through this creative construction of experience that we become aware of those experiences we have not yet formulated. The realisation of this gives rise to newly emergent ways of non-verbally recognising, and/or verbally articulating, our experiences (see Stern, 2019). Over time, we might better be able to give a shape, meaning, articulation or verbalisation to these formally unformulated experiences. The incorporation of unformulated experiences into narrative about our life, allows for therapeutic processing of unconscious psychological processes and provides cognitive and emotional frameworks for making sense of the confusion.

In essence, the ideas about unformulated experience are a modernised psychoanalytic expansion of the phenomenon of *Nachträglichkeit* in relation to trauma. In the case of psychological trauma more specifically, Stern (2010: 137) suggests that we need to find a way of recognising and articulating the unformulated or preformulated experience by relating it to current experiences. He notes that even when people can recall factual details about a traumatic event, the feelings, meanings and the 'part it plays in *our* story' can remain elusive in our unconscious (ibid. my emphasis).

Stern suggests that this is because people who experience trauma can remain unaware of the co-occurrences (i.e. the actual and metaphorical similarities) between an unformulated traumatic experience and an experience in the present (ibid.: 139). This lack of awareness arises from dissociation of the unformulated experience as being something the traumatised person themselves has experienced (ibid.: 140). One can already begin to see the clinical application of these ideas in working with people who have significant confusion over, for example, unformulated preverbal experience of childhood neglect and sexual abuse. By working with co-occurrent present 'me' experiences, a meaningful formulation of the experience, emotional overwhelm and relevance to the life narrative can emerge.

War neuroses and the origins of traumatic symptoms

There was a continued interest in the realities of traumatic experiences through the study of 'war neurosis' in the First and the Second World Wars. During the First World War, renewed attention was placed on conversion, somatic dissociation (a sense of detachment from your body or a body part), and psychobiological states of arousal, vigilance and stress. This expanded clinical practice away from hysteria's long primary association with women, with some theorists shifting focus to a perceived deterioration of 'willpower' in male soldiers being treated (van der Kolk, Weisaeth & van der Hart, 1996: 50). As such, interventions focused on motivating soldiers to re-engage in active service through external stimulation and suggestion. However, it led to a diagnostically separate genesis of what were to become 'traumatic-stress'-related disorders (van der Hart et al., 2001).

The impact of war could be less readily denied, and leading neurologists and psychiatrists began to debate the commonalities between injured and/or returning soldiers and their childhood experiences. This was spurred on by the observations of psychiatrists from across Europe, the United Kingdom and the United States of America that trauma experienced in infancy and childhood was beginning to surface within the phenomena of war neurosis and war shock (see Ferenczi et al., 1921 [1919]).

The American psychiatrist Abram Kardiner (1941) detailed his experience of working with veterans of the First World War. He notes that many of the somatic presentations seem to directly relate to the actual traumatic experiences of war and the resulting psychological elaboration and perceptions of the solider. Within this he suggests there are significant alternations in the soldier's perception and 'conception of the outer world and his conception of himself' (ibid.: 82, 84, 184), and further his 'conception of his own capacities to deal with [the traumatic situation and its consequences] have undergone a profound change' (ibid.: 232). Fundamentally, Kardiner notes that the trauma of war creates a relational fracturing with other people and the world around the soldier (see also ibid.: 86). He writes:

> The new adjustment is erected on the ruins of what was once a rich reciprocal relation with the outer world [...] The quality of [the person's] contacts with the world are coarser, and the individual is always on the verge of wanting to get away from it.
>
> (Ibid.: 184)

In the United Kingdom, the Scottish psychoanalyst Ronald (W. R. D.) Fairbairn described in detail the phenomena of flashbacks and dissociations. He saw recent 'traumatic situations' (i.e. experience of loss, a car accident or exposure to violence or war) as new 'traumatic factors'. Moreover, these new factors serve to 'precipitate a psychopathological reaction through the activation of *pre-existing*, but hitherto latent [contained in the subsidiary egos], psychopathological factors' (Fairbairn, 1994 [1943b]: 257, emphasis added). Thus, he described ways in which the lived experience of trauma stays with the person and impacts on their everyday life. In the language of Fairbairn, this would be the traumatic release and *return* of bad objects (Fairbairn, 1994 [1943a], 1994 [1944]). In this psychoanalytic context, the bad objects are emotionally neglectful parents, who do not transmit their unconditional love and attuned relationality. It is in these emotional or developmental traumas of neglect that Fairbairn locates the original trauma, which creates the conditions for emotional reactions to newly traumatic situations.

A Hungarian psychiatrist, Sándor Ferenczi, who was himself a close associate of Freud, returned to the reality of experiences of trauma in clinical presentations of war neuroses. Building on the emerging Freudian psychoanalysis, Ferenczi (1926 [1916/1917]: 133, emphasis added) writes:

> It appeared that these patients [the soldiers] had repressed into the uncon-scious the affective reactions to certain *psychic traumata* [...] and that these continued from the unconscious to influence their activities, and on any threat of repetition of the pathogenic [traumatic] experience led to the develop-ment of anxiety. The patient then learns to escape these anxiety states by avoiding every activity that would in any way lead to the repetition of the pathogenic situation.

In his exploration of the phenomena of war neuroses, Ferenczi (among other European psychiatrists[6]) played a significant role in making the case for their psy-chogenic basis, disrupting what had been until then a dominant framework of somatic and neurological dysfunction or injury.

Like Fairbairn, Ferenczi used his understanding of the realities of the trau-matic situations that soldiers faced, and the psychogenic origin of presenting symptoms to inform his later work on psychopathological understandings of childhood traumas. In his most renowned psychoanalytic address and subsequent paper, Ferenczi (1949 [1932]) detailed what Freud had abandoned – namely, the reality of interpersonal violence in children's lives. He reflected:

> Even children of very respectable, sincerely puritanical families, fall victim to real violence or rape much more often than one had dared to suppose [...] The real rape of girls who have hardly grown out of the age of infants, similar sexual acts of mature women with boys, and also enforced [meaning non-consensual] homosexual acts, are more frequent occurrences than has hitherto been assumed.
>
> (Ibid.: 226)

He continued, in a more cutting critique of Freud: 'The immediate explanation – that these are only sexual phantasies of the child, a kind of hysterical lying – is unfortunately made invalid by the number of such confessions, e.g. of assaults upon children, committed by patients actually in analysis' (ibid.).

Anna Freud: developmental (re)turns in psychotraumatology

In the inter- and post-war periods, there was a sustained interest in the develop-ment of emotional trauma resulting from relationships between children (espe-cially in infancy) and their parents, caregivers and other adults in their lives. During this time, a major split within psychoanalysis took place,[7] which is best typified by the infamous debates between Anna Freud (Sigmund's daughter) and Melanie Klein: the so-called controversial discussions. Klein had been seen as a leading authority in Britain on the emerging field of psychoanalysis, until the Freuds themselves were forced to immigrate to the United Kingdom because of the anti-Semitism of the Nazi regime. Anna Freud's and Klein's work created diverging psychoanalytic, psychodynamic and object-relations traditions. These traditions differ in the interpretation of intrapsychic mechanisms, how these were developed over time (and especially in infancy and childhood) and the significant emotional and relational impacts of this on the lives of children and adults.

Anna Freud (1967) advocated for a more restricted definition focused on seeing 'psychic trauma' as an experience that disrupts the internal functioning of the development of the ego, resulting in pre-ego modes of relating to self and others in children. She describes a number of presentations that would indicate this mode in the child, including feelings of numbness, inaction or temper tantrums.

Building on the earlier work of her father, Anna Freud (2018 [1936]: 109–121) further describes that when children face a threat from another person, they take on a form of identification with the aggressor. The child might display aggression towards others, use the physical or moral stance or style of their adult aggressor or attempt to replicate the symbolic power dynamics they have witnessed and/or experienced in relating to the aggressing adult. According to Anna Freud, this is an 'assuming', 'impersonating' or 'imitating' by the child of what they have experienced (ibid.: 113). This form of defence is used by the child as a way of becoming active and thus enabling them to 'assimilate unpleasant or traumatic experiences in infancy' by an adult, or manage the anticipation of further threat or punishment for the act(s) done to them by the adult (ibid.: 113–118). As such, the child 'transforms himself from the person threatened into the person who makes the threat' (ibid.).

Klein, Fairbairn and Ferenczi: traumatic object-relations

In contrast, Klein's work on childhood trauma is somewhat more elusive, despite Ferenczi being her first psychoanalyst, and the influence of Fairbairn's theories on the development of her own thinking. For Klein (1998 [1975]: 338–340), and many subsequent Kleinian psychoanalysts, the focus is less on the realities of traumatic experience itself, but rather the way the infant or child integrates this as part of their establishment and experience of their *object-relations*. Latterly agreeing with Fairbairn (1994 [1943a]: 59–61; 1994 [1944]: 82–85), Klein sees our primary drive as seeking human contact and relationships. The most important of these are seen to be with the parents, and in her writings, first the mother and then father. According to Klein, the infant and child creates their sense of self, world and other through their relationship with the *parents* (external objects), and the *representations* of their parents, and relationships with them in their internalised world (internal objects).

Klein (1997 [1975]: 4–5) suggests that dealing with anxiety is a 'prominent' or 'primary' and early function of the ego. Importantly, she sees anxiety as arising from the death instinct and being realised through a felt fear of 'annihilation' (death itself) and 'persecution' (the possibility of annihilation or destruction by the other). This is played out in the fear of the uncontrollability of an external object (a parent) or its internalised form (a representation of the object). Fear of annihilation arises from 'the trauma of birth', or rather the anxiety of being sep-arate from the mother, and frustrations in bodily needs within infancy, both of which are experienced as being caused by the objects (ibid.: 4–5; 43, 49, 61–64, 238). If a person, at any point in their life experiences doubt about the goodness of their objects and the existence of goodness in their world, it can undermine their ability to reintegrate their self or overcome adversity. Klein (ibid.: 104) suggests that this is especially the case when the 'belief and trust' in the goodness of objects is 'shaken' at a high 'intensity' and for a long 'duration'.

The relationship between trauma and a person's object-relations is somewhat illustrated in her clinical discussion of a returning soldier. In Klein's analysis, the war itself was not the trauma, nor the poor treatment and nursing care by his land-lady. Rather, it was that these experiences reactivated the earlier infantile 'trauma' of weaning, and the anxiety situations surrounding this. Further, without a suffi-cient internal object of the 'good mother' from his own childhood, this resulted in a 'breakdown' (ibid.: 259). Here, the 'trauma' is defined by the lack of internal resourcing of a good internal object of the mother to protect against future anx-iety situations.

Building on Klein's work, Wilfred Bion (2004 [1962]): 90–98), a soldier in the First World War and psychiatrist in the Second World War, describes the ways in which a parent (by which he also meant the gendered role of a mother) can act as a container for the distress of a child or infant. The infant experiences overwhelming emotional states and through projective identification the parent (mother) can take these into their (her) own mind, make sense of them and return them to their child in a more tolerable and understandable form. The infant and then child learn that this emotional exchange represents the parent's (mother's) care towards them, and through the internalisation of this they are able to give meaning to the emotional experiences they are having. In this way the parent (mother) provides containment for the overwhelming emotional feelings the infant is having. Vitally, the parent (mother) needs to tolerate the infant's emotional distress, render it something that is tolerable for the child and over time help them make meaning out of it. If the parent (mother) is experiencing overwhelming emotional distress, and/or is unable to tolerate the distress of the child and/or provide a containment of it, then the child is left with a 'nameless dread' (ibid.: 96), leading to further emotional terror and possibly psychosis (see also Levin & Brown, 2013).

Both Fairbairn and Ferenczi were practising during this time, and more readily stayed with the realities of traumatic experiences, and their emotional impacts on the people they worked with. Ferenczi (1949 [1932]) describes the impacts of sexual violence towards children from adults, including incestuous abuse by parents. He suggests that these traumatic experiences breach the tenderness and emotional playfulness that a child needs during its development. According to Jay Frankel's (2004) reading of Ferenczi, it is the emotional abandonment of both the parent/adult who abuses the child, and the other that denies or silences the reality of what has happened, that leads to a state of 'traumatic aloneness' (Ferenczi, 1949 [1932]: 227; 1988 [1932]). The emotional abandonment by the child of the parents/adults causes the child to disassociate (distance themselves) from their own, overwhelming feelings of pain.

In some situations, Ferenczi (1949 [1932]: 228) notes that there can be a 'traumatic progression, of a precocious maturity', in which the child attempts to take on the role or function of an adult for the abuser. He describes children being caught between a 'passionate love and passionate punishment', which is the 'terrorism of suffering' in which the child assumes responsibility for repairing or restoring the fracture that has been made through the sexual violence (ibid.: 228). Caught in this bind, the child is left with introjected feelings of guilt that belong to the abusing adult, and shame for taking on the role of the adult. He describes the ways in which a child or young person, taking on the role of an adult or becoming precisely what an attacker needs them to be, will collude with the aggressor in order to survive in their environment (ibid.: 225, 227). This, he suggests, can lead to confusion and a fundamental loss of trust.

Michael Balint introduced and translated many of the works of his mentor Ferenczi into the English-speaking world, and to the emerging field of British object-relations. Balint (1969) extended Ferenczi's theories of the confusion of tongues to focus on emotional trauma, in which a parent is emotionally unresponsive or unattuned to the needs of their child, and suggests that an infant has a primary need to relate to a human object and its environment. Balint (2015 [1968]: 18–23) continues that, if there is a disruption in the two-person relationship between child and parent, then the child experiences a 'basic fault'. This basic fault can remain with them throughout their later life and is accompanied by a need to be resolved, healed or be 'put right' (ibid.: 21, 29). When this disruption occurs to a more significant degree, or where there is a lack of emotional connection between parent and child, in modern parlance we might think of this as emotional neglect.

Donald Winnicott: when parenting isn't 'good enough'

Donald Winnicott, a British paediatrician and psychoanalyst, is perhaps one of the most explicitly existential of the independent object-relations theorists and practitioners. Winnicott (2018b [1965]) developed a psychological model of human development, which describes a trajectory from an infantile dependence to independence. This maturation involves the development of psychological mechanisms and processes that move from a subjective-conceptual world, to an objective-perceptive one (ibid.; 1953; 1974: 104).

Foundational in Winnicott's model is the physical and symbolic importance of the parents' presence in enabling the child to develop their sense of self, world and other, within their experiences of time and space. He proposes a 'good-enough' state of environmental and parental conditions, which are required to support a child and person's emotional and interpersonal development (Winnicott, 1953; 2018b [1965]: 9, 37–55). An important part of this is the parents' (by this he primarily means the mother's) role in introducing the reality of the world to infants in small doses (Winnicott, 1991 [1964]: 69–74).[8] For this reason, his work places a significant emphasis on the positive role of play, illusion and fantasy in children's lives.

Both the child and the parents are seen to go through different interrelational stages of adaptation in order for the child to develop a healthy sense of self and relationships with others (see also Loparic, 2002). Boldly, Winnicott (2018a [1965]: 145) asserts that 'trauma belongs to dependence [...] [and] is a failure relative to dependence'. By this, he means that we can only understand what constitutes 'trauma' for the child or adult by first understanding the specific vulnerabilities to trauma that emerge from the emotional (staged) development of a child and their relative dependency on their parents.

Winnicott eloquently summarises the entirety of developmental trauma as

> the destruction of the purity of individual experience by a too sudden or unpredictable intrusion of actual fact, and by the generation of hate in the individual, hate of the good object, experienced not as hate by delusional as being hated.
>
> (Ibid.: 147)

In this way, trauma begins with a breakdown in what the child can reliably expect from an 'average expectable environment', meaning the emotional and relational expectations a child can have of 'good-enough' parenting (ibid.).

Trauma can continue with the family not being able to mitigate the child's exposure to the reality of their environment, and thus leaving them unable to fully adapt to it. Here, Winnicott suggests there is a possibility for both a normative and more pathological traumatisation by the family. From the perspective of adaptation, a parent (mother) and family are normatively and perhaps universally traumatising for the child. This is because they are responsible for finding ways to slowly expose the child to the reality of their environment, and thus disillusioning them of their childhood omnipotence and dependency (ibid.: 146). As we have previously noted, the early or unmitigated exposure of the reality of the environment to the child by the parent is seen to be more substantively traumatising. For Winnicott, the overexposure to the reality of the environment seems to be where he draws the clinical line in seeing 'trauma' as a psychopathological, rather than normative, phenomenon.

When a child experiences an unreliable holding environment and is exposed to the reality of their situation too early or quickly, it can affect their faith in a parent's ability to be a protective and good object in their life. Winnicott (ibid.) notes that when a parent or family has broken a child's capacity to 'believe in' them as a good object, it can result in anger and rage towards the parental objects. The breaking of a child's capacity to believe in the goodness of their parent is seen as a universal experience of trauma resulting from the need for the growing child to find independence from their parental objects.

In situations where the child can express 'appropriate' anger to the parental object and is tolerated by them, this remains within a normative level of trauma, which can be incorporated by the growing ego into the child's sense of self and others. If the 'appropriate' levels of anger and rage cannot be expressed or tolerated, then the child will experience this as persecution by the family and parental objects. It is these feelings and experiences of persecution that further (psychopathologically) traumatise the growing child and influence their experiences of self and of the sense that other people are persecuting them in their environment (ibid.: 146–147). Through an exploration of traumatic bereavement in childhood, Winnicott (ibid.: 134–136) further notes how pointing out relationships between the original past trauma and present situations can be additionally 'traumatic' for the client. This is seen especially to be the case when the client is disillusioned of a perceived 'persecutory' experience, which seemingly brings the relational experience of the past into present situations, and into the therapy room.

The more that the child develops and 'integrates' their inner world, the more they can be 'hurt' or 'made to suffer' through traumatisation (ibid.). 'Good enough' parenting allows the child to have the 'interrelationships' and experiences necessary for the development of psychic mechanisms (including projection and introjection). The development and experiencing of these physic mechanisms, according to Winnicott and other object-relations theorists, enables the child to form an 'inner physic reality' and fantasise about their relationships with parental objects. We can infer from this that the potential 'hurt' and 'suffering' arise from the experiences that a child has of their parental object during this time of integration. The extent to which these experiences of the parental object are traumatic are integrated into the inner physic reality of the child, and as such forms part of their fantasised and actual experiences of their environment. The hurt and suffering in this regard are the internalised traumatic experiences of the interrelationships between parental objects and the child.

Through the case of an adolescent girl with a disability, Winnicott joins others from the independent tradition within psychoanalysis in re-emphasising the reality of more explicitly, non-developmental, traumatic experiences. The girl had experienced a sexualised attack by a visiting adult male stranger while she was residing in the children's ward of a hospital. Initially, Winnicott was drawn to a more Freudian or Kleinian reading of her account, bringing a clinical suspicion of the fantasy of her experience (ibid.: 130). Later he abandoned this to return to the reality of the girl's experience. He notes the importance of her sharing this account with him, given that the girl seems to have actively withheld the experience from her parents and the hospital staff.

In an honest reflection, Winnicott discloses that he found it difficult to encounter the reality of her experience. He describes how many of the other children on the ward also had a generalised sense of danger in their environment, which were articulated as a fears or nightmares. In contrast, the girl seemed to understand the specific danger she faced from the visiting 'male pervert'; a 'man being nasty' (ibid.: 131–132). Winnicott suggests that he, and many other clinicians, are torn between an understandable denial of the experience and 'frenetic reactive activity'; it being difficult to tolerate the idea that a child could be subject to a sexualised attack in a supposedly caring and protective environment (ibid.: 131).

Through further disclosure and reflection, the hospital eventually took action to protect the girl and the other children on the ward.

In this specific case of hospitalisation, Winnicott sees the family as being protective of sexual trauma, in that the taboos of incest protect against sexual assault within the family. This role as a protective environment is meant to transfer to the hospital and its staff in constructing a family-like environment within the hospital (ibid.: 131). Clearly, Winnicott sees the girl's experience of sexual trauma as a failure of the hospital environment, but maintains that in the family environment the protection would have been sustained.

I feel immediately and viscerally irritated when reading this account. It is possible that avoiding hospitalisation would have protected the girl from exposure to sexual violence. And yet, Winnicott's seeming faith in the strength of the taboo of incest generally protecting against sexual trauma in the home feels overly simplified. In previous cases of trauma discussed in this chapter, we have seen the frequency of sexualised threats and attacks from within the family and from strangers.

Winnicott (ibid.: 132) suggests the girl had a trusted relationship with both him and her family, and this was also protective, in that her 'innocence' was not spoiled. In this statement, Winnicott seems to contradict the wider observations that the girl did not feel able to share the experiences with her family. Moreover, Winnicott frequently cites the girl's specific recognition of the sexual danger the man poses and outlines the relational consequences and re-enactments in the girl's seeming over-attunement to the presence of a male therapist, and changes and movements within the therapeutic environment (ibid.: 133). In good faith, I take Winnicott to mean that the fact that he, the family and the hospital acknowledged the reality of the girl's traumatic experience, took action against the offending individual and offered the girl therapeutic support was seen to be protective against further traumatisation.

Within therapy with this child, and other patients, Winnicott notes a 'staging' of 'minute' relational traumas within the therapeutic relationship. He proposes that these are actively introduced by the client in order to make sense of a traumatic experience they have had, and to work through a lingering sense of relational danger resulting from it (ibid.: 134). This observation relates more directly to his wider ideas about the importance of play in making sense of the reality of situations. Here, Winnicott is not judging the client's 'staging' of minute traumas within the therapeutic relationship, but rather is noting the ways in which this 'staging' has a value in the client's meaning-making and relational healing.

Trauma, using the variable conceptualisations above, can result in a primal anxiety, which Winnicott considers to be the threat of annihilation – somewhat paralleling Klein. More specifically, and existentially, this threatens to interrupt the 'continuity of being' (Winnicott, 2018b [1965]). For Winnicott, 'being and annihilation are the two alternatives' (ibid.: 47). Therefore, the parent–child relationship (the 'holding environment') can mediate and minimise the potential for an interruption in the 'continuity of existence' (ibid.; see also 1991 [1971]: 97). And thus, the need for an infant to react to a threat with the 'annihilation of [their] personal being' (Winnicott, 2018a [1965]: 147). It is in this way that the family is seen as protective for the child against traumatisation (see ibid.: 139, 143–144).

Winnicott (2006 [1965]: 11) writes that by the first year an infant has begun to organise their inner reality, seeking to preserve what is felt to be good and strengthening their sense of self (ego). Further, they are isolating what is felt to be 'bad', including those things 'injected from external reality without acceptance (trauma)' (ibid.). This enables them to also preserve a space within their psychic reality for their internalisation of the interrelational world with others.

The threat to the continuity of being is located within an existential paradox. The paradox is expressed in the reality of being both 'joined' to, and 'separated' from, others. In the process of making sense of this paradox, the infant, child and then adult, must make sense of the 'potential space' that can exist for a sense of self (c.f. Winnicott, 1991 [1971]). For the growing human child, 'there can be no separation, only a threat of separation; and the threat is maximally or minimally traumatic according to the experience of first separations'; that is, the separation from parental objects (and for Winnicott specifically the mother) (ibid.: 108). Therefore, emotional neglect removes the protection of good enough parenting, resulting in the 'experience [of a] break in life's continuity' (the 'unthinkable anxiety' of annihilation), traumatic (confused and disintegrated) emotional states and internalised models of human relationships (ibid.: 97; see also 2006 [1965]: 200; 2018a [1965]: 138–140; 2018b [1965]: 139). In short, it is when a parent is in a situation where they are able to provide good enough care, when the parent threatens the child's continuity of being or actively exposes the child to danger that the protective potential of the family is transformed into harm and trauma.

In a posthumously published paper, Winnicott (1974: 106) outlines a new direction in understanding the consequences of interruptions in the continuity of being. He writes that when a child is in a state of dependence on the parental figure (mother), the child can face 'primitive agonies' (ibid.: 103).[9] Rather than focusing on ego defences, Winnicott encourages us to see a variety of 'unthinkable' states of 'agony' that exist behind the defences. These include feelings of falling forever, a loss of psychosomatic dwelling (being in one's body), and a loss of a sense of reality (ibid.: 104). The child, and later the adult, experience these primal agonies as a form of 'phenomenal death', 'annihilation', 'emptiness' or 'non-existence' (ibid.: 106–107).

In this view, psychic defences are protective against encountering the rawness of a primary agony. Rather than the fear of a 'breakdown' being the anticipation of a forthcoming traumatic state, Winnicott suggests it is a sensing of a past primary agony (ibid.: 104). He suggests that the experience of the primary agony can only enter the experience of the past if it is incorporated (through present-time experiences) into the control of the ego. There is, however, a significant challenge in bringing the 'unthinkable' primary agony into the present, as the original experience(s) of the agonies precedes the maturation of the ego and its functions.

Without a clear location in the past, our unconscious searches for the (already experienced) primary agony in the future. The experience of the primary agony is projected forwards, 'looking for the past detail which is *not yet experienced*' (ibid.: 105, emphasis added). Temporally, the 'fear' of the past is compulsively projected into the future fear of breakdown, which for Winnicott is a reversal of the maturation process (ibid.: 103, 105).

For Winnicott, the adult needs to 'remember' the experience of the primary agony, and it is here that the temporality of the phenomena of 'fear of breakdown' provides a challenge (ibid.: 105). Given the person cannot remember the past experiences of agony, they relocate them in the future, as if the experience of the agony has not yet taken place. The task of the therapist is to work with the client to understand the 'queer truth' that *the experience they fear and search for in the future is in reality an unthinkable phenomenon of the past* (ibid.). In this way, Winnicott says that the therapeutic relationship in the present can become a safe relational space to re-experience the primal agonies and create experiences akin to remembering them (ibid.: 106).

John Bowlby: fear-arousing situations and adverse attachments

Like Winnicott, the psychiatrist John Bowlby worked alongside the diverging schools of British psychoanalysis and object-relations in a more independent manner. His well-known theories of attachment focus on a central concern about a child's experiences of loss and separation from their primary caregiver (he initially means the gendered role of mother) over time. This preoccupation is illustrated in his jointly authored letter to the *British Medical Journal* (BMJ) during the Second World War, to raise concern about the impact of separating children from their mothers during wartime evacuation and resettlement.

Bowlby, along with Winnicott and child psychiatrist Emanuel Miller, write that a child's 'capacity to experience and express sadness marks a stage in the development of a child's personality', and this establishes the basis for the kinds of social relationships the child will have over their lifetime (Bowlby, Miller & Winnicott, 1939: 1202–1203). Their critique is that wartime social policies promoting child evacuation, do not adequately address the developmental importance of acknowledging and responding to parental separation and feelings of loss that the child will experience. Bowlby, Winnicott and Miller warn that neglecting this developmental consideration could lead to 'radical [psychological] harm' and significantly 'impact [the] relationship[s] and social roles' that children will go on to have, and consequently societal problems may emerge (ibid.).

Bowlby was keen to better understand the lives of the children (predominantly boys and young men) he was working with, who were seen to be socially and pathologically delinquent. To do this he drew on his early clinical experience, examination of case histories and work as deputy director of the Tavistock Clinic in London. Building on more Kleinian and Fairbairnian orientations, Bowlby (1955: 587) rejects a contemporaneous popular notion that children are 'spoilt' by their emotional connections with their parents. Alternatively, he states that children have a 'primary socially-orientated drive', which needs to be met (ibid.). He suggests that the 'need for attachment' is at the heart of human dependency, independence and mental health (ibid.: 588).[10]

Bowlby (ibid.: 589) identifies a unique 'special characteristic' within the human experience. We form a primary attachment to one specific parental object (in his model, it is the mother), even in situations where the parent neglects or treats us badly (ibid.: 589). Thus, his interest is in both this primary attachment, and the impact of the quality of the attachment. For Bowlby, it is the trajectory of this attachment over time, as the child matures and explores their independence, which determines their outcomes. He argues that 'unfavourable outcomes' can result from a too intense or too weak attachment between child and caregiver, which affects the child's relationships with other people and environments as they develop (ibid.: 590–591).

The value of the 'biologically rooted' attachment between a child and their caregiver (mother) is that it is essential for human survival (Bowlby, 2005 [1988]: 6, 30, 33). Bowlby notes that the emotional communication and bonds of attachment are the original means of communication between the primary caregiver (mother) and the infant. Therefore, the attachment provides a means of protection for the infant, and a basis on which to develop their understanding of the world around them (ibid.: 136).

Continuing with a gendered and heteronormative frame of the Western nuclear family, Bowlby suggests that the child builds an internal 'working model' of the attachment patterns (communication and behaviours) of the parent (mother) towards the child, and then a 'comparable' model of the other parent (father) towards the child (ibid.: 135–139, 146). The working model of the child is based on 'real-life experience(s) of day-to-day interactions' with their parents (ibid.: 146). Subsequently, the working model the child develops of themselves reflects the image the parents have of them, which is communicated through the experience of the attachment bonds and related treatment, behaviours and actions of parents towards them (ibid.). The extent to which the working models of the self, parents and wider environment are 'updated' by the child over time depends on the pattern of attachment established between parents and their children (ibid.: 146–149). If working models of the parents and children are not updated over time, it can lead to significant breakdowns in communication interaction, with either or both the child and parents using outmoded forms of relating to one another (ibid.).

In contrast to Fairbairn or Bion, for Bowlby it is not the mother per se who regulates the world of the child, but rather the proximity of the mother to the child (ibid.: 68–69, 90–93). For Bowlby, the mother acts as a 'safe base' from which the child can explore the world, engage in play and return when they experience distress or threat in their environment (ibid.: 50–51, 68–69). As such, separation of the mother or attachment figure gives rise to separation anxiety (ibid.: 33–34), and preferably (in Bowlby's eyes) would be resolved by the child returning to the secure base of the parent (mother).

We can better understand the role that attachment plays in the survival of the infant or child by delving deeper into Bowlby's ideas about what constitutes danger in a fear-arousing situation. Reviewing first non-human animal studies and then human studies, Bowlby (1973: 98–118, 123–137, 160–165) describes a range of situations that arouse fear in human infants and children. Across the data he presents for all ages of childhood (up to around five years), fear-arousing situations include: (a) *sudden change in stimulation*, of sound, light, movement (especially approaching), distance and height; (b) *strangeness* of people, places, objects and situations; (c) the presence, appearance or behaviours of *non-human animals*; (d) *darkness and being left alone* (especially being alone in the dark).[11] These fear-arousing situations can be experienced singularly or at the same time, which he terms 'compound situations' (ibid.: 112–113, 117).

Importantly, none of these changes in stimulus, and situations, are intrinsically seen as being dangerous; rather, they indicate an increased risk of potential danger (ibid.: 137–138). We have evolved genetically, cognitively, relationally and behaviourally to sense and respond to these 'natural cues' in order to mitigate the raised potential risk of danger, and thus survive in our environment (ibid.: 131; see also 1979: 122). Within this order of 'natural cues', we have both the initial fear resulting from change in stimulus and 'situational' fears (i.e. strangeness, darkness, aloneness, non-human animals). These situational fears are conceived of as 'derivatives' of the natural cues of change in stimulation (Bowlby, 1979: 150).

In addition to natural cues, Bowlby (1973: 152) suggests the child acquires, in their second or third year, 'cultural cues' of the risk of danger. These are 'learnt by observation' of adults in the infant's environment, through which they build a repertoire of behaviours. These behaviours imitate the culturally determined responses adults have to potentially dangerous situations. Initially, the child imitates these behaviours 'without insight into the nature of the danger being avoided' (ibid.: 150). Over time, Bowlby claims, the child develops cognitive understanding into the cultural clues and behaviours being observed and imitated. Cognitive insight enables them to discern the potential risk of danger relating to these kinds of clues.

Cultural cues further give rise to the development of cues based on the lived, social experiences a child themselves has. These experiential cues are both learned and used by the person in order to assess the risk of danger, and behaviours that might avoid it (ibid.: 152). Depending on the capacity of the adult, a child can witness and imitate both positive and negative models of what danger looks like and how to respond to it (ibid.: 158–160).

Bowlby suggests that all forms of cueing have a survival value. They enable the person to act quickly to maximise safety and minimise the risk of danger (ibid.: 151–152). As such, he proposes that we should not discount, nor dismiss, the complexity of anticipation and assessment of danger as forms of neurosis (as he sees many of his fellow psychoanalysts doing). Rather, he invites us to investigate the ambiguities that arise from our 'imperfect capacity to comprehend' the reality of a dangerous situation (ibid.: 154).

The ambiguities of potential danger relate to valid questions that emerge for the child, and later for the adult, about the nature of danger. These questions include where the boundaries of danger are drawn (whom to be concerned about); what causes injury; and what (based on our emerging working models) might be the best means of response to avoid, mitigate or attend to the perceived danger (ibid.: 134;

153–155). Questioning and discernment are illustrated in the text using the more nuanced example of determining whether one faces a danger when confronted by a specific dog, as compared to a generalised working model of a dog, or a more naturalistic cue of the potentiality of dogs (as a non-human animal) as dangerous. Likewise, Bowlby describes the challenges in assessing whether or not we might get food poisoning, and within this the multiplicity of relevant factors – some visible (like the state of the food) and some invisible (the intentions of the cook) – that play into this.

Bowlby suggests that underestimation, overestimation and misunderstanding of situations should be expected as our childhood working models do not have fully formed understandings of the nature of a potential danger (ibid.: 155–156). The misattribution of potential danger to non-dangerous situations arises from our attempts to fit a new cue or situation into an existing working model of the risk of danger and this leads to the misattribution of, for example, whether a person is the source of threat (ibid.: 168–173).

Bowlby points to the protective factor of 'companions' in reducing feelings of fear (ibid.: 165–167; 1979: 123–125). Relating this more substantively to his theory of attachment, Bowlby explains that when the child experiences a clue to the risk of danger, they seek out the proximity of the caregiver for protection. The parent can help the child assess whether a situation presents a risk; in this sense the attachment figure is 'accessible' to the child (Bowlby, 1973: 177). In situations where a parent is 'inaccessible', absent or unresponsive, the child is unable to rely on the attachment figure to protect them from the threat or risk of danger. Bowlby terms situations where the attachment figure is temporarily unavailable as 'separation', and permanently unavailable as 'loss' (ibid.). Given that aloneness can often naturally cue a heightened risk of danger for children, Bowlby (ibid.: 177–181) hypothesises that the 'basic [survival] adaptive response' of the infant is to fear the inaccessibility (through separation or loss) of the primary attachment figure (mother).

The accessibility, or inaccessibility, of the attachment figure(s) is incorporated into the evolving working model of the infant or child. These models are used by them to forecast the potential availability of the attachment figure when they encounter a fear-arousing situation. The 'forecast' is based on both the actual availability of the attachment figure, and the level of confidence a child develops over time as to whether the attachment figure will be available to them at a time of potential danger (ibid.: 202–204). Rather than having a single working model and forecast, Bowlby suggests that the developing child has a number of working models cognitively available to them. The multiple working models have a dynamic relationship with how the child sees themselves, and the availability of the attachment figure (ibid.: 204–208).

Bowlby attempts to provide us with a way of differentiating between the world as we experience it through our 'feelings' (anxiety, alarm and fear), and the potentially dangerous 'world as it is'. Our feelings of fear can be balanced with 'feeling secure', and danger can be mitigated by a 'secure base' (ibid.: 181). Ultimately, the caregiver (mother) can act as a 'secure base' for the child, by making themselves available to the child when they sense or experience fear-arousing situations (Bowlby, 2005 [1988]; see also 1979). The risk and potential for trauma is located in the form of attachment a child has with their caregiver (their availability to the child), and the extent to which this attachment mitigates or promotes exposure to feelings of danger. In situations where a child is less securely attached to the mother, the child can experience significant separation anxiety (see also the experimental account offered by Salter Ainsworth et al., 2014 [1978]; and Waters et al., 2000).

In situations where the parent (mother) is not a safe base, there is an increased potential that the child will be exposed to both fear arousal and danger. Instability of the base (the primary attachment) can emerge from a child's prolonged separation from the primary carer (see Bowlby, 2020 [1933–1983: 50; 83–86), and/or the caregiver themselves being threatening (Bowlby, 1973: 156–157), unsafe or actively exposing the child to danger (Bowlby, 2005 [1988]: 114; see also Main & Solomon, 1990 for the expansion of D (disorganised/disoriented) forms of attachment).

Ever critical of Freud's 'disastrous volte-face' in abandoning the seduction hypothesis, Bowlby (2005 [1988]: 87, 199) was frustrated at the greater focus placed on repression and fantasy by psychoanalysts at the time he was writing. Consequently, Bowlby tasks himself with revisiting the relevance of 'real-life experiences […] and events' behind psychopathology, and the ways in which a child can be the 'target for the violent words and violent deeds of one or both of [their] parents' (ibid.: 87). As such, he suggests that Freudian, and other forms of psychoanalysis are met by a 'blanket of silence' presented by the family, which covers the true extent to which children are experiencing adversity from the parents (ibid.: 112). Further, the psychoanalyst can easily collude in the secrecy around adverse experiences in the family, by actively discouraging children and parents from expressing the reality of the experience, and thus maintaining their silence (ibid.: 119, see also 127).

Exploring the silencing and secrecy within families, Bowlby describes situations where parents seek to 'discredit' or 'ridicule' the child, in order to 'disconfirm' an experience, emotion, cognition or memory a child has about an adverse event (ibid.: 115–118). He gives the example of parental suicidality, where a parental figure or other adult seeks to confuse the child's understanding, or disconfirm their memory of the event, by suggesting the death was by another means (despite the child's direct exposure to the suicide), or challenging whether or not the child should be crying (ibid.: 118–120).

Bowlby further describes a secrecy of language that is developed between a child and parent with the context of incestuous abuse (ibid.: 118–119, 128). He writes of the ways in which a parent might induce knowledge to a child of the sexual assault through secret forms of communication, such as looks or gestures. Among other families, he notes that there is no reference in the daytime behaviour of the parent to the night-time sexual abuse, and in this way the secrecy of incest mirrors the split ways in which the family present themselves to the therapist and the world. Inevitably, these secret and silent incestuous behaviours within the family create significant confusion in the child. Confusion not only relates to the reality of the abuse, especially when it is split off to a particular moment of the night or state of the parent, but also the seemingly unacknowledged behaviours by the wider family to others in the environment. The secrecy and silence of incest intensify the confusion the child faces over the reality of the abuse, and can lead to terror, vigilance and make their experiences of themselves, others and the world feel unreal (ibid.).

Bowlby also sees the reversal of emotional availability, within the parent–child attachment, as resulting in psychopathology. He cites the situation where a parent will attempt to protect against their own depressive feelings or memories about their own traumatic childhood by continually demanding positivity and happiness from their child (ibid.: 121). Here the parent is not seeking to be available for the child at a moment of emotional distress, but rather insisting that the child become a substitute primary attachment figure for them. This can be seen as enduring rejection by the parent of the child's emotional needs, and a repetitive contempt for the child's need for parental availability (ibid.: 128).

Other psychologists, such as Jennifer Freyd (1994: 309–321; 1996) have proposed that the 'betrayal of trust' experienced by a child in intra-familial abuse creates 'a conflict between reality and the need to maintain trust in caregivers'. She suggests that while there is an evolutionary advantage of being attuned to these social and relational betrayals, in the case of incest and child abuse the more adaptive response could be to block the cognitive processing (i.e. incorporating it into their autobiographical memory) or to forget (i.e. through psychogenic amnesia) these betrayals (Freyd, 1994: 312–319).[12] Following a similar vein to Bowlby, Freyd says this forgetting would enable the child to retain an attachment to their parent or caregiver and ultimately survive in their environment (ibid.: 310, 318). Like Bowlby, Freyd suggests that the motivation for children to forget emotional, psychological and sexual abuse in childhood can come from explicit threats and demands for silence, or reality-defining statements by the caregiver (ibid.: 322).

Adverse situations like those just described result in what Bowlby (2005 [1988]: 115) describes as 'grave distort[ions]' in the communication between a child and their parent. Moreover, having their thoughts and feelings disconfirmed by attachment figures and other significant adults, makes the child insecure about the reality of their perceptions and understanding of the world around them. It further creates complexity in the discernment of the risk of potential danger and can give rise to feelings of being or living in a world that is unreal (ibid.: 116), or locating the fear arousal or danger in imaginary monsters (ibid.: 129–133),

Bowlby (ibid.: 41) neatly summarises his perspective in observing that

> adverse childhood experiences have effects of at least two kinds. First they make the individual more vulnerable to later adverse experiences. Second they make it more likely that he or she will meet with further such experiences. Whereas the earlier adverse experiences are likely to be wholly independent of the agency of the individual concerned, the later ones are likely to be the consequences of his or her own actions, actions that spring from those disturbances of personality to which the earlier experiences have given rise.

If we unpack this paragraph, we can first see how Bowlby proposes that 'adverse childhood experiences' increase the risk and likelihood that a child will experience more adversity in their lives. Second, and possibly more importantly, Bowlby distinguishes between the levels of agentic participation a child has in earlier and later experiences of adversity. Whereas, the earlier adversity is done unto the child, in later experiences there is an active co-creation of the adversity by the growing child or grown adult. Moreover, the co-creative agentic potential of the person's engagement in later experiences of adversity are seen by Bowlby to arise from the impacts that the earlier experiences have on their personality, attitudes and behaviours.

The consequential impacts of earlier adversity on later actions in adulthood are illustrated by Bowlby's discussion of familial violence. In the case of women who physically and emotionally abuse their children, Bowlby notes that this arises from anxious forms of attachment with their own parents (ibid.: 93). Further, he suggests that there are repeated threats, and actual experiences, of separation or abandonment in these women's childhoods, which resulted in them being unable to turn to their own parents (mothers) for emotional support (ibid.: 96–104). Likewise, men who 'ill-treat' their female partners, are seen to have experienced poor attachments with their own parents and been subject to adversity themselves (ibid.: 104–107). It is the combination of early exposure to adversity, and the impact that it has had on their personalities, which gives rise to physical, emotional and sexual abuse, and coercive and controlling behaviour (ibid.).

Bowlby takes this model of the consequential impacts of adversity further, in suggesting that both the men and women who experience later adversity actively seek out the patterns of attachment and forms of emotional intimacy they experienced in a childhood adverse experience of home (ibid.: 105, 107). Moreover, he notes that despite their adverse experience of the other, each of the partners says they need each other, and Bowlby puts this down to earlier experiences of separation anxiety that relate back to their childhood attachments (ibid.: 107). Bowlby describes how these 'adverse experiences with parents' go on to impact the mental health of their children, and to forms of attachment that exist between the parent and child (ibid.: 112). His conclusion is that abusive relationships and parenting are the consequences of earlier adversity within parental attachment or the wider environment.

Bowlby (1955: 590–591) is recognising here what he sees to be an intergenerational cycle of unfavourable outcomes resulting from adversity. The 'emotional disturbances' of one generation of parents are seen to have their origins in the attachment problems they experienced in childhood with their own parents (ibid.). It is the disturbed patterns of parental attachment in their own childhood that are passed on to the next generation of children (see also Bowlby, 2005 [1988]: 40–41, 112, 150–152).

The intergenerational effects of attachment are echoed in more recent attachment research suggesting that the unresolved fear of parents can be transmitted to the child through more disorganised forms of attachment, where the parent exhibits frightened and/or frightening behaviour (including aggressive forms of interaction) to the child (Hesse & Main, 2006; Lyons-Ruth & Block, 1996; Main & Hesse, 1990). These transmissions of disorganised attachment are seen to substantively impact the behavioural, attentional and relational strategies a child develops and uses over their life (c.f. Hesse & Main, 2000). Furthermore, there is an intensification of frightened and frightening responses in parents who come to believe their child is dangerous, or who locate the threat of danger within them (Hesse & Main, 2006: 323–325). That said, Bowlby (1955: 591; 2005 [1988]: 19, 154) clearly advises against a deterministic or fatalistic attitude, suggesting that with support this 'vicious cycle can be broken'.

As Lyons-Ruth and Spielman (2004: 319–320) suggest, attachment theory represents a significant departure from the Freudian, Kleinian and independent psychoanalytic theories of human development. Its focus and emphasis on fear arousal, and the ways in which the child's fear (and the risk of danger itself) is 'modulated' by relational attachment with the parent provides an alternative framing of how trauma might arise both developmentally and situationally in the lives of children and adults. As Hesse and Main (2006: 311) note, the paradox of Bowlby's model is that a child will seek proximity to the primary attachment figure to resolve fear-arousing (of in their terms frightening) situations, even when the parent is the source of the fear or danger. While Bowlby focuses primarily on the language of fear, danger and adversity, the repetition of the adverse patterns of attachment and the re-experiencing of adverse impacts on personal and relational worlds is equivalent to the psychological wounding expressed in other psychoanalytic and object-relations definitions of 'trauma'.

Feminist perspectives on early psychotraumatology

A long-standing debate continues to rage between scholars (c.f. Masson, 1984), feminists (c.f. Rush, 1996 [1977]), historians (c.f. Esterson, 2001) and psychotherapeutic practitioners about the extent to which Freud and Freudian psychoanalysis actively moved away from the reality of traumatic experiences of abuse and sexual violence in his patients' lives. Peter Fonagy 2001: 48) suggests that it is more complex than it might first seem. He proposes that Freud moved away from the 'naive realism' of his early theories, while continuing to emphasise in later cases the 'pathogenic significance of seduction experiences' (ibid.).

Whatever the truth of the matter, it is clear that Freud's shift in thinking resulted in the notion of infantile sexual fantasy becoming the dominant theme within the earlier clinical development of talking therapies and Freudian psychoanalysis (Kitzinger, 1996). Further, the move away from Freud's initial understanding contributed to the silencing of the traumatic origins and realities of people's distress within psychiatry, psychology and psychotherapy for generations to come (following Herman, 2015 [1992]). This was coupled with silencing of the prevalence of childhood abuse in institutional and family care within psychiatric and wider Western social thought throughout the majority of the twentieth century.

In contrast, the prominent psychoanalyst Alice Miller was heavily critical of the role that psychoanalysis had played in the suppression of the reality of people's traumatic experiences. Having survived the Second World War and the horrors of the Warsaw ghetto, Miller initially trained as a psychoanalyst in Switzerland. Drawing on her wider appreciation of and training in philosophy and sociology, she heavily critiqued the psychoanalytic tradition for its contribution to a 'poisonous pedagogy' (Miller, 1984 [1981]: 40; see also 1990 [1988]). Her critique led her to eventually reject psychoanalysis as a coercive and retraumatising psychotherapeutic method (c.f. Miller, 1984 [1981]: 181–189).

Miller sees the Freudian abandoning of the seduction thesis as being part of a wider practice of manipulating children's emotional worlds through coercive and harmful practices. Critical of the psychiatric theory and practice of the time, she is concerned by the increasingly 'ingenious methods of humiliating patients […] [and] silencing [their] coded language' about the reality of the trauma they have experienced (ibid.: 130). In her analysis, she shows how the child, the parent(s), the analyst and the wider society all collude in the denial of the reality of trauma within children's lives (ibid.: 41). More pointedly asking, 'Why is the truth so scandalous?' she accuses Freud of complicating people's trauma by dismissing his discovery of the reality of sexual trauma in the lives of his patients, and misdirecting attention away from the notion that adults and even parents were abusing their children (ibid.: 109–116).

The reformulation of child sexual abuse into a generalised theory of 'infantile sexuality' is deeply problematic for Miller. She accuses this reformulation of failing to understand the facticity of a child's dependence on their parents (ibid.: 3). If there is 'no sympathetic or supportive person' available to the child with whom they can share their trauma, they are forced to repress it to survive in their familial or social environment (ibid.: 6). This accounts for the investment some children have in covering up, keeping secret or blaming themselves for the traumatic experience they have had (ibid.: 7).

By relocating the reality of the child's abusive experiences into the notion of infantile sexuality, Freud preserves the idealisation of the parent and the child's dependence on them, and renders difficulties as forms of defence by the child (ibid.: 113–119), making the child's mind the site of pathology and disorder, and presenting a more palatable version of reality to the public and the potential parents of psychoanalytic patients. Miller strongly challenges the denial of the analyst in their suggestion that all ideas about trauma are located in the fantasies or intra-psychic worlds of the child's mind. She contends that the psychoanalyst is retraumatising the child or adult client, by insisting that it does not matter whether the traumatic experience is real or imagined as it only has meaning through the lens of the Oedipal drama (ibid.: 42–43). The insistence of the fantastical nature of sexual abuse is part of an unconscious resistance of the psychoanalyst, who does not want to confront societal taboos (ibid.: 175). Rather, they find solace in taking 'the side of the adult and blame the child for what has been done to him or her' (ibid.: 216). This solace constitutes a historical denial of what has been done to the child, and serves to maintain the societal dogma of 'thou shalt not be aware' (ibid.: 316, 326). The dogma permits parents to destroy the lives of their children with 'impunity', with the only thing that is truly forbidden to break the silence and scandal of childhood neglect and abuse (Miller, 1990 [1988]: 22–26, 35–36).

For Miller, it is the adult gaze that reverses the reality of the situation, the adult 'wishfully' hopes that the child shares their abusive desires, and thus it is the adult intentionality of sexual contact that is being projected onto the child's need for proximity, intimacy, play and tactile connection (ibid.: 69, 129). The more explicit focus on the realities of sexual abuse enables her to bring closer attention to experiences of intra-familial abuse, neglect and incest, and stranger violence, and these forms of violence can be accepted, or tolerated, by some parents because of their own history of sexual abuse (ibid.: 40–41, 62–67; 1984 [1981]: 125–127, 153–154). More challengingly, Miller (1984 [1981]: 154–155) proposes that parental acceptance and the allowance of sexual abuse could be a way in which the parent takes revenge on the world for their own traumatic experiences in childhood. She suggests that by understanding the experiences of one child, we might be better able to understand the traumatic backgrounds of the other children or adults who perpetrate abuse.

Miller's own trauma theory leads her to focus on connecting to the traumatised child she senses within the client. She aims to become their advocate within the therapeutic relationship (ibid.: 55, 59). As an 'enlightened witness' and therapeutic 'advocate', Miller seeks to understand the experiences of humiliation in the life of her clients (when they were children), and how this relates to the drama of being a child who has been traumatised by experiences (ibid.: 66–67; 1990 [1988]: 174–175). The drama is still present, within this model, in later adult behaviours and relationships that are repetitions and re-enactments of the childhood trauma experiences (Miller, 1984 [1981]: 76, 83).

Vitally, Miller gives us an alternative way of understanding the function of fantasy and unreality in children's lives and sense-making around sexual trauma. She suggests that children's stories, play, dreams and screen memories are both conscious and unconscious means by which the early experience of childhood trauma is symbolically understood. The forms of fantasy 'serve to conceal or minimise unbearable childhood reality for the sake of the child's survival: therefore so-called invented trauma is a less harmful version of the real, repressed one' (ibid.: 317). Here we can see a clear commonality with the object-relations theorists Bowlby and Freyd. Miller places an emphasis on the actuality of the child's need to survive its environment and immediate relationships (see Miller, 1990 [1988]). As such, the use of fantasy, or the augmentation of the reality of traumatic experiences, enables the child to creatively survive.

Miller's contribution to understanding the reality of abuse in the child's life, and her advocacy of breaking the silence that surrounds it, was exceptionally powerful. It ran contra to many of the prevailing psychoanalytic approaches at the time and offered hope for many who felt psychiatry and psychology were becoming complicit in a permissive culture surrounding the abuse of children (Miller, 1990 [1980]).[13]

Beyond the world of psychoanalysis, second- and third-wave feminist thinking had a significant impact on the classical theories of psychotraumatology and the practice of psychotherapy. Feminist scholars and practitioners addressed head-on the silencing of actual experiences of trauma within psychoanalysis, psychiatry and society at large (c.f. an important edited collection by Burgess, 1985); they sought to more explicitly address the structural and relational impact of patriarchal power on girls' and women's experiences of trauma (Brown, 2004).

Many feminist therapists saw psychotherapy as a way of unwittingly entrenching the traumatic impact of patriarchal and heteronormative oppression through psychiatric and psychological discourse (c.f. Brownmiller, 1975), for example, the way in which earlier concerns raised by Breuer on the issues of rape within marriage, Ferenczi on the rape of infants, and Bowlby on the silencing and secrecy around child abuse, were overshadowed by the intra-psychic relevance of infantile sexuality in mainstream Freudian psychoanalysis.

Most notably in the case of rape and sexual abuse, feminist theorists and practitioners have been instrumental in repositioning interpersonal sexual violence as a social problem; a social problem that has traumatic consequences for all genders. Through detailed social and clinical inquiry and description, feminist scholars demonstrated that sexual violence (in all its forms) requires both psychological support for the survivor and social interventions to address structural and institutional inequalities that promote and reify cultures of violence against women and girls (c.f. Burgess & Holmstrom, 1974; Harvey, 1996).

For example, the work of the feminist psychiatrist Judith Herman was instrumental in challenging prevailing assumptions about the rarity of child sexual abuse. In a groundbreaking clinical study of father–daughter incest, Herman (1985; Herman with Hirschman, 1981) exposes the secrecy and shame surrounding incest and challenges the culture of blame, shame and denial in families and society that surrounds the realities of father–daughter incest. She details the psychological and traumatic impacts of this abuse on girls and young women, including nightmares, flashbacks, insomnia, bed-wetting and dissociation. Herman notes how the family constellations contain a relatively normative, unquestioned patriarchal dominance and paternal authority, which enables the abuse and silences the disclosure or recognition of it.

In her later works on wider forms of interpersonal violence, Herman distinguishes more explicitly between a single incident and the significant and enduring responses that arise from early and repeated experiences of trauma. Focusing primarily on these more complex forms of traumatic experiencing (including domestic violence, child abuse and torture), Herman (1998, 2015 [1992]) proposes three stages of trauma recovery: establishing safety, retelling the story of the traumatic event(s) and reconnecting with other people. Her therapeutic model strongly advocates providing treatment for people that is most appropriate to their stage of recovery. Importantly, Herman increasingly uses the term 'survivor' to provide people with a sense of meaning and enabling the empowerment of the person through their journey of trauma recovery.

Feminist critiques of interpersonal violence were further extended by authors drawing attention to the wider culture of violence in which sexual abuse and rape were taking place (c.f. critiques of Brownmiller by Dworkin, 1974, 1993 [1989]; and hooks, 2015 [1981]: 77–78). Within such critiques, feminist theorists have also drawn attention to the ways in which societies enact violence upon men, and they in turn participate in this cycle of violence towards others (c.f. hooks, 2015 [1984]: 75, 124, 150–153). The philosopher and political activist Angela Davis (2019 [1981]: 155–181) echoes this sentiment. She notes how efforts to raise public consciousness of cultures of rape within the United States of America were infused with mythical representations within journalism, legal cases and public discourse about the prevalence of dangerous and highly sexualised black, Hispanic/Latino and native men. Davis draws attention to how these gendered and racialised representations of rape culture frequently obfuscated and marginalised the experiences of black women, and women of colour, and the crimes of white perpetrators.

The feminist scholars explored above provide an important insight into the situatedness of interpersonal trauma, and how the sociocultural and political context and understanding can frame the reality (or denials of reality) of a traumatic situation or event. I will return to wider feminist critique and insights about the reality of traumatic situations in subsequent chapters of this book. Having outlined some of the foundational ideas in early psychotraumatology in this chapter, I will now turn to consider the commonalities that emerge from these accounts. In the next chapter, my focus will be on highlighting for the reader some of the main paradoxes that arise out of these earlier ideas, and what they might reveal about the structure of human experience.

Notes

1 Those readers wanting a more comprehensive genealogical analysis of trauma within psychoanalysis, would benefit from consulting Leys (2000).

2 In the second edition of his book *L'État Mental des Hystériques* (1911), Janet uses the term *l'esprit*, which in the context of the writing can be simultaneously translated as 'spirit' and 'mind' (c.f. ibid.: 6).

3 Much of Janet's contribution to defining the unconscious and the study of dissociation was overshadowed by the work of Freud, until it was revived in the 1970–1980s by psychotraumatologists who saw the significance of the observations he made. See, for example, the repopularisation of Janet's work through Ellenberger (1970).

4 For a more substantive discussion of the impact of Janet's ideas about dissociation on contemporary understandings of trauma, see the important papers by Putnam (1989) and van der Kolk and van der Hart (1989).

5 See also Freud's earlier articulation of this in his discussion of the case of Katharina (Breuer & Freud, 1982 [1908]: 133–134).

6 For a more detailed discussion of the change in psychiatric thought in Germanic, Austro-Hungarian and wider European contexts, see Brunner (1991).

7 I do not provide here a detailed description of the debate and differences within the (Anna) Freudian and Kleinian traditions, but refer the reader to King and Steiner

(1991) and Likierman (1995) for a good overview. For the purposes of openness within this debate, more specifically I have always been more drawn to the resonance of Fairbairn's writing, notwithstanding my use of existential alternatives to psychoanalytically based formulations of intrapsychic mechanisms.

8 See also Winnicott (1953) for his discussion of the infant's experiences and relationships with transitional objects and phenomena as part of illusionment/disillusionment and reality testing. Within this we can understand how the use or destruction of transitional objects within childhood trauma can have an additional psychological impact on the person's sense of threat, reality and continuity of existence.

9 This is in contrast to the anxieties that arise from the Freudian primal states.

10 Those readers looking for a comprehensive treatment of the history and genesis of attachment theory, and its potential relationships with psychoanalysis, should consult the work of Peter Fonagy (2001).

11 Bowlby is dismissive of physical pain as a natural cue of potential danger. The delayed onset of pain feelings and sensations (usually after a danger is experienced) suggest for Bowlby that they should be seen as a natural learning mechanism, by which we refine our more distal clues of potential danger (Bowlby, 1973: 140–141).

12 Those wanting a balanced account of the debates within psychiatry over the reality of 'recovered memories' might consult the series of papers written by Solinski (2020a, 2020b, 2020c) in *Frontiers in the Psychotherapy of Trauma and Dissociation*.

13 In a memoir, which includes letters written by his mother, Martin Miller (2018) sets out what he sees to be the inconsistencies in Alice Miller's relationship to her own traumatic past, specifically, the impacts of abuse at the hands of her mother and experiences of Nazi persecution in the Warsaw ghetto. He notes that, in reality, she was caught in a cycle of violence that she never broke the silence of. Further, he suggests that Alice Miller only acknowledged her own, and more violently her husband's, emotional and physical abuse of their children at the end of her life. Martin Miller writes that breaking the silence on his mother's own abusive behaviour should not diminish or negate 'the merits of her books and the importance of her theories' (ibid.: 19). Moreover, he is seeking to show the incongruence between her research and theories on childhood trauma, and the ways in which she 'split off this from her real existence' (ibid.).

2 Paradoxes and tensions

Paradoxes arising from early psychotraumatology

The previous chapter sought to re-examine the early accounts of psychological trauma in neurology, psychiatry and psychology. These accounts reflect the sociohistorical context in which they were written. It is likely that many readers will be frustrated by the gendering of familial roles, the overemphasis on mothering, the seeming idealism and centrality of a nuclear family in Western culture and the heteronormative and racialised discourses advocated within psychotherapeutic solutions and interventions. From our current standpoint, we can see that the early psychotraumatologists did not appreciate the full complexity of contemporary human relationships, familial patterning and non-familial attachments. That said, there is still value in understanding how these theories and practices have gone on to shape Western psychiatry, psychology and psychotherapy, and what they might tell us about the nature of traumatic experiencing.

The aim in this chapter is to discern the paradoxical features that arise out of these early psychotraumatological formulations, and to begin to build a thematic synthesis of what they might disclose about the nature of human and traumatic experiencing. In the thematic synthesis that follows, I will outline, and draw attention to, some fundamental tensions and paradoxes. No doubt the reader will have identified other tensions within the early writings, and my synthesis here is not conclusive or exhaustive. Rather, I am focusing on the core paradoxes that we will return to in a different form throughout the subsequent chapters of this book.

Confrontations with reality

Within the above accounts of interpersonal trauma, we find a paradoxical sentiment. The paradox centres around the need for people to see the reality of the traumatic situation they have experienced and/or are currently experiencing, and the recognition that perceiving and experiencing the world as it truly is, is too overwhelming and terror-inducing for the person to tolerate.

While divergent on the intra-psychic mechanisms and interpersonal dynamics and defences at play, all the early psychotraumatologists emphasise the ways in which people need to (consciously or unconsciously) find ways of relating to the

DOI: 10.4324/9781003181675-4

traumatic realities of the world and human relationships. Janet's (1901) notion of the disaggregation of the consciousness and the forgetting of traumatic experiences, and Fairbairn's (1994 [1943a]) return of bad objects illustrate the ways in which the reality of a situation can elude our own understanding.

The confrontation with the reality paradox is one of the reasons an emphasis is placed on parents and caregivers (in a child's life) and psychotherapists (in a person's life) to mediate the reality of the traumatic potential of the world and to protect against traumatic experiencing. Bion's (2004 [1962]) notion of the parent as a container for the child, Bowlby's (2005 [1988]) focus on the proximity of the parent and Winnicott's (1991 [1964]) hope that good enough parenting introduces small doses of reality to the child are clear examples of this. However, as we have seen, the family and indeed the psychotherapist themselves (see feminist contributions in Chapter 1) can be the source of overwhelming exposure and disclosure of the reality of a traumatic situation.

Bowlby (2005 [1988]), Herman (1998) and Miller (1984 [1981]) all vividly illustrate the lengths to which families will go to deny the reality of a traumatic situation: the regimes of secrecy, silencing, splitting off and threatening mobilised by family members to augment the reality of what has, or is, occurring in the person's life. Ferenczi (1988 [1932]), among others, reminds us that these denials, suppressions and augmentations of reality represent forms of active communication about interpersonal trauma. Whether it be in the confusion of tongues, knowing glances in the view of others or unspoken terror in the morning after the night before, they all communicate the extent to which the reality of the interpersonal trauma can be acknowledged, recognised and confronted in the present moment. Even the confusion around the unformulated experiences that Stern (2003) describes, and the anxious attachments Bowlby (2005 [1988]) noted, are active expressions of the interpersonal trauma and ways of articulating the paradox of confronting traumatic realities.

Fixed origins and changing meanings

There is a further paradox contained within the seeming causalism of some of the early psychotraumatological accounts. The psychopathological standpoint of neurology and psychiatry at the time primarily resulted in a focus on the aetiology of psychological trauma and its intra-psychic and somatic manifestations. For Freud (1963 [1940]), Breuer (Breuer & Freud, 1982 [1908]) and Janet (1901), the traumatic original experiences might be responsible for all dissociations and splits within the person's conscious mind that presented in their clinics.

The causal focus of aetiological inquiry comes from an understandable human desire, as well as a professional one, to find certainty about the origins and causes of so-called psychopathological phenomena: the flashbacks, intrusive thoughts, memories and/or sensations, somatic responses, dissociation, states of fear and terror that clinicians encounter in their experiences with their clients. The causal model acknowledges the presenting symptom and seeks to understand how it emerges from an *original* trauma. In some of the models, the causal explanation seeks to demonstrate how this original trauma is a breaching of the 'normal' progression of human, psychic and relational development.

If we follow the later causal model of (S) Freud, we are encouraged to trace the origins of the Wolf Man (for example) back to the trauma of either the real or unconscious phantasy of the primal scene (Freud, 1953 [1914/1918]). If we recall the traumatic phenomena expressed by Fairbairn's war-experienced soldiers (Fairbairn, 1994 [1944]), we are urged to see the return of early bad (parental) objects. According to the Bowlbian model (Bowlby, 1955), the cause takes us beyond the interpersonal trauma of the person we are working with, to the intergenerational attachment patterns of their parents and grandparents that pre-existed them.

Likewise, within the feminist frame, the traumatic origin is located both within the specific interpersonal dynamic of human relationships, and the wider socio-cultural systems in which they are situated, giving us a more multifactorial and dispersed causal origin. As Miller (1984 [1981]) and Herman (1998) note, while trauma may emerge from a specific relationship in a person's life, it can be seen as a manifestation of the wider cultures of permission and silencing around (for example) abuse and violence, and the power relations enabling these (c.f. hooks, 2015 [1984]). Similarly, Bowlby et al. (1939) in their letter to the BMJ, are contextualising the risk of psychological and developmental impacts of maternal deprivation within the context of a policy of evacuation during the Second World War.

The *causal (perhaps linear) fallacy*, the idea that any one human experience has a single cause, echoes the influence of Cartesian dualism within Western thought and psychiatric genealogy. The artificial distinction between body and mind (moving in medicine and psychiatry from spirit to psyche) posits a worldview where somatic phenomena are *caused* as an after-effect of the *causal* psychic and intra-psychic experience. Somatisation, in the early psychotraumatological frame, is an embodied response or displacement of the psychic experience of traumatic events and situations. That said, we can see in Janet (1901) how there is a resistance to the body–mind dualism, suggesting (for example) that Janet's notion of the fixation and synthesis of ideas is a mode of being that incorporates both body and mind as a co-occurring coenesthetic cognitive generality.

Within early curative and fixative models of psychological trauma, there is an insinuation that the broken psyche or forms of relating (or attachment) need to be healed, resolved or recovered from. The framing of this frequently involves a form of mental time travel, in which the clinician and the client find ways in the present of returning to the splits and breaks in consciousness of the person in the past. Here, blame for traumatic experience can easily be ascribed to the person perpetrating the act(s) or enactment of violence, or equally to the lack of psychological robustness, will or resilience of the person who experienced the violence, rending them implicitly guilty for not moving beyond the causal event, situation or relations.

The notion that all presenting, manifesting or perceived phenomena (clinically seen to be symptomology) exhibited by a client can be reduced to a single event, or set of relationships, is problematic. It does not account for the changing meanings of experiences and situations over the course of a person's life. Despite this, in my own clinical work and that of colleagues, many clients come to psychotherapy with a want or intention for an *explanatory singularity*, echoing the certainty that the early psychotraumatologists themselves sought.

Within the aforementioned traditions, there is at times a tacit complicity between psychotherapist and client in finding a *retro-causality*, an *explanatory singularity*. The chronological focus is on a causal event or relationship that could give all meaning to the ways of experiencing and relating the person has in the present. This is echoed in the ways in which many clients seem to be compelled to return to, and re-experience, the features of the *retro-causal explanatory singularity*, akin to the fixity described in Janet's (1901) accounts, and the cycle of violence within Bowlby's (1955) formulation.

If we return for a moment to Freud's (1966 [1895]) own descriptions of *Nachträglichkeit*, retro-causality as a chronologically linear explanatory mechanism becomes problematic and paradoxical. While Freud maintains the linear causality of traumatic events and symptoms, they are mediated through a retro-causal dynamics with the changing meaning of an event. For example, in the case of Emma (discussed in Chapter 1), her sexual abuse as the original traumatic event only has relevance and meaning through the subsequent experiences of shops and shopkeepers, and associated memories and sensations that arise. The causal singularity of Emma's original trauma becomes traumatic through the retro-causal remembering and change in meaning ascribed to it.

The *causal-retro-causal paradox* weaves back into the *paradox of confrontations with reality*, as it calls into question the experiential and therapeutic relevance or reality of an external, interpersonal precipitating event or situation. The causal-retro-causal paradox and the privileges given to meaning-making risks the facticity of the experience (both its actuality and its perception by the person) being subsumed into intra-psychic machinations. This, worryingly, can position people within the psychotherapeutic gaze as being self-traumatising subjects, seemingly abstracted once again from the relational worlds in which the trauma took place or is taking place. If we take the example of torturous treatment, whatever causal meaning we, or the client, ascribes to the event and/or relationships, there is facticity in the reality of the experiences. The bruised flesh, the voice of the torturer, the blood-stained clothes, are all testament to the reality, however and whether we confront its meaning or not.

We can see the tensions of *retro-causality* in the questions that I, and other psychotherapists, encounter in the therapy room. I am frequently asked by my clients whether 'who they are' is singularly caused and determined by an event or relationship they have had in the past. In this moment they are seemingly unaware or uncurious about the totality of their lives, the creative ways they have adapted to the changing situations, relationships and worlds they have lived in. The search for an explanatory singularity, a retro-causality, takes precedence over all other explanatory meaning.

The tension around a want for a retro-causal, explanatory singularity becomes a bind for the psychotherapist and client. In affirming a retro-causality, the therapist and client can bind all of their explorations within the explanatory singularity. It also becomes an existential paradox for the client, as their life can only be understood in terms of retro-causality, and thus the person who presents in the therapy room is someone whose being is located in the past moment. Alternatively, in disaffirming the retro-causality, the therapist and client can be lost in attempting to find an autobiographical narrative and understanding that enables the client to make sense of themselves and the world around them. As we will see in forthcoming chapters of this book, the temporal–spatial experience of trauma requires a deeper reconsideration, and I will offer a more existential basis for understanding it.

Human interdependency and survival

Although articulated in different ways, the early psychiatric and psychological formulations of interpersonal trauma describe how these experiences and emotional responses disrupt our connection with ourselves, other humans and human systems (i.e. families and communities). Klein (1998 [1975]) describes the loss of trust that results from familial abuse and neglect. Similarly, Freyd (1994; 1996) explains how the erosion of trust is experienced by the person as a betrayal. Experiences of loss and betrayal result in forms of traumatic aloneness (as described by Ferenczi, 1949 [1932]), within which we paradoxically find ourselves isolated emotionally and relationally from others, and at the same time inexplicably trapped within our relations with the traumatising other.

Further, the early phenomenological descriptions of Janet and Freud describe the ways in which we are betrayed by ourselves to others, that betrayal being expressed through the disclosure of our distress within, for example, seemingly uncontrollable somatic phenomena and sensations (i.e. shaking, sweating, gasping), distancing experiences from our consciousness (dissociation) and our relational adaptations and responses (i.e. withdrawing from social contact, searching our environment for threat).

Underlying the loss of trust and betrayal in ourselves and in the other is the facticity of interdependency on other human beings. Miller (1984 [1981]), Herman (2015 [1992]) and Bowlby (1973) all show how the child (and later the adult) has to adapt to the contingency of their environment, the immediacy of their dependency on their parent(s), and find ways of relating and attaching to them – even in situations where the parents are the source of danger, neglect or harm to the child. Even when we live beyond the moment of a traumatic event, flashbacks, intrusive images or thoughts, memories and dreams all bring us back into contact with the traumatic other. We continue to live in relation to them, even in situations where they are no longer physically present or proximate to us.

The reality of our interdependency discloses a foundational risk of interpersonal danger and harm within the structure of our human experience. As we have seen, Klein (1997 [1975]) saw the other as a potential source of risk and endangerment, and (A) Freud (2018 [1936]) noted the importance of recognising threats posed by another, not just the actual bodily harm caused by them. Bowlby (2005

[1988]) and Salter Ainsworth (Salter Ainsworth et al., 2014 [1978]) more substantively demonstrated how the presence and absence of the other can mediate or intensify fear-arousing experiences. Even when the traumatic person or experience is abstracted or dissociated into a generalised perception of fear arousal or threat in our environment, we remain psychologically related to the impact of the interdependency with the other.

The reality of our human interdependency, and the possibility of interpersonal threat as part of the foundation of human existence, leads us to see the centrality of survivalism and adaptation to human experiences. Illustrating this, Bowlby (1973) suggests that people's attunement to cues of danger, attachment patterns and working models are the basis of them surviving in relation to others and their wider environment. For Janet (1901), dissociation enables people to distance themselves from the conscious reality of their situation and survive their experiences. Similarly, Miller (1984 [1981]) suggests that repression of memories of traumatic experiences enables children to survive their dependency on their parents and other abusive adults in their life. Ferenczi (1949 [1932]) describes how children subject to abuse and neglect will collude with the people abusing and neglecting them in order to survive the relationship.

In bringing our attention to the centrality of survivalism and adaptation to human experiencing, I do not seek to reopen debates over psychoanalytic drive, instinct or will theories, nor the evolutionary psychology of human development. Adaptation and survival in the context of the early writings on psychological trauma have two intertwined existential values. The first is making sense of the paradoxical nature of human interdependency – albeit in traumatic circumstances. That is the existential paradox of finding a space to exist within the tension of being connected to, and separate from, others. The second value is how we find agentic potential through being able to (and having the existential capacity to) adapt and survive a traumatic situation or relationship(s).

While sometimes sidelined or left as tacit acknowledgements within some of the early psychotraumatological writings, the agency of the child or adult person is a central tenant of interpersonal interdependency. Freudian accounts of childhood trauma are frequently misread as stripping the human child of their agentic potential; however, the child of Freud's writings exists in more than a constellation of complexes, defences and repressions. A human child, as Bowlby (2005 [1988]), Winnicott (2018a [1965]) and Herman (2015 [1992]) suggest, is co-creative and agentic in their environment, actively making sense of the relationships, environment and traumatic experiences they are exposed to. The agentic potential of the child and person enables them to find meaning, attitudes and ways of surviving or adapting that transcend the immediate moment, and make them more than products of their immediate world.

Finally, this leads us to a philosophical problem relating to human interdependency. The co-creative nature of traumatic interpersonal relating leaves us with the question of where to *locate* the psychological trauma: is it within the subjective experience and agency of the traumatised person, between the persons involved in the traumatic encounter and/or the interpersonal relationships the traumatised person has beyond the encounter – their parents, family, friends, children or in the wider society around them? The ambiguity disclosed within the reality of our human interdependency will be something we will explore in more depth in subsequent chapters of this book.

3 Interpersonal traumas as psychological and social pathologies

In the previous chapters, I explored some of the foundational early accounts of psychological trauma within psychiatry, psychology and psychotherapy. I went on to draw attention to a number of the paradoxes and tensions that arise from these writings and practices. In this chapter, I set out the ways in which the impact of interpersonal trauma on the person has been constructed as a psychiatric, psychological and social pathology. Focusing on the rise of post-traumatic stress, and the ways it is incorporated into psychiatric diagnoses as a sociocultural artefact arising from specific sociohistorical events. As such, I suggest that these diagnoses disclose more about the cultures from which they arose than the lived phenomena of interpersonal trauma that they seeks to describe.

Subsequently, I turn to examine the more recent rise of the adverse childhood experiences (ACEs) movement. In this, I suggest that researchers and public health professionals draw on specific ideas about risky subjects to relocate the potential danger of psychological and social pathology in the person who has experienced adversity. In doing so, professionals legitimise their power to intervene in people's lives to prevent a possible future of adverse outcomes and the intergenerational transmission of adversity.

Post-traumatic stress as a psychiatric disorder

Within contemporary psychiatric diagnostics, the focus is not primarily on the event or situation, but rather the continuing emotional and neurocognitive impacts on the person. In the clinical literature, the continuing psychological impacts of trauma have been incorporated into models of anxiety and stress. *Post-traumatic stress* is the term used to describe the ongoing psychological, physiological and emotional stress that arises after the traumatic incident or experiences.

The notion of post-traumatic stress and its incorporation into psychiatric diagnoses owes much to the significant influence of Mardi Horowitz's (1976) stress response theory. While the exact diagnostic formulation of post-traumatic stress has changed over time, a number of descriptive features have endured.[1] The enduring features of the diagnostic formulation of post-traumatic stress, as a psychiatric disorder, are explored in what follows, and continue to build on Horowitz's

DOI: 10.4324/9781003181675-5

stress response theory. The incorporation of Horowitz's theory into discussions on psychological trauma emerged from a psychiatric debate over the causality of a traumatic event. The debate centred around tensions resulting from the afore-mentioned retro-causal paradox in early psychiatric formulations of psychological trauma (see Chapter 2).

Psychiatrists in the 1960s and 1970s were increasingly using experimental and clinical research to interrogate whether it was the traumatic event itself that resulted in psychiatric symptoms, or whether there were predisposing individual personality or (so-called) 'vulnerability' characteristics that resulted in psychiatric symptoms – through the exposure to the traumatic event. Horowitz's (1976) psychodynamic research on emotional stress led him to conclude that all humans respond to stressful events, and while there is variance in the forms of response, the experience of the stressful event or environment itself is the foundational factor in observed psychiatric symptoms.

Horowitz (1976, 1986) suggests that our responses to stressful situations and life events oscillate between intrusive repetitions of the event expressed in our emotional responses, thoughts and behaviours, and responses that seek to deny or avoid these repetitions. His model includes five phases of post-stress response (Horowitz, 1993: 49–54). These include in the normal response: (1) an outcry and realisation of the event, leading to feelings of rage, fear and sadness; (2) denial and avoidance of the memory of the event; (3) intrusions, where thoughts, memories and emotions of the event unconsciously arise; (4) working through and facing the reality of the event and experience; and finally (5) completion, involving an incorporation of the experience into one's life.

Between each of these phases is a potential for what Horowitz sees as psychopathological responses to a traumatic life event. These include: (1) being overwhelmed by the immediate emotional reaction to the event; (2) becoming panicked or exhausted by escalating emotional reactions; (3) engaging in extreme avoidance to deny the pain of the event; (4) entering a flooded state where the person is overwhelmed by persistent and disturbing images, memories, thoughts and sensations of the event; and (5) a psychosomatic response resulting from the overwhelming emotional distress. These five psychopathological responses can result, for Horowitz, in long-term distortions in the person's thinking, memory and behaviours. While adopting a phased model, Horowitz is clear that in practice the model may not be sequential and there might be overlaps and movement between and within these five phases.

Turning now to consider recent psychiatric constructions of post-traumatic stress, we can see the legacy and influence of the early psychotraumatologists and the stress response theory. The latest version (fifth edition) of the *Diagnostic and Statistical Manual of Mental Disorders* (*DSM-5*) (APA, 2013) describes the symptoms and suggested treatment for post-traumatic stress disorder (PTSD). It includes a new 'dissociative subtype' of PTSD, which focuses on feelings of disconnectedness and detachment from one's body or experiences (c.f. Lanius et al., 2010). Furthermore, it notes that many people who experience PTSD will have at least another co-occurring diagnosable condition related to the traumatic experienced they have had. This might include anxiety, eating disorders, adjustment disorders, conduct and personality disorders, somatic disorders or the problematic misuse of substances.

According to clinical studies, almost a third of young people born in England or Wales are exposed to a form of trauma by the age of 18 years (Lewis et al., 2019; see also Chandan et al., 2019). Research further suggests that around 16 per cent of children and young people exposed to these experiences go on to develop PTSD specifically (Alisic et al., 2014). International studies have indicated that this might be a conservative estimate of prevalence, with some finding between 56 per cent and 68 per cent of young people experiencing trauma (Copeland et al., 2007; Landolt, 2013; McLaughlin et al., 2013) – although contextual socio-political factors may account for these higher estimates.

The World Health Organisation's (2019: 6B40) *International Classification of Diseases (ICD-11)* contains a specific description of PTSD, which has a similar aetiology and symptomology as the diagnosis in the *DSM-5*. The *ICD-11* also includes a second diagnosis of 'Complex PTSD' (ibid: 6B41). Complex PTSD has a higher threshold of traumatic exposure, and occurs following exposure to an event or prolonged series of reoccurring events that are 'extremely threatening or horrific nature' and from which 'escape is difficult or impossible'. This includes experiencing traumatic disasters, or an enduring possibility of death and exposure to life-threatening situations, which would include torture, slavery, genocide, prolonged domestic violence, and repeated childhood abuse (see also Maercker et al., 2013). The inclusion of a new classification of Complex PTSD follows advocacy by leading clinicians (c.f. Herman, 1992) about the intensification of post-traumatic stress symptoms among people who have experienced prolonged and repeated interpersonal trauma.

The psychiatrist Bessel van der Kolk (2014) has proposed the introduction of 'developmental trauma disorder' (DTD) into the *DSM-5*. DTD would specifically recognise trauma resulting from traumatic experiences in childhood (Schmid, Petermann & Fegert, 2013). Despite being considered for the most recent revision of the *DSM-5*, and significant support from researchers and practitioners, it was not included as a new classification (Bremness & Polzin, 2014).

The *DSM-5* (APA, 2013) additionally includes the diagnosis of acute stress disorder (ASD), which is seen as being within a so-called *normal* range of psychological responses to traumatic experiences. These symptoms of acute traumatic stress are said to usually develop within a month of an event or situation. ASD can involve a wide range of trauma-related responses, including intrusive memories or thoughts, nightmares, flashbacks, psychological distress when play resembles the traumatic event, a persistent negative mood, dissociation, problems sleeping or concentrating, unprovoked aggressive behaviour or continuous scanning for threats in the immediate environment. The main difference between ASD and PTSD is that one needs to experience fewer symptoms to get an ASD diagnosis, and they tend to subside after a month, whereas more of the symptoms are present in PTSD and they persist for a much longer period of time.

PTSD as a sociocultural artefact

While these psychiatric classifications portray a sense of clinical certainty and authority about the nature and impact of psychological trauma, we must hold them lightly. It would be remiss of me not to mention here the ongoing sociological concerns about the expansive medicalisation of human distress, and the ways in which classifications like PTSD, Complex PTSD, DTD and ASD bring more of our human experiencing into the auspices of psychiatric and psychological power. Diagnosis can increase professional control over the everyday lives, thoughts, bodies and relationships of people, rendering professional assessment the validating authority on the legitimacy of a person's distress and access to social and emotional support (c.f. Foucault 1979, 1990 [1984], 2009 [1961]).

Medical anthropologists and sociologists, such as Allan Young (1995), suggest that PTSD emerges as a social construct (using the words of Latour, 2005) arising from specific American and Anglo-American sociohistorical events. For example, the experiences of First and Second World War veterans significantly impacted psychiatric classification in early Anglo-American psychiatry, and the social movements of Vietnam veterans and their allies increased pressure on society and psychiatry to develop further classifications and treatments for PTSD in the American context (Horwitz, 2018; Leys, 2000; Young, 1995). The adoption and stimulus of PTSD as a psychiatric diagnosis within private markets and consumerism in mental health and psychiatric care have led to significant popularisation within both professional and lay communities, which in turn has reinforced the legitimacy and power of psychiatric diagnosis (following Frances, 2013; Horwitz & Wakefield, 2007). As such, trauma-related diagnoses are socially constructed behavioural phenotypes, used by professionals to locate forms of distress and to legitimise intervention in people's lives. In reality, the marketisation and structural operations of trauma-related diagnoses within social networks lead to a reductive and overly deterministic framework, which is convenient for clinical classification, but fails to understand the complexities of traumatic experiencing and response.

As we saw earlier, the contribution of feminist clinicians and researchers illuminated the ways in which permissive cultures around rape, abuse and incest (for example) enabled the structural and interpersonal power relations and conditions for these traumatic experiences. Further, these same sociocultural power dynamics shaped the experiences that are seen within society and psychiatry as being legitimate forms of human suffering and distress to intervene in, and offer treatment for (following Hacking 1991; 1999; Illich, 1976; Smith, 2014; Zola, 1982). This explains in part Herman's advocacy for the inclusion of Complex PTSD in psychiatric classification, and that of van der Kolk for DTD. The phenomena described within psychiatric diagnostics clearly exist at an experiential level. Here, I am drawing the reader's attention once again to the proposition that the psychiatric and diagnostic features and characterisations of traumatic experiencing are socially and historically produced. As such, the classifications disclose as much (if not more) about the genesis of Anglo-American societies as they do about the experience of any one person who has lived through an interpersonal trauma.

Transdiagnostic features of psychological trauma

Over the last decade (2010s), there has been a more substantive transdiagnostic turn in psychiatry and psychology, following the increased popularisation of biopsychosocial models of health and illness (see Dalgleish et al., 2020; Ehrenreich-May & Chu, 2014). Rather than focusing on condition-specific aetiology, pathways and treatments, many psychological clinicians and researchers have turned their attention to the common factors that underlie many of the condition-specific symptomologies (Conway et al., 2018; Debanné & Nolte, 2019: 30–31 on the p factor). Within this movement, psychological trauma is seen as a transdiagnostic risk or vulnerability factor, resulting in a diverse range of mental health outcomes and implicated within a wide number of mental health phenomena and diagnoses (Luyten & Fonagy, 2019: 82; Teicher & Samson, 2013), from depression to psychosis (Hoppena & Chalder, 2018; Schierholz et al., 2016; Varese et al., 2012).

Leading neuroscientists and clinical psychologists suggest that early experiences of adversity (e.g. childhood neglect and maltreatment) result in changes to people's neurocognitive systems. Neurocognitive and neurobiological alterations reflect the ways in which a child adapts to survive in their harmful environment. These neurocognitive adaptations include changes in the way people process threat, reward or autobiographical memories, and how they regulate their emotions (McCory, Puetz et al., 2017; McCory & Viding, 2015; Weissman et al., 2019). The argument is that neurocognitive adaptations in the longer term are maladaptive and can contribute to the development of a wide range of mental health conditions, social connectedness (McCrory, Gerin & Viding, 2017) and accelerated biological processes, including puberty and cellular ageing (McLaughlin et al., 2020).

While transdiagnostic research and understanding of psychological trauma continue to grow in influence in psychology and neuroscience, in reality condition-specific conceptualisations continue to dominate clinical understanding within psychiatric, psychological and psychotherapeutic practice. For the most part, the legacy of a pathological model of the impact of traumatic experiences has endured within psychiatric nosology.

Intergenerational transmissions of trauma

Within contemporary psychotraumatological research there has been a renewed focus on the intergenerational (or transgenerational) transmission of interpersonal trauma (c.f. Fitzgerald et al., 2017; Widom, 1999). This renewed focus extends beyond the aforementioned observations within psychodynamic, object-relations and attachment-based theories about the intergenerational consequences of patterns of relating from one generation to subsequent generations. More recent neuroscientific and genetic research into trauma-related parental stress has extended the earlier psychotraumatological ideas through investigating the epigenetic, intergenerational impacts of trauma on people's neuroendocrine and neuroanatomical structure and functioning (c.f. Dashorst et al., 2019; Yehuda & Bierer, 2008; Yehuda, et al., 2016; Youssef et al., 2018). However, limitations of the methodologies and frameworks used means that firm conclusions about the impacts of trauma on people's neuroendocrine and neuroanatomical system cannot be drawn (Bowers & Yehuda, 2016).

Yehuda, Lehrner and Bierer (2018) encourage us to understand intergenerational transmission at a genetic and psychological level as a form of sociobiological learning, where one generation transmits its understanding about how to survive in an environment to the next. In this, they warn against adopting a biological determinism, clarifying that their research contributes to a wider field of how interpersonal biological systems are impacted by traumatic stress, and how from this, systems can also build resiliency in, adaptability to and mutability within their environment.

Much of the focus of study within transgenerational trauma research has been at the community level, which is beyond the scope of the discussion in this book. Transgenerational researchers have explored how collective experiences of war, famine and genocide impact community coherence, collective values and meaning-making, and give rise to trauma-based coping strategies, which are transmitted through the generations (c.f. Bezoa & Maggib, 2015).

That said, the intergenerational transmission of PTSD symptoms has proven more complex. For example, a meta-analysis of studies on the intergenerational consequences of the Holocaust found that traumatisation of the first generation did not necessarily lead to more complex psychiatric consequences in the second generation of children of survivors (van IJzendoorn, Bakermans-Kranenburg & Sagi-Schwartz, 2003). Similarly, a Portuguese study (Castro-Vale et al., 2019) concluded that the children of male veterans of wars (with Angola, Mozambique and Guinea between 1961 and 1974) experienced higher psychological distress; however, they concluded that this related to the 'intensity' of the father's 'exposure' to the war rather than the father's PTSD symptomology.

Increasingly, social psychiatry and public mental health frameworks are focusing on community violence reduction theories to explore impacts of cycles of abuse and/or violence on lived experience and outcomes. This follows the idea that what is passed on to the next generation is not the PTSD (or other diagnostic) symptoms per se but rather the patterning of traumatic relating and adaptations (c.f. Hulette, Kaehler & Freyd, 2011; Pat-Horenczyk et al., 2020; Roth, Neuner & Elbert, 2014; Song, Tol & de Jong, 2014).

The renewed focus on intergenerational consequences of traumatic experiences is not a recent concern. In Chapter 1, we saw how Bowlby, among others, described how an intergenerational transmission of trauma could occur within family systems, emerging from interpersonal traumas and the resulting disorganised patterns of attachment. Within these accounts we see again the tension between the actual traumatic experience, the individual subjective experience and the adaptive responses of the person over time (in part described psychopathologically).

Beyond the realms of PTSD and post-traumatic stress, the research on the intergenerational transmission of interpersonal trauma intersects with a broader social notion of intergenerational cycles of violence. The idea that people who have experienced interpersonal trauma (childhood abuse or neglect) will become adults who are more likely to maltreat their own children was a dominant narrative within psychological research during the 1950s and 1960s in particular. You might recall that Bowlby (2005 [1988]) portrayed situations where mothers and fathers who had experienced interpersonal trauma in childhood were more likely to re-enact these experiences in their own caregiving (see also Crittenden & Ainsworth, 1989).

To date, there remain conflicting empirical findings as to whether parental experiences of abuse and neglect in childhood are associated with a greater risk of them abusing or neglecting their own children, or engaging in intimate partner violence in adulthood, and the factors that might mediate any relationship (c.f. Berlin, Appleyard & Dodge, 2011; Kaufman & Zigler, 1987; Pears & Capaldi, 2001; Renner & Slack, 2006; Sidebotham et al., 2001; Widom, Czaja & DuMont, 2015; Zuravin et al., 1991). Cathy Spatz Widom (1989a, 1989b) has sought to interrogate the evidence surrounding the cycle of violence hypothesis. She suggests that there are significant methodological limitations underpinning it (see also Thornberry, Knight & Lovgrove, 2012). Despite this, her own large prospective cohort studies (Maxfield & Widom, 1996; Widom, 1989a, 1989b; Widom & Osborn, 2021) conclude that experience of childhood abuse and neglect does significantly increase the likelihood of adult criminality and violence within the family and community.

Adverse childhood experiences (ACEs)

The popularisation of PTSD and intergenerational transmission of trauma has been complemented by social policy and public health frameworks that have presented interpersonal trauma as a social pathology, which requires population-level surveillance, prevention and intervention. The initial return, within the public health models, to the experience of the event(s) or situation enables the language of trauma (as an event or experience and potential psychological impact) to take another form.

Since the early 2000s, there has been rapid growth in clinical and political discourse around adverse childhood experiences (ACEs), especially within epidemiology and public health disciplines. The reader may recall that Bowlby extensively used the terms 'adverse experiences' in childhood; however, these recent reconceptualisations draw us away from his meaning and epistemological framework. While the terms 'adversity', 'childhood adversity' and 'adverse experiences in childhood' have been present within clinical and social research since the early decades of the twentieth century, the idea of ACEs has a specific conceptual meaning in contemporary psychotraumatology.

The recent reconceptualisation of childhood adversity as ACEs was codified through a set of studies undertaken by the Centers for Disease Control and Prevention (CDC) and the Department of Preventive Medicine at Kaiser Permanente (KP) in the United States of America. Vincent Felitti and colleagues (1998) sought to understand the relationships between childhood adversity, health risk behaviours and wider health outcomes in adulthood. The original study surveyed 9,508 Californian adults, who were privately insured by KP, in two waves between 1995 and 1997. In addition to a general medical screening, the survey enquired about people's exposure to seven categories of ACEs. The seven categories were more broadly described as forms of 'childhood abuse' and 'household dysfunction'. The forms of childhood abuse and household dysfunction included in the original study were psychological, physical or sexual abuse; violence against mother; and living with household members who misuse substances, are mentally ill or suicidal, or have ever been imprisoned.

Analysis of the CDC–KP study (Felitti et al., 1998) suggested a graded relationship between the number of categories of childhood adversity a person had been exposed to and poorer adult health risk behaviours and outcomes. Poorer health outcomes and riskier health behaviours included alcoholism, substance use, suicidality, psychopathology and severe obesity. More specifically, those participants who had exposure to four or more categories of ACEs were reported to have the poorest psychological and mental health outcomes, health risk behaviours and social outcomes. The findings of the original CDC–KP study popularised the notion of a graded and cumulative dose-response relationship between the ACEs scores (the number of ACE categories exposed to) and outcomes in adulthood. As a result, the CDC and KP used the studies to advocate for increased focus and funding for preventative public health interventions.

The dose-response relationship between ACE scores and adult outcomes recorded in the original ACE studies has been replicated across the world (c.f. Amemiya et al., 2019; Bellis et al., 2014; Bellis, Ashtoni et al., 2015; Bellis, Hughes et al., 2015; Hughes et al., 2016). The country-specific studies have drawn similar conclusions in relation to exposure to ACEs and adverse behavioural, health and social outcomes in adolescence, adulthood and later life. Consequently, there have been efforts by the World Health Organisation (2018), among others, to standardise international definitions and questionnaires on ACEs, and to agree on the basis of preventative and early intervention in relation to ACE exposure.

Increasingly, researchers have sought to diversify the various definitions and measurement frameworks used to describe what experiences constitute an ACE, and the various mental health and social outcomes resulting from them (Bethell et al., 2017; Burgermeister, 2007; Mersky, Janczewski & Topitzes, 2017; Quigg, Wallis & Butler, 2018). For example, Peter Cronholm and colleagues (2015) are critical of the restricted socioeconomic and racial profile of participants included in the original and subsequent ACE studies. The authors have critiqued the primary focus on so-called household dysfunction within the 'conventional' measures of ACEs, and have investigated a number of 'expanded' community-level ACEs. These community-level measures aim to identify those children experiencing adversity beyond the home, who may not be identified through the conventional measures. The expanded measures include witnessing violence, living in an unsafe neighbourhood, experiencing bullying, living in foster care and experiencing feelings of discrimination (see also expanded UK definition in Bush [Boaz], 2018b). As such, when we write of ACEs in lay, policy, clinical or research terms, we are not by any means describing the same conceptual construct (Science and Technology Committee, 2018). Nor are we drawing on consensus or validated methods of measuring and investigating the experiential phenomena associated with ACEs (Early Intervention Foundation, 2020).

ACEs as a sociocultural artefact

ACEs are underpinned by a developmental and life-course risk model. The model suggests that exposure to ACEs increases the likelihood of disrupted neurodevelopment; social, emotional and cognitive problems; and increased morbidity and even premature and avoidable mortality from the leading causes of adult deaths from natural causes, including heart disease, respiratory disease and cancer (c.f. Brown et al., 2009; Kelly-Irving et al., 2013).

The prospective psychosocial risk model is a compelling sociopolitical narrative within public health, mental health, epidemiology and social policy. Identification of potential risk provides fertile ground for social and mental health interventions in people's personal and family lives. Furthermore, the uncertainty regarding which specific person will exhibit PTSD, post-traumatic stress or wider mental health symptoms as a result of ACEs, enables public health, social policy, psychological and psychotherapeutic professionals to take the mere existence of these interpersonal event(s) or situations into a professional gaze. This renders anyone (or any family or community) who is exposed to an ACE, or who is profiled as having the potential to be exposed, as being legitimately within the scope of understanding and professional power through the exercise of public policy, public health and psychotherapeutic interventions (following Foucault, 1979, 1983, 2003 [1963], 2009 [1961]).

The CDC–KP model emerges out of the US context of private insurance underpinning access to psychiatric, psychotherapeutic or psychopharmacological provision and treatment. Private insurers in the United States of America have a financial incentive to find ways of reducing the lifetime cost of mental health treatment, and where possible preventing escalations and additional complexity in needs (Frances, 2013). The marketisation of mental health insurance and treatment (including through private, Medicare and Medicaid schemes) in the United States of America has been subject to changing political interests in investigating preventative and early treatment models. The social justice philosopher Michael Sandel (2012) questions whether the very presence of consumerism and marketisation in mental healthcare *corrodes and corrupts* the very social, psychological and emotional values required to meaningfully provide interpersonal care and support.

The focus on early intervention gained significant political and public support beyond the United States of America, with the concept of ACEs now playing a major role, for example, in UK policymaking. This is especially the case in Wales

(Public Health Wales, 2018) and Scotland (Scottish Government, 2017), where it is embedded in the governments' National Health Service (NHS) and public health frameworks (albeit with a less marketized and consumerist framing). While the UK nations do not primarily operate on a private insurance model for mental health treatment, the NHS has its own financial, social and operational incentives to reduce the duration and perceived severity of psychiatric conditions, and in turn lower the lifetime costs of mental health treatment and care, not least because it is ultimately the NHS (through its commissioning and procurement structures), and wider state social support system (through welfare provision), which is responsible for meeting the cost of mental health outcomes in adulthood.

ACEs, risk and the potentiality of danger

As interpersonal sociopsychological phenomena, the enactment of traumatic experiencing occurs within the social domain of existence. As such, our understanding of it cannot be abstracted from the social world and meanings that weave through, and around, these enactments. In the context of public health and social policy, the meaning of an event cannot be abstracted from systems of professional power/knowledge (following Foucault, 1990 [1984]) and social interpretations (following Latour, 2005). These systems frame the identification of risk and social intelligibility of interpersonal trauma through the categorisation of experience (renamed using the empirical 'exposure') as ACE phenomena.

The population-level public health framing of ACEs creates an ambiguity as to where to locate the 'pathological' aspect of the traumatic experiencing. The location of the *risk* of psychopathology depends on the values, attitudes and beliefs of the organisations and persons engaging in the ACEs discourse. In practice, ACE research and advocacy err closer to a naive realism, suggesting an objective universal reality of childhood adversity that 'exists and can be measured independently of social and cultural processes' (following Lupton, 2013a: 49). At best, social and cultural processes are deemed to be mediating factors within the ACE phenomena, rather than ACEs being framed more explicitly as emerging from, between and within sociocultural and interpersonal processes.

In addition to being a public health mechanism for describing adversity and (potentially) traumatic events and situations (through the use of tools, scores, data and concepts), the ACEs framework and its operation as a research and professional paradigm for intervention is also highly sociopolitically situated. Thus, it is open to significant influence and (re)appropriations by wider political discourses (Foucault, 2000 [1970]; 1979). The medical sociologist Deborah Lupton (2013a), among others (see Douglas, 1986; Douglas & Wildavsky, 1982), has demonstrated how the identification, assessment and communication of risk has become a central cultural construct in Westernised societies. She describes how the concept of *risk* within public health discourse has become intertwined with the idea of *potential danger*.

Within the ACEs framework, exposure to an ACE creates a *risky subject*, who is imbued with a new danger, that is, not merely the danger of exposure to an

ACE, but also the potential danger of psychopathological and other adverse outcomes. The risky subject of the ACE-exposed person becomes the legitimised site of professional governance and sociotechnological investigation and intervention (see Lupton, 2013a: 113–171 for a more detailed analysis). Moreover, the potential danger of the intergenerational transmission of adversity and trauma is also located within the risky subject. Intervention in their lives and personhood within the ACEs framework, transforms the person into a site for prevention of the intergenerational transmission of interpersonal trauma.

The focus on increased likelihood of *potentially dangerous outcomes* within the ACEs model operates as form of risk technology, which has been taken up, through abstraction, by the use of *ACE scores* within the ACE advocacy movement and public campaigns aimed at lay audiences. There are various websites where people can now calculate their own ACE score. Further, ACE training organisations hand out different modified checklists at professional conferences, asking attendees (as a warm-up exercise) to calculate their ACE score. Within the popularised forms of ACE scores, public health technology loses its epidemiological formula and meaning. There is a transformation of the adversity to better correlate with the wider sociocultural framing of risk as a potentiality and futurity of danger. The proximate danger Bowlby (1982 [1969], 2005 [1988]) spoke of is no longer the possibility of engagement by the other but rather transformed into the possibility of adverse psychological (and other health) outcomes.

In the ACEs campaign movement, the equation becomes akin to: the level of cumulative exposure (*number of ACEs*) x risk of danger (*likelihood of poorer health outcomes*) = level of intervention required and justified to prevent future potential danger (*psychopathology and other adverse outcomes in the person and future generations*) from occurring. The movement from an epidemiological, population-level construct to an individual, personal, explanatory construct is concerning as it loses all the evidential nuance contained within the original and subsequent ACEs research. Researchers using and investigating the ACEs frame are clear that ACE exposure does not determine an outcome trajectory. Furthermore, the technological reductionism of the ACE score is cautioned against within the original research. The majority of ACE research states that the pathways between exposures and outcomes are uncertain and mediated by a range of as yet underinvestigated factors. That said, the technological reductionism is understandable. In crafting ACE scores as a proxy for human experiencing, the risk (potentiality and futurity of danger) becomes seemingly concrete, unambiguous and intelligible to the person, especially as the self-ascribed score derives (in part) from their own assessment and recollections of their exposure to the categories of ACEs (following Lupton, 2016; Tulloch & Lupton, 2003).

Lupton (2013b: 638) suggests that risk, 'because it involves an incipient rather than a realised threat or danger, is about projecting ideas into the future, about imagining the consequences of an action or event'. Imagined future and potentiality of danger within the ACEs model have an important function in personal and collective meaning-making. Our human anxiety regarding the emergence of adverse psychopathological outcomes (including increased morbidity and mortality) leads to the need for a sense of certainty and containment (albeit a false sense). In retrospect, many people socially, and in a therapeutic environment, long for an explanatory mechanism for poor health, social and economic outcomes. The transformed reductionism in parts of the ACEs advocacy movement enables people to locate all signs and realisations of potential danger (presence of emotional distress, relational difficulty, illness, substance use etc.) as having their origin in the exposure to ACEs. The person's own agentic adaptation to their exposure to ACEs is rendered a phenomenon of personal resilience or incorporated into narrative advocacy, demonstrating the possibility of adverse outcomes without psychological or psychotherapeutic intervention.

At a sociopolitical level, uncertainties regarding risk, potentiality and psychopathological futurity of ACEs (and resulting psychological traumatisation) are compelling and attractively ambiguous collective narratives. In my own experience of working in a social policy context in the field of ACEs, I have seen the same ACEs evidence and tools used to advocate for diverging, conflicting and contradictory social and psychological interventions. The political malleability of the ACEs discourse reflects the ways in which conceptions of risk and potentiality can be used by social actors, institutions and movements as evidential artefacts conveying a model of danger to the person and wider society (Lupton, 1993).

By way of illustration, I have worked with conservative moralists in the United Kingdom who use the ACEs framework and evidence to critique the liberalisation of social welfare reform and attribute this reform to the rise of ACE phenomena and health risk outcomes. Others have spoken to me of the perceived erosion of the nuclear family, the networks of support seen to be supporting this and the perceived consequences for interfamilial dynamics, and the rise of disorganised patterns of attachments and poorer mental health outcomes. In contrast, I have also worked with more liberal commentators who have taken up the ACEs discourse to challenge what they see to be a socially pathological nature of systemic injustices. They challenge, for example, the perceived conservative moralising and silencing of social problems, like violence against woman and girls, and institutional abuses of power. In doing so, they proffer policy reform and social intervention measures that aim to prevent ACE exposure, reduce the stigma associated with it and advocate for greater support for those who have experienced interpersonal trauma.

I am drawing attention here to the sociocultural context of risk within public health and social policy narratives so that the reader can reflect on the ways in which they themselves take up these frames and discourses within their own use of the ACEs framework. Through professional practice we may end up ascribing and assigning particular kinds of people a status as *risky kinds of people* who contain within them latent potentialities for psychopathology. If we are going to move away from deeply reductive and pathological frames, as professionals we need first to be aware and cognizant of our own potential to take up pathologising frames of reference and unwittingly reapply this within our own professional practice.

Adversity, trauma and subjectivity

The meaning of psychological trauma as both an event and an incorporated impact upon the person is taken up in the usage of ACEs. This has led to the continuous slippage between the terms 'adversity' and 'trauma' within the public discourse around ACEs. The original, and subsequent, public health applications of ACEs tend to be explicit in stating that not all ACEs are experienced by the person as traumatic, and that not all mental health consequences of exposure to adversity are trauma related (and/or more specifically, result in PTSD phenomena). However, in application, many ACE- and trauma-informed training providers and professionals use the terms 'trauma' and 'ACEs' interchangeably, as if they delineate and signify the same phenomenological experience. The interchangeable use of trauma and adversity, and its reduction to an ACE score, leads to confusion over what is being described and intervened in. I have attended and observed workshops where the professionals have been asked to briefly reflect on their autobiographies, and have latterly concluded that (in light of the ACE discourse and presentation provided) that they, and the majority of the room, are now traumatised adults.

The conflation between the event(s) and the incorporated impact on the person takes us back to the tensions I explored in relation to early psychotraumatology, specifically, in relation to the paradoxical nature of the search for the origins of psychopathology, and the changing meaning of event(s) and situation(s) to the individual. By locating the potential danger in the futurity of a person's psychopathology, the ACEs framework loses sight of the richness of interpersonal experiencing and the emergence of the traumatic encounter. The translational limitations of the ACEs framework create a simultaneous, and paradoxical, opening up and closing down of the complexity of lived and subjective realities of interpersonal trauma. The traumatic event, or ongoing situation, is flattened into a knowable social descriptor, and the persons involved into artificial risky subjects, filled with potentiality of danger (psychopathology, including post-traumatic stress and PTSD phenomena). The meta-epistemological reduction of mitigating potential danger into preventative or early intervention in pathological social phenomena and/or the lives (and sometimes framed as the minds) of risky (potentially psychopathological) subjects, strips humans of the agentic reality of their existence.

The ACEs framework and the concept of post-traumatic stress share a commonality: the adverse interpersonal experience, which is seen as a prerequisite for the psychopathological traumatisation of the person. The potentiality for psychological trauma is bound up with the reality of the actuality of a social experience. The interpersonal enactments described as ACEs could therefore be understood as social facts – in that an adverse encounter occurred and has been socially codified through a network of social systems and actors. In reality, the complexity surrounding the emergence of the specific interpersonal moments, the changing descriptors and meanings ascribed to the encounters or enactments, and the ways in which these are incorporated into the person's ways of living in the world are agentically and dynamically situated within intersubjective experience.

For this reason, in my work with YoungMinds and NHS Health Education England, I attempted to bring back some of the important framing of childhood adversity and traumatic experiencing from the early traumatology to the extent it was possible and permissible in this context. Through a consensus description (Bush [Boaz], 2018b: 28), the contributing authors proposed that professionals should move away from pathologising understandings of health risk behaviours and mental health outcomes. In their place, we suggested that professionals could think of presenting behaviours and ways of thinking, and remembering, as creative adaptations and creative adjustments that represent people's attempts to

> survive in their immediate environment [...], finding ways of mitigating or tolerating the adversity by using the environmental, social and psychological resources available to them, establishing a sense of safety or control, making sense of the experiences they have had, the community or family that they are growing up in and the identity they are forming.
>
> (Ibid.)

Emphasising the intersubjective elements of people's responses to adverse experience was an attempt to bring the active and agentic realities of traumatic experiencing back into view within the ACEs discourse.

The centrality of intersubjective experience to understanding the lived realities of ACEs and interpersonal trauma is echoed in recent research suggesting that subjective memory and experience mediate between an experience of ACEs and adverse outcomes. Notably, in a systematic review and meta-analysis of the evidence base, J. R. Baldwin and colleagues (2019) found that prospective and retrospective measures of childhood adversity (using maltreatment definitions) identified different groups of people. While both prospective and retrospective reports of childhood maltreatment were associated with psychopathology by 18 years of age, the strongest associations were found when maltreatment was retrospectively self-reported. As such, this meta-analysis concludes that people who recall experiences of being maltreated as a child are at higher risk of psychopathology (ibid.; see also Newbury et al., 2018; Reuben et al., 2016). Furthermore, Andrea Danese and Cathy Spatz Widom (2020) have suggested that the subjective experience of ACEs mediates the development of post-traumatic stress phenomena. In cases where the experience is both objectively and subjectively appraised as traumatic, this is associated with the highest levels of reported PTSD symptoms and phenomena (Boals, 2018).

In this chapter, I have explored the ways in which traumatic experiencing is contextualised and constructed as a psychological and social pathology in contemporary societies. In doing so I have highlighted the ways in which the person is transformed into a risky subject, whose personhood and futurity are taken into the social and professional gaze for exploration and intervention. In Chapter 4,

I will build on my discussion above to describe the ways in which contemporary psychologies and psychotherapies understand traumatic experiencing and aim to respond to it.

Note

1   I have refrained from rehearsing here the full genesis of the diagnostic categorisation, and refer readers to the works of Herman (2015 [1992]) and van der Kolk et al. (1996) for a fuller analysis.

4 Contemporary trauma-focused psychotherapies

In the previous chapter, we explored the ways in which interpersonal trauma has been constructed within psychiatric diagnosis and public health discourse as a psychological and social pathology. I now turn to consider some of the prominent contemporary trauma-focused psychotherapies. The aim is to provide the reader with an orientation to the ways in which contemporary psychology and psychotherapy are responding to people's experiences of interpersonal trauma. This chapter by no means provides an exhaustive description and analysis of contemporary trauma-focused psychotherapies, but rather some more dominant frames in current practice. Further exploration of contemporary psychotherapies as they relate to existential concerns is continued in the final section of this book.

Neuroscience and contemporary psychotraumatology

Contemporary psychotraumatology has followed a wider turn towards neuroscience within the social and psychological sciences. Increasingly, psychological and psychotherapeutic research and training are synthesising and combining diverse insights from neurobiology and neurophysiology with the practical techniques within their orientation (c.f. Balchin et al., 2019; Northoff, 2011; Schwartz, 2016; Solms, 2004). Much of the evidence base is drawn from neuroscientific theoretical and experimental studies, and particularly utilises hypotheses, observations and visualised explanations from neuroimaging technologies, including the growth of functional magnetic resonance imaging (fMRI), computed tomography (CT) and positron emission tomography (PET) scans in psychotraumatological research.

The turn to neuroscience within psychology and psychotherapy is seemingly a new evolution in contemporary disciplines. However, in many ways it is more useful to see the presence of neuroscience as an attempt to bridge the diverging and meandering developments of psychiatry, psychology and neurology over the course of the twentieth century (see e.g. the work of Hebb, 1949; Kandel, 1998, 2006, 2013). Neuropsychiatry is not a new phenomenon, but rather a revisiting of the psychoneuroses that Freud, Breuer and their contemporaries hoped would be explained through the emerging disciplines of psychoanalysis, and the eventual insights of psychiatry and neurobiology (Rose & Abi-Rached, 2013: 116–117).

DOI: 10.4324/9781003181675-6

Neuroimaging technologies brought about new ways of theorising and empirically investigating the relationships between psychological phenomena and specific regions, neural messages and neurochemical interactions within the brain.

Today, the incorporation of neuroscientific theory and research into contemporary psychotraumatology aims to provide greater understanding about the underlying neurobiological mechanisms that are involved in, and impacted by, the social, emotional, cognitive and somatic experiences of interpersonal trauma. The popularised applications of neuroscience in contemporary psychotraumatology are dominated by the theorisation and investigation of threat perception, detection and processing and the ways in which this dysregulates the person. The theory and research seeks to describe our *neurobiopsychosocial* responses[1] to perceived or actual threats in our environments (c.f. Lucero, 2018). The neuro-focused turn in psychiatry, psychology and psychotherapy proffered a possible reframing of intrapsychic impacts of trauma as being intertwined with the experience of the human person as an embodied being.

The hope for a post-Cartesian and non-dualistic conception of the body and mind was not fulfilled through the turn to neuroscience in contemporary psychotraumatology (also see Dennett, 1991: 101–138). While many of the proponents of neuro-focused psychologies and psychotherapies aim to better situate our so-called psychic life within our neurophysiological and somatic embodiment, the descriptions of the impact of interpersonal trauma frequently retain many of the hallmarks of dualistic and mechanised ideas or descriptions of the body, and functional body–mind processing. By some accounts, the psychic world of the person is significantly diminished, with the primacy given to the explicit or implicit psychological machinations of our bodies. The mechanistic descriptions of the traumatically embodied person are best disclosed and articulated in the titles of well-known recent texts on interpersonal trauma, including Robert Scaer's (2014) *The Body Bears the Burden*, Bessel van der Kolk's (2014) *The Body Keeps the Score*, Gabor Maté's (2019 [2003]) *When the Body Says No* and Babette Rothschild's (2000) *The Body Remembers*.

Neuropsychotherapies and the 'triune brain'

The influence of neuroscience and neurology, and latterly immunoendocrinology (c.f. Sherin & Nemeroff, 2011) has resulted in notable attention being given to the impact of experiencing trauma on our autonomic nervous system. Among some theorists and practitioners, this manifests in significant theorisation about the role of the vagus nerve and our parasympathetic responses to stress and trauma (see Stephen Porges's work on the polyvagal theory, 2003, 2009, 2011). The focus on the responses of specific regions of the brain and autonomic nervous system has led to biomechanical descriptions and explanations of traumatic experiences, and the observed post-traumatic phenomena in clinical and psychotherapeutic work. The biomechanical formulation of traumatic experiencing has been popularised most notably through neuropsychiatrist Daniel Siegel's formulation and application of *interpersonal neurobiology*, and the practical psychotherapy guides created by the leading *sensorimotor* psychotherapists (see, in particular, Minton, Ogden & Pain, 2006; Ogden & Fisher, 2015).

In broad terms, interpersonal neurobiology and sensorimotor psychothera-peutic models suggest that traumatic experiencing alters our neuroception both in the moment and in subsequent interpersonal encounters. Our neuroception is our automatic detection of whether or not there is a threat in our environment or in an interpersonal situation. The focus on threat detection and our neuroceptive responses puts an emphasis on our states of hyperarousal – a heightened state of alert and priming oneself to fight or flight – or hypoarousal – a state of freeze where one feels emotionally numb, dissociated or paralysed from the actual or threat of threat or danger. Associated with the states of hyper- and hypoarousal are the person's hyper- or hypovigilance. The former means the person's overattuned or overactive identification and detection threats in their environment, and the latter an underattunement or underactivity (Siegel, 2006; van der Kolk, 2014).

The alterations in threat detection and our neuroceptive responses emerge from the emotional impacts of traumatic events, relationships and situations. The experience of the events or situations overwhelm and dysregulate the person to the extent they are unable to incorporate and cope with the emotional states evoked by the experience. The neurophysiological and neurocognitive mechanisms involved in dysregulation in the moment of the trauma(s), are seen to have a lasting impact on the person's emotional regulation, threat detection and neuroceptive response over time.

The therapeutic response within the sensorimotor psychotherapy, in par-ticular, focuses on enabling the person to find methods for bringing themselves back into a state of self-regulation, and functional arousal and vigilance. Self- and bodily regulation is the foundation required within the sensorimotor models for neurocognitive explorations in making sense of these traumatic experiences and the person's responses to them. Indeed, the term 'sensorimotor' refers specifically to the sensorimotor – meaning bodily (in contrast to emotional and cognitive) forms of processing traumatic stress and dysregulation. Sensorimotor processing relates directly to the mechanistic ways in which sensorial information is integrated into motor responses in our central nervous system. The focus on threat reactivity is clinically uncontentious; however, it is unclear whether stating that the autonomic nervous system is implicated adds substantively to neuroscientific understanding or to the specific ways in which trauma impacts and disrupts (for example) memory and reward functioning or interpersonal relationality and learning (for a sensori-motor description, see Ogden & Minton, 2000).

The neurophysiological model of the brain used within sensorimotor psychotherapies is of a 'triune brain' (see Ogden & Fisher, 2015: chap. 9). The theoretical hypothesis of the triune brain was developed by the neuroscientist Paul MacLean (1990).[2] MacLean described a hierarchical structure of evolutionary functioning in which three distinct neuroanatomical structures developed through the course of animal (human and non-human) evolution. The three areas of the triune brain within MacLean's model are the reptilian complex (the *basal ganglia*), the paleomammalian complex (the *limbic system*), and the neomammalian complex (the *neocortex*). The model proposes that cognition is layered on top of more prim-ordial emotional processing, and beneath this an instinctive survival-focused neural circuitry. In addition to a Cartesian distinction between mind and body, the triune brain model creates an abstracted separation of cognition from emotional processing, stating that emotions regulate or dysregulate the person's cognition.

Among advocates of the triune brain hypothesis within sensorimotor psychotherapies and psychotherapy more broadly, significant attention is given to the operations of the limbic system and its relationships with experiences of trauma.[3] The limbic system is associated with threat perception and acts as an early warning signal to suggest that a threat is close by. Within the limbic system, the amygdala is seen within the triune model as being the centre for emotions, emotional behaviour and motivation in the brain. The amygdala is attuned to perceive and recognise a threat, and is responsible for triggering our 'fight, flight or freeze' responses, be they in the moment, in memory or in the re-experiencing of trauma.

Within the triune brain metaphor, once an 'alarm' is raised by the amygdala, a neural message is sent down the spinal cord to the adrenal glands to release a surge of adrenaline and noradrenaline into the bloodstream, which prepares the body for urgent action (fight, flight or freeze) and causes our hearts to beat faster. At the same time, the hypothalamus (which receives information through our senses) also sends a signal to our pituitary gland at the bottom of the brain, telling it to release a stress-mitigating hormone called cortisol. This hormone helps the body enact the fight, flight or freeze response, ensuring that muscles get a temporary increase in the energy they will need to respond, and surpassing the immune system to enable this.

Sensorimotor psychotherapies draw attention to the role of the hippocampus (also part of the limbic system) in controlling our emotional and hormonal response to a threat. The hippocampus is seen as relaying new information it receives about a present threat to our memory of past traumatic experiences and feelings, before passing the information on to other parts of the brain responsible for controlling our behaviour. Overexposure to stress hormones can suppress the response of the hippocampus (affecting both memory and behavioural responses) and significantly impact brain development and neurocognition, including the prefrontal cortex that is responsible for making sense of executive thought.

Pat Ogden and Janina Fisher (2015: 243–252) describe three phases of trauma-focused sensorimotor psychotherapy. The first focuses on developing resources to enable the person to self-regulate and manage their states of arousal and vigilance (ibid.: 253–432). The second entails addressing and making sense of memories of the past (ibid.: 433–582). The third involves exploring relationships with other people and finding ways to move on from past experiences of trauma (ibid.: 583–568). The phased model suggests a linear progression, although the authors note that the psychotherapist and client could use the phase structure to find the best way of applying the model to the client's goals and aims for their therapy. These three phases of sensorimotor psychotherapy broadly reflect its association with the structure of the triune brain model. Each phase seemingly builds from the instinctual and survival, through emotionality to the cognitive and meaning-making. The theoretical organisation is focused on sensorially and somatically resourcing the person so that when traumatic response states are triggered in the present, people can find ways of bringing themselves back to a state of somatic, emotional and relational regulation (c.f. Sharpe Lohrasbe & Ogden, 2017).

The sensorimotor psychotherapy approach is explicitly psychoeducative, aiming to provide the client with clarity and certainty about the sensorimotor, neuropsychological, neurobiological, neuroceptive and neurocognitive basis of the traumatic experiencing. The significant use of psychoeducative tools, diagrams, exercises and visualisations makes it a popular resource for trauma psychotherapists, trauma-focused trainers and clients alike.

One of the most well-known and impactful conceptual visualisations is that of the 'window of tolerance',[4] which is used extensively within sensorimotor psychotherapy (Ogden & Fisher, 2015: 219–242; see also Minton, Ogden & Pain, 2006), and has its origins in interpersonal neurobiology. Daniel Siegel (2020: 341) describes the window of tolerance as the parameters in which 'various intensities of emotional arousal can be processed without disrupting the functional system'. Within sensorimotor psychotherapies (c.f. Ogden & Fisher, 2015: 227, 231–235), and their influence elsewhere (c.f. NICABM, 2019), the most frequent application of this is the depiction of a zone of hyperarousal and a zone of hypoarousal, which are situated above (former) and below (later) a window of tolerance (or 'optimal arousal zone'). By Siegel's assessment, the use of the window of tolerance to denote a midpoint between high and low arousal is useful; however, he regards it as less neuroscientifically accurate than his preferred use of the concept.

In his preferred use, Siegel describes an integrated 'harmonious' form of human functioning that exists between more 'chaotic' and 'rigid' mental states. He suggests that internal and external factors influence the 'width' of this window of tolerance and thus the extent to which emotional states can be processed by the person in an integrated, regulated and harmonious way (Siegel, 2020: 342–349). In both the sensorimotor and interpersonal neurobiology applications of the window of tolerance model, the psychotherapist is encouraged to work with the client to expand the window of tolerance, so the person can more easily integrate their emotional processing. This is achieved through learning techniques to self-regulate emotional states and bring them within the boundaries of the window of tolerance (ibid.: 349–350; Ogden & Fisher, 2015: 219–242). The focus on expanding the window of tolerance is further used as a basis for establishing greater harmony and relationality with others in the person's environment.

Similar approaches to the sensorimotor psychotherapies have been developed by psychiatrists and general family practitioners in the United States of America. For example, Bruce Perry (2009; Perry et al. 1995) and the ChildTrauma Academy (c.f. Hambrick, Brawner & Perry, 2019) have created and popularised a 'neurosequential model' of trauma psychotherapy within the United States of America in particular. Perry draws on his clinical experience and a neurobiological model to suggest that trauma disrupts the sequential development of brain functioning. In a similar way to sensorimotor psychotherapy, Perry proposes that psychotherapeutic responses to trauma need to first address lower-brain function disruptions (i.e. of physical touch, regulation and arousal), before attempting to work with higher-brain functions (i.e. emotional regulation) and higher executive functions (i.e. attachment, concrete and abstract thought and meaning-making). For this reason, Perry frequently advocates establishing safety through proximity and building titrated tolerance for touch through massage before proceeding to building emotional regulation and meaning-making around the traumatic experience (c.f. Perry with Szalavitz, 2011, 2017).

Likewise, Maté (2019 [2003]) explores the clinical presentations of autoimmune and inflammatory responses to traumatic stress in his patients. He proposes that there is a transdiagnostic impact of relational distress and trauma in the aetiology, genesis and prognosis of the autoimmune and inflammatory conditions he works with. Maté advocates interventions focused on self-regulation and self-soothing, and couples this with a more phenomenological interest in the person's meaning-making around the illness or condition. As such, he suggests that medical and psychotherapeutic clinicians should be using the presentation of illness as a phenomenological entity to be inquired into, in order to understand the systemic (and potentially interpersonally traumatic) distress that is being communicated through the person's embodiment.

Within sensorimotor therapy, and other neuropsychotherapies, there is an inappropriate equivalence between neurobiological phenomena and proposed treatment responses. Sensorimotor theory and psychotherapeutic practice continually risk a neurobiological reductionism. Asserting that there is a correlation between neurobiological phenomena and traumatic responses does not mean that relationship is necessarily causal. Reducing traumatic phenomena to concrete and discrete brain regions and neurobiological processes is misleading, as neuroscientifically the complex relationships involved in the phenomena remain at best neuroscientifically uncertain and frequently unknowable. Further, the reductionism contained within neuropsychotherapies leads to a targeting of interventions based on specific autonomic and regulatory processes. The use of neuroscientific framing of the intervention does not in reality tell us anything meaningful about the efficacy of the intervention, nor the neuroscientific accuracy of the forms of neurobiological targeting.

Despite the neurobiological reductionism, neuropsychotherapies offer a powerful explanatory system for psychologists, psychotherapists and individuals in therapy (Rose & Abi-Rached, 2013: 6). This is primarily because the seeming certainty of the structure and operations of a triune brain, primacy of threat reactivity and self-regulation offers a compelling narrative for psychoeducative understanding and intervention. It proffers a neurobiomechanical illustration of the impact of interpersonal trauma on the way we think, act and relate to ourselves and others. The enduring influence of the triune brain, and its more stable home within the rapid growth of sensorimotor psychotherapies, is reflected in the proliferation of thousands of psychology and psychotherapy books, texts and trauma-informed training around the world now using this neurobiologically reductive explanatory model of human brain functioning and traumatic experiencing. While seemingly reductive in neurobiological focus, the proponents of the triune brain are in many ways expansionist in that they adopt medicocultural and social practices that have previously enabled psychiatry and psychology to colonise areas of human life, distress and experiencing as legitimate sites for psychological investigation, explanation and/or intervention (building on Rose & Abi-Rached, 2013: 9).

Trauma-focused movement practices

The influence of threat detention and somatic processing has transcended the more specific treatment frameworks and plans used within triune brain-informed neuropsychotherapies. Popularised versions of sensorimotor information and threat processing, emotional and somatic dysregulation have been incorporated into a wider resurgence in somatic and movement practices within Western culture, and led to the increasing interest in the benefits of Eastern somatic insights within cultures of wellbeing. The integration within, and between, trauma-focused neuropsychotherapies and trauma-informed somatic and movement practices has drawn significantly more attention to the notion of an embodied mind, a form of consciousness that can only be understood and processed through bodily wisdom, movement, articulation and expression.

The diverse modalities and forms that could broadly be described as trauma-focused movement practices place a significant emphasis on processing the relationships between somatic, sensorial, perceptive, emotional and relational embodiments of traumatic experiencing. The focus on embodiment is present within the utilisation, for example, of grounding techniques (Tord & Bräuninger, 2015), rhythm and rhythmic experimentations within dance therapy (c.f. Boyd, 2007; Gray, 2017; Levine & Land, 2015; Pierce, 2014), and the exploration of proximity (Stanek, 2015), including touch (c.f. Cristobal, 2018) within biodynamic body psychotherapy (c.f. Arnault & O'Halloran, 2015; Carroll, 2002; Smith, 1998). Through these somatically expressive and experiential modalities, people are encouraged to explore post-traumatic forms of embodiment and relationships with others (following Steenkamp, 2012; Totten, 2015).

In the European and Anglo-American context, the last two decades have seen significant growth and popularisation of trauma-informed yoga (Cramer et al., 2018; Emerson, 2015; van der Kolk, 2006, 2014), somatic experiencing (Andersen et al., 2017; Brom et al., 2017; Levine, 2010; Levine with Frederick, 1997) and, increasingly, trauma release exercises (TRE) (Berceli, 2005, 2008, 2015). These practices are seen as mainstream therapeutic adjuncts to more clinical trauma neuropsychotherapies, with many psychotherapists and psychologists actively encouraging clients to explore these new ways of experiencing their bodies.

The aim of these practices is to support people to release traumatic states and responses that are stored in the body, and enable them to re-experience positive forms of proximity, touch, breath, interpersonal safety and a greater connection with the present moment. For example, TRE is a standardised set of exercises aiming to slightly fatigue muscle sets in order to induce neuro- and psychogenic movements, which are said to safely release stress, tension and trauma (Berceli, 2005, 2008, 2015). The content and interpersonal descriptions related to the trauma are blind to the facilitator, and therefore verbal instructions focus primarily on the inducement, therapeutic holding and phenomenological description of sensations and movements during the practice. Most TRE practitioners hold a debriefing at the end of the session and are encouraged in their training to hold a boundary between the experiential practice of TRE, and psychotherapeutic exploration of the memories, encounters, relationships or situations that may relate to the somatic shaking, trembling or tightness witnessed and experienced.

Similarly, trauma-informed forms of yoga (following Emerson, 2015; van der Kolk, 2006, 2014) are modelled predominantly on Hatha yoga, which can take both active and more gentle forms of movement. It uses clinical insights about traumatic stress to shape and structure the forms of yoga offered, the verbal instructions given and the physical and proximate interactions with participants. Emphasis is on using the yoga as a method of exploring and moving the body, making different shapes and also unlearning traumatic memories or assumptions about what it means to move or not move around other bodies. Within this, consideration is also given to the ways that verbal cues are used to ensure that the instruction does not induce what are seen to be trauma-related responses (i.e. freeze or fold responses in Shavasana – a resting posture). A greater emphasis is placed on mindfulness practices that promote kindness, body awareness and attunement, and the regulation, modulation or tolerance of emotional and physiological states (including hyper/hypoarousal and hyper/hypovigilance), feelings and sensations (i.e. pain or discomfort) through movement and breath.

There remains an active and lively debate within the yoga practice community as to whether it is necessary to craft trauma-informed yoga out as a specific and distinct practice. Notably, the leading clinical psychotraumatologists researching yoga did not specify the need for trauma-informed training; rather, they focused on the benefits of the practice to the person and their processing of traumatic embodiment (see van der Kolk, 2006, 2014). Those advocating for a distinct trauma-sensitive yoga practice have created thematic frameworks and lists of postures for responding to the embodiment of traumatic experiences. One of the most well-known examples has been developed by David Emerson (2015), a yoga instructor who collaborated with contemporary psychotraumatologists (including van der Kolk) to develop the Trauma Centre yoga programme and a 'trauma-sensitive' approach to yoga. Emerson describes the ways in which yoga can be used to increase people's interoception, and thus rediscover their capacity to somatically and emotionally regulate themselves (ibid.: 41–58).

Emerson, along with clinical psychologist Elizabeth Hopper (Emerson & Hopper, 2011: 39–57), propose four core themes that guide trauma-sensitive yoga classes and practices. First, is the experience of the present moment, in using physical cues and breathwork to support people to connect to their interoception, and greater awareness of their somatic experience and orientation in the space around them. Second, is making choices, where the person is able to practise ways of choosing to move and express their body in new ways, and in doing so address the traumatic sense of fear or helplessness in relation to somatic experience. Third, is taking effective action, which builds on the first and second theme by emphasising the person's own ability to take effective action for themselves. This can take the form of small and micro movements and self-adjustments to better articulate a posture, through to seeing the progression of their yoga practice over time and through the development of their own action.

Finally, the fourth theme focuses on creating rhythms. Emerson and Hopper note how experiences of interpersonal trauma can fracture the synchronous relationships we have with our body, with other people and the world around us (i.e. through dissociation). Trauma-sensitive yoga, for Emerson (we might say all yoga practice), addresses the traumatic isolation by connecting people to their own rhythmic embodiment, and in time to connect synchronically to the collective movement and rhythm of the class or practice, and the wider environment in which they are moving. When explaining this final theme in my own papers, seminars and workshops, I tend to additionally describe the importance of proximity and cultivation of a shared experience, where people increasingly find both the capacity for moving themselves as an active agent and moving with others as a relational rhythmic and synchronic experience. I am in agreement with Emerson and Hopper that the re-establishment of synchronic movement and rhythm provides the ground for new meaning and experience of a personhood and world that moves beyond traumatic experiential states.

Beyond the limitations of the 'triune brain'

The separation of rational, emotional and bodily processes described in the triune brain theory is grounded in a wider philosophical fallacy shared by some of the contemporary neurosciences. The philosophic fallacy is one of Cartesian dualism, and the idea that mental and physical processes are distinct and different substances, which interact within the person. The psychologist and neuroscientist Lisa Feldman Barrett (2017a, 2021) has contended that the creation, and applications, of the triune brain are based on a philosophical hypothesis that human rationality is what marks us out from other non-human animals (see also Smith, 2010). The philosophical perspective suggests that rationality and emotionality are distinctive and separable parts within the human mind and consciousness. Further, the separate rational and emotive parts are also in some way distinct from our more primal animalistic body. Rational thought is seen to be a newer evolutionary neuro-architectural structure built on top of older animalistic drives and emotional responses (Cesario, Johnson & Eisthen, 2020; Evans, 2008).

Within neuroscientific and triune brain discourse this leads to what the cognitive and computational neuroscientists Liad Mudrik and Uri Maoz (2015: 211) describe as a 'double-subject fallacy'. The doubling of subjectivity is a result of the abstraction of the person's personhood from their brain, which becomes the site for neuroscientific description and investigation. The advent of neuroimaging technologies has spurred efforts to locate the specific neuroanatomical regions of the brain associated with rational thought and emotional processing. Broadly, locationist neuroscientific approaches to emotion seek to identify specific neuro-anatomical locations that produce activity that consistently produces the same emotional experience or category of emotions. The sociologist Nikolas Rose and medical historian Joelle Abi-Rached (Rose & Abi-Rached, 2013: 79) remind us that despite their 'apparent realism', the locationist 'claims to account for the phenomenology of mental states in terms of these simulated functions localized in the living brain require an act of faith', as there is significant unknowing, uncertainty and ambiguity present in all 'elements on which the image is premised'. Ultimately, the neuroscientific truth that the locationists seek to demonstrate is 'a matter of dispute' (ibid.: 79).

Constructionist approaches of the neurophysiological and neurobiological basis of mental states critique locationist endeavours for their emotional reductivism. Feldman Barrett (2017a: 82), for example, reminds us of the complexity of human emotional experiencing, describing how the human brain is 'anatomically structured so that no decision or action can be free of interoception [our conscious or non-conscious sense of the physiological condition of the body (see Craig, 2003, 2015)] and affect [emotion]'. Within the constructivist neuropsychological model, our physicality, emotionality and cognition are interwoven, and emotional experiencing and responses emerge out of neurobiological, psychological and relational processes that are not specific to one emotion.[5] This means that emotions emerge within and between a networking of basic neuropsychological and neurobiological operations, which are not specifically localised to functionally produce that emotional state or group of emotional experiences (see Lindquist et al., 2012 for a relevant meta-analysis).

For psychological constructionists, emotional responses and experiencing are thus contextualised with the existing meaning and memories we have made from previous experiences of the world. As such, the physicality, rationality, emotionality and personhood cannot be separated, abstracted or localised from each other within neuroscientific theory and practice. As Feldman Barrett (2006, 2009, 2017a) demonstrates, our experience of emotion is produced through an act of categorisation, which itself is guided by our embodied and contextual knowledge about emotionality, our experiences and the world we find ourselves in (see Siegel et al., 2018).

When applied to traumatic experiencing, psychological constructionist accounts would see the emotional experience, meaning-making, memory recall and somatic responses all being constituted through, and contextually activated by, the contextual appraisal of a new situation or event to embodied features of the traumatic one(s). In part, the constructivist perspective provides insight into the broad range of psychological outcomes associated with trauma in the psychiatric and neuroscientific literature (from heightened anxiety and depression to post-traumatic stress disorder (PTSD) or schizophrenia). Identifying the basic neuropsychological operations that contextually contribute to our traumatic experiencing could provide more insight into the role neurobiology plays in emotional experiencing and meaning-making in relation to interpersonal trauma.

However, we should here heed the advice of British psychologists John Cromby and Penny Standen, who suggest we should note 'the influence of phenomenal, hormonal, anatomical and physiological factors, but to do so without falling prey to either deterministic essentialism or Cartesian dualism' (Cromby & Standen, 1999: 153). The activation of specific regions clearly plays a role in our embodied responses to interpersonal trauma, albeit without this meaning that specific emotional states are functionally located there. Utilising the seemingly neat and overly simplistic triune brain theory within psychotraumatology does not accurately reflect the complexity of somatic, emotional and cognitive processing, nor does it appreciate the contextual importance of the person's lived phenomenological reality in constructing their specific form of traumatic experiencing and the responses they exhibit.

Despite the above critiques of dualistic and localised accounts within contemporary neuroscience, we should not dismiss the explanatory potential of these models out of hand. In particular, the insistence of sensorimotor psychotherapies on focusing on sensorimotor information processing can be used to draw our attention to sensorial and movement-focused dimensions of traumatic embodiment. As the early psychotraumatologists frequently noticed, what is re-experienced and remembered of traumatic experiences can be non-verbal articulations and visceral reactions to traumatic situations. Used in a more constructionist way, some of the sensorimotor psychotherapeutic exercises and resources could be used to explore these non-verbal remnants and reminders of interpersonal trauma, which operate beyond a clear verbalisable articulation, conceptualisation or expression. Further, as the constructionists suggest, not all contextualised meaning-making is verbalised, nor does it necessarily have a coherent verbalisable cognitive conception.

Cognitive-behavioural turns in contemporary psychotraumatology

Paralleling the neuroscientific focus on somatic and bodily states, there has been a rising dominance of cognitive-behavioural modalities in psychiatric, psychological and psychotherapeutic practices. These were particularly notable within the Anglo-American context from the late 1950s, 1960s and 1970s (e.g. Beck, 1963, 1964; Ellis, 1957, 1963), and have been burgeoning internationally from the close of the twentieth century. While significantly varying in focus, cognitive-behavioural psychologies and psychotherapies share common features. These commonalities include the use of psychoeducative direction and interventions to build practical problem-solving, and wider skills for understanding cognitive, emotional and behavioural states (see Rachman, 2015 for a useful summary). Some of these models emphasise cognitive restructuring or reframing of understandings of past or present experiences. Others emphasise self-compassion and perspective-taking in relation to our beliefs about ourselves, others and the world around us. The influence and dominance of cognitive-behavioural therapy (CBT) within the UK context, combined with its strong commitment to empiricism, has led to CBT forms of practice being recommended by the National Institute for Health and Care Excellence (NICE) for the treatment of PTSD in England (NCCMH, 2019; NICE, 2018).

While seemingly different to psychoanalytic and attachment-based orientations, CBT is interested in the subjective experience of the person in relation to lived situations, and how meaning is made cognitively, emotionally, behaviourally and sensorially. It is easy for psychologists and psychotherapists who have had negative experiences of working with CBT-based organisations and structures to be dismissive of the contributions CBT could make to our understanding of interpersonal trauma. For example, many of my colleagues and clients have an understandable aversion to CBT because of their interaction with the reductionist, mechanistic, target-driven and overwhelmed operationalisation of trauma-focused CBT within the NHS in England's Improving Access to Psychological Therapies (IAPT) services.

With adequate resourcing and the ability to meaningfully work with clients, CBT practitioners dynamically see the person as an active agent in constructing their own worldview, and in their encounters with others. Establishing one of the foundational perspectives in CBT, Arron Beck (1963, 1964) proposes that it is not the event itself that determines the person's emotional and behavioural responses, but rather the cognitions and attributions we have around the event or situation that gives rise to our responses. The directive, at times formulaic and manualised, approach in CBT is taken by the psychologist or psychotherapist to build the person's self-efficacy. Setting out existing automatic thoughts, core beliefs and adaptive or compensatory strategies, enables a dialogue around understanding the consequences of experiencing and responding in a particular way, and offers ideas and paths to new ways of experiencing, understanding and responding to life situations. Through Socratic questioning, the CBT practitioner supports the client to describe and understand their cognitive appraisals and emotional or behavioural responses to events, and collaboratively challenge and reframe these in the present and for the future.[6]

Notwithstanding my experience of Keres's reframing of my own interpersonal trauma (see the Introduction), there is clear therapeutic value in opening up the ways we think about and respond to our experience of events and situations, and how we use this questioning and inquiry to stimulate alternative ways of understanding and responding. Like all forms of therapeutic intervention, CBT is a fundamentally political act, in that it promotes a facilitated and educative (epistemic) change in a person's understanding of themselves, others and the world around them. The power wielded by a CBT psychologist and psychotherapist needs to be clearly held by the practitioner, understanding that promoting self-realisation, awareness and understanding is a more ethically valuable and humane focus for psychotherapy than a radical insistence on an alternative (and psychopolitical) perspective. In my encounter with Keres, it was her offhand and immediate denial of my confrontation with reality, and her want to reframe and dismiss the reality, that triggered a post-traumatic stress response from me. Given the short-term, high caseload and target-driven culture of NHS IAPT (and equivalent) services, CBT practitioners must be significantly attuned to the political power of epistemic reframing and the consequences of not collaborating with the client in world- and meaning-making.

Trauma-focused cognitive-behavioural psychotherapies

A summary review and discussion (Schnyder et al., 2015) of leading psychotherapies – founded in CBT and focused on PTSD – identified six key commonalities between the models. If we take any of the recommended NICE (2018) psychological treatments for PTSD in England (for example), we can see the commonalities between the models at play within the operations of eye-movement desensitisation and reprocessing (EMDR) therapy (Shapiro, 2018), prolonged exposure therapy (Foa, 2011; Foa, Chrestman & Gilboa-Schechtman, 2009), narrative exposure therapy (Schauer, Neuner & Elbert, 2011), and cognitive therapy for PTSD (based on the model of Ehlers & Clark, 2000).

The identified commonalities within CBT focused on trauma (following Schnyder et al., 2015) included the use of psychoeducation; the building of capacity and skills for emotional regulation; and imaginal exposure to feared thoughts, beliefs, images, memories, situations and environment. Building on the cultivation of skills to cope with dysregulation and gradual exposure to traumatic experiences and memories is an emphasis on cognitive processing, restructuring and meaning-making around the post-traumatic symptoms, the relationships with the experienced situation or event and person's responses to these. Although referred to in different ways, the processing of traumatic memories and the establishment of a coherent narrative around this is a core part of these CBT-focused trauma psychotherapies. Changes in memory and meaning (including the person's trauma narratives), allow more space for emotional expansion and for addressing difficult emotional states underpinning trauma-related cognitions and behavioural responses to be explored (including fear, shame and guilt).

For the purposes of further illustration, let us turn to consider another of the NHS-approved models within CBT for working with trauma and PTSD. Judith Cohen, along with her colleagues, clinical psychologists Anthony Mannarino and Esther Deblinger, noticed some of the limitations of earlier forms of CBT in working with clients who had experiences of trauma (Cohen, Mannarino & Deblinger, 2017). Drawing on their clinical experience (primarily with children and young people), the authors devised trauma-focused cognitive behavioural therapy (TF-CBT). TF-CBT has more specific criteria for treatment, including the presence of a remembered trauma, presentations of trauma-related emotional or behavioural responses and an exclusion for treatment where the client's parents are the source of the trauma.

Utilising the biopsychosocial model of mental health, the focus of TF-CBT is on re-regulating the person's domains of experiencing (emotional, behavioural, biological, cognitive and social) that were impacted by trauma. This re-regulation is organised around three phases of treatment, including stabilisation, trauma narration and processing, and integration and consolidation (for a useful overview, see Cohen & Mannarino, 2015; Cohen, Deblinger & Mannarino, 2018). The first phase focuses on psychoeducation aimed at describing common responses to trauma, how reminders of these can arise in everyday life (through emotional, behavioural, biological, cognitive and social cues or experiences), and at connecting these to the experiences of the client. Second, through dialogue the person is encouraged to describe increasingly challenging details about their experiences of trauma. This enables the person to process and find ways of articulating their trauma, with the therapist attending to and addressing maladaptive cognitions that arise from the recalling and retelling of these experiences.[7] The final phase is an optional component, aiming to establish in vivo mastery of the traumatic response. In contrast to the imagined exposure in the second phase of the trauma narrative, this third phase involves a graduated exposure to reminders of the traumatic experience in the traumatic environment, for example, the school, workplace or street that the person fears and avoids. It could also take the form of sensations (i.e. smells or touch through massage) in order to build a gradual *mastery* through facing the feared situation.

TF-CBT advocates a commitment and adherence to the clinical sequential model of these phases across the course of the time-limited treatment to be effective (for an overview of effectiveness, see Lewey et al., 2018; Morina, Koerssena & Polletc, 2016). Especially in the final phase, it incorporates a professional judgement of the graduated exposure to traumatic reminders and triggers. In the case of children and young people, therapists share with the parents and family members the formulation and progress of the therapeutic phased journey and co-opt them into mirroring and reinforcing the purpose of each phase. In the final phase, this culminates in conjoint sessions between child and parent or caregiver, to integrate and consolidate the stabilisation, processing and gradual exposure that the child (and as a consequence the family as a whole) has worked through.

There remains within humanist and existential schools of psychology and psychotherapy a high level of scepticism about the dominance of, and mistrust around the use of, CBT within contemporary psychotraumatology. I do not share this aversion to the models and practices of CBT. Elsewhere (Bush [Boaz], 2019), I have sought to describe the significant compatibility and translational potential in between (for example) the use of Levinasian existential psychotherapy for fatigue within CBT environments. While CBT, existential and humanistic practitioners epistemologically understand and describe the world in fundamentally different ways, in practice the forms of intervention and engagement with clients can bear striking resemblance (see also Corrie & Milton, 2000; Edwards, 1990; Mirea & Hickes, 2011, on meaning; Heidenreich et al., 2021, on the presence of existential givens in CBT).

We could take Viktor Frankl's logotherapeutic (existential) technique of paradoxical intention as an example. Frankl (1960, 1975) uses paradoxical intention to encourage a client to actively do the thing they fear, or paradoxically wish for it to occur. In the case (for example) of someone avoiding a street they were attacked on because they fear freezing, trembling or shaking, Frankl would encourage them to intentionally walk down the street with the aim of freezing and shaking uncontrollably. In Frankl's clinical experience, the paradoxical intention of the client actively intending to do the thing they feared, disrupted both the fear and avoidance. If either freezing or shaking happened, Frankl would explore these in subsequent sessions, with the ability to reflect on the real-world experiment, rather than imaginal exposure. Such an approach is clearly resonant with the forms of exposure advocated in the latter stages of TF-CBT, as well as the in vivo (rather than imaginal) mastery exposure experiments advocated in a number of the afore-mentioned trauma-focused forms of CBT. Indeed, many CBT practitioners have incorporated paradoxical intention as a therapeutic method into their research and practice over the years (see the efforts of Ascher, 1981, 1989; Ascher with Schotte, 1999).

Mentalisation and the loss of epistemic trust

Alongside the growth of somatic and sensorimotor psychotherapy practices, there has been a social turn within neuroscience. Social neuroscience aims to under-stand the relationships between complex social and interpersonal experiences and neurobiological processes. The turn towards social neuroscience within psychotraumatology interacted with continued elaborations of attachment-based theories of human relating and development (building on Bowlby, 1982 [1969]; Salter Ainsworth et al., 2014 [1978]). These attachment-focused theories of social neuroscience underpin many contemporary trauma-focused psychotherapies used in the United Kingdom and internationally. Most of the attachment-focused trauma psychotherapies have brought together the clinical research in child attachment patterns with developments in interpersonal neurobiology and neuro-science (Hughes, Golding & Hudson, 2019; Insel & Young, 2001; Shah, Fonagy & Strathearn, 2010; Siegel & Solomon, 2003).

Peter Fonagy, Anthony Bateman and Jon Allen (among others) have proposed a new model of how we attend to our own mental states, and the mental states and behaviours of others. Updating Bowlbian attachment theories with a syn-thesis of contemporary attachment and neuroscientific research, Allen, Fonagy and Bateman (2008: 4) use the term *mentalising* as 'imaginative perceiving or interpreting behaviour as conjoined with intentional mental states' (see also Allen, 2001: 53–54). The authors here are describing our capacity to interpret the pos-sible intentionality of the mental states and behaviours of others in our envir-onment. Mentalisation theorists suggest that the capacity to mentalise about the cognitive and emotional states of other people is not localised within a 'fixed set of specialized brain region[s]' (Fonagy & Bateman, 2019: xvi). That said, they maintain, in part, the locationist sensibility that the neural circuits involved in mentalisation can be identified and hypothecated (Luyten & Fonagy, 2015; see also Frith & Frith, 2006).

Congruent with wider social neuroscience and attachment-based theory, our capacity to mentalise is seen to emerge from the attachment and interactions with caregivers. It is through the attuned attention and secure responses of caregivers that the child becomes reflexive about themselves, the intentions of others and their environment. Mentalisation is the way in which the child comes to understand themselves and others as having minds and intentionality. Through this mentalisation, the child comes to know their world, regulate their emotional responses to experiences and build a sense of safety and trust in the minds and actions of others (Allen et al., 2008: 76).

The experience of trauma can result in the child experiencing their mind as being alone and isolated from the intentional mind of the caregiver. As such, the child is unable to use the mind of others (and specifically that of their caregivers) to mediate and understand the meaning of frightening traumatic experiences or relationships (following Allen et al., 2008: 102; Fonagy & Bateman, 2016; Luyten & Fonagy, 2019: 86). Echoing the early attachment researchers, in mentalisation theory, children may actively avoid mentalising about the mind of an abusive other (see Allen, 2013: 161–212). Further, abusive parents, caregivers or others in the child's relational system might actively discourage the child from reflection or discussion about mental states or actions of an abusive other (ibid.). The discouraging person aims to discourage the child's mentalisation in order to avoid the confrontation of the reality of the traumatic experiences and the emotional states resulting from them for the child (Allen et al., 2008: 247).

When a child is subject to abuse, neglect or other forms of interpersonal trauma, it leads to mental disconnection and isolation from the minds of others. The isolation from other people's minds undermines the child's developing capacity to mentalise. With an impacted ability to mentalise the intentional mind and actions of others, the child experiences enduring fright and confusion over both the abusive or neglectful experiences they have had, and the wider experiences they have with other people (following Allen et al., 2008). When the active and developing capacity to mentalise is compromised by trauma, the child can revert to *autonomic (or prementalising) modes of mentalising* (the fight, flight and freeze responses previously mentioned), to enable the child to survive its environment (Luyten & Fonagy, 2015, 2019: 84–85).

Alternatively, when a child or adult is unable to mentalise because of the experience of trauma, they might develop *non-mentalising* modes of experiencing their subjectivity (Fonagy & Bateman, 2019: 13–15). Non-mentalising modes of experiencing include a loss of internal and external reality (psychic equivalence), pretend mode (dissociation and unreality), and taking a teleological stance (using actions such as self-harm or substance use to alter emotional dysregulation). Additionally, it could result in *pseudomentalising*, which includes intrusive thoughts or beliefs about others knowing what you are thinking; *hypermentalising* about the intentional mind of another, in excessive detail, but detached from emotional reality of the other person; and destructively inaccurate mentalisations – where the person denies the internal states of others and asserts their own understanding of the other person's mental state (ibid.; Luyten et al., 2019: 49).

Non-mentalising and autonomic modes of mentalising can lead people to subjectively experience everyday relational disappointment as traumatic. This is because the experience of interpersonal trauma threatens and undermines interpersonal trust and the sense of safety and capacities for empathy related to it (Luyten & Fonagy, 2019: 84). A lack of interpersonal trust results in *epistemic mistrust*. Epistemic mistrust means that people who experience trauma lose the foundational trust required to learn from others that a person, situation or environment is safe. The epistemic mistrust resulting from interpersonal trauma leads people to be suspicious of both their own perceptions of a new person or situation, and the information and social cues they receive from others (Fonagy & Allison, 2014). Without epistemic trust, the person cannot synthesise or incorporate the new learning about a person, situation or environment into their mentalising (Luyten & Fonagy 2019: 90–91). The lack of incorporation of new learning into our mental states leads to an *epistemic vigilance* or *epistemic hypervigilance*, where the person searches for the perceived intention behind a person's mistrustful and suspicious information (Fonagy & Allison, 2014). Consequently, the person does not have a 'relational referencing' to aid them in the cognitive reframing of adverse experiences, and therefore is left in non-mentalising or autonomic modes of mentalising, and with a level of epistemic vigilance (c.f. ibid.: 85). For me, Fonagy and colleagues', formulation of epistemic trust and mentalisation provides an alternative articulation of the phenomena of fixing and disintegration of ideas in the work of Janet.

Within mentalisation theory, an inability to synthesise or incorporate new relational information about people, situations or environments can lead to re-enactments of attachment traumas (Allen, 2001). These re-enactments can manifest as forms of re-victimisation, in which the person seeks out new relationships that are characterised by abuse and neglect. Alternatively, the person may engage in re-enactments of neglect, defined by a hypersensitivity to, and misperceptions of, relational difficulty and actions of others as signs or cues of neglect. Further, there may be re-enactments of attachment trauma within their own parenting behaviour, as the parent is emotionally triggered by the emotional states and actions of their own children (Luyten & Fonagy, 2019: 88–89).

Mentalisation-based therapy (MBT) has developed out of mentalisation theory and research to address relational distress, loss of epistemic trust and capacities to mentalise, and the emotional regulation related to this. Luyten and Fonagy (2019: 94–95) have described the MBT approach for working with clients who have experienced interpersonal trauma. They suggest a staged approach to MBT trauma psychotherapy, beginning with psychoeducation about the impacts of trauma on mentalisation and human relationships, in order to foster the client's understanding of their own mental states and the impact that trauma has on their understanding of the intentionality of other people's mental states.

The authors (ibid.) next turn to psychotherapeutic validation and normalisation of the client's feelings and mental states in the present moment. The validation and normalisation aims to provide the client with an empathetic understanding of their own experiences and emotional world, and to build epistemic trust between the client and psychotherapist. The building of epistemic trust enables the psychotherapist to support the client to mentalise about the interpersonal traumatic experiences they have had, and to explore the impact they have had on their understanding of their own mental states and the mentalisation of the intentional mental states and actions of others. Additionally, the psychotherapist works with the client to build strategies for regulating their emotions and emotional responses to the traumatic experiences and memories. This is similar to the focus on emotional regulation used within the sensorimotor psychotherapy. Finally, the psychotherapist works with the client to foster changes in their interpersonal relationships, through addressing their re-enactments and epistemic vigilance.

Practising as an existential psychotherapist within CBT environments I have found that MBT can provides for an honest and relational orientation for exploring traumatic phenomena and the relational world of my clients. In CBT settings, I find myself being drawn to MBT as a pragmatic bridge between the more structured clinical models within attachment-focused CBT and the more Socratic and/or phenomenological methods of humanistic existentialism. In my own practice, MBT has been instrumental in building and maintaining therapeutic relationships and making sense of the impact of interpersonal trauma in people's lives. In the therapy room, my clients frequently describe the inability to comprehend the intentionality of the actions to which they were subjected. Epistemic vigilance understandably arises within the dialogue between us, with some clients proffering intentionality to my behaviours, questions or silences. By disclosing the intentionality behind these interpersonal phenomena, we are able to build epistemic trust and make the intentionality of the other knowable and understandable. Often the therapeutic relationship creates an alternative model to that of the traumatic experience, and when a traumatic state is triggered (and the relational contact is not incorporated by the client), it provides space and impetus for the therapist and client to deepen their relating and unpack issues of epistemic mistrust between them.

When using mentalisation in my practice, I augment the original theoretical stance of Fonagy and Bateman (2019) by considering and emphasising the ways in which epistemic vigilance and mistrust can be cultivated and activated beyond the relational transmissions of an attachment figure. While always contextual in nature, mentalisation theory falls short of understanding the ways in which epistemology and trust are held not only between people, but between networked structures and cultures within any given society. A lack of epistemic trust resulting from traumatisation might just as likely (simultaneously) arise from our contextual mentalising about the cultures in which we live, participate and elaborate. Working with clients to understand the cultural meanings that contextualise interpersonal epistemic trust is of equal importance as those transmitted from attachment figures or the traumatising other. The need for this augmentation occurred to me not only from my own background in sociology, but also because many of the client groups I have worked with (especially from the lesbian, gay, bisexual, transgender, queer or questioning and others (LGBTQ+), autism and learning disability communities) have been subject to epistemological frameworks, models and treatments that contest their personhood or the value of their humanity and/or existence. These sociocultural experiences interweave with attachment-focused, and internalised mystifications of intentionality of the other.

If I draw on examples from my own life history, I understand as a young person how my exposure to British societal narratives around rape culture and gendered norms about human sexuality might have contributed to transferring this cultural-epistemological stance onto my own attachment figures and peers, preventing the epistemic trust required for my earlier disclosure of sexual coercion and assault. This interacts with continual exposure to governmental communications and public health messaging in the 1980s and 1990s in Britain about the AIDS pandemic, typically communicated as 'AIDS = death' (see Dowset, 2009 on AIDS and moral panic; building on Cohen, 2002 [1972]). Overlying this were socio-cultural narratives about the immorality of homosexuality, and the subsequent government-enforced prohibition on the so-called promotion and existence of homosexuality or homosexual practices in schools. These wider social narratives also contributed to my own loss of epistemic trust required to disclose my sexuality or incorporate my consensual and non-consensual homosexual experiences into my identity. As such, what is seen as personal or interpersonal mentalising capabilities within MBT, might also be imaginative renderings of meta-contextual accounts or epistemological stances of human intentionality, cognitive and emotional states arising from collective or structural sociocultural discourse.[8]

Contributions and limitations of contemporary trauma-focused psychotherapies

In the previous subsections I have sought to provide the reader with a general overview of contemporary trauma-focused psychotherapies. In doing so, the aim has been to orientate the reader to some of the dominant neuropsychological frameworks being used across psychiatry, psychology and psychotherapy. I have drawn attention to the philosophical and epistemological features that frame the dominant models and forms of interventions. I will now turn to reflect on the contemporary trauma-focused psychotherapies included above, to identify some common limitations and important contributions they can make to our understanding of supporting people who have experienced interpersonal trauma.

First, fixative and curative models continue to dominate contemporary trauma-focused psychotherapies. If we look back across the dominant frameworks already described, within sensorimotor psychotherapies and CBT there is an explicit framing of the person (or human organism) as being in a state of dysfunction – be this alterations in their threat perception or information processing about interpersonal intentionality. The professional is positioned as a psychoeducator who brings these dysfunctions to the attention of the person. While the epistemological orientation and method of intervention vary significantly, the psychologist or psychotherapist works with (possibly on) the client in a fixative and curative manner, in order to return them to a state of personal and interpersonal functioning. The desired state of personal and interpersonal functioning, more often than not, is a product either of the psychoeducative materials, the prescribed protocols and procedures of the given method, or a transmission of the personal, organisational or sociocultural politics of the person delivering the intervention.

Second, the dominance and popularisation of neuroscience within contemporary psychotraumatology is reductive in terms of its formulation of human subjectivity. The neuroscientific models in operation frequently use organic and mechanical metaphors as a way of explaining complex interpersonal systems. While useful to the psychologist or psychotherapist as a psychoeducative tool, the effect is that there is an oversimplification of the person's experiential existence and phenomena. At the extremities, the application of locationist neuroscientific attitudes creates neurobiological essentialism, where more deterministic rhetorical myths (such as the triune brain) are incorporated by the client into their own meaning-making about the embodied nature of their experience. The focus on information processing at a somatic or neurocognitive level is frequently rendered into diagrammatic illustrations or is accompanied by extracts of neuroimaging, which do not illustrate a neurobiological reality. Rather, the inclusion of neuroimaging is used as a technological and explanatory device to make abstracted theoretical assumptions more concrete for the clinicians and client (building on Foucault, 2003 [1963], 1983; Latour & Woolgar, 1979).

The misuse of neurotechnological determinism gives rise to a translational fallacy within contemporary psychotraumatology. First, the client's attention is rarely brought to the difficulties in using lab-based, animal and even adult-focused studies to draw conclusive psychotherapeutic statements about the neurobiology of human minds developmentally (over time), and in interaction with their socio-cultural environment (building on Abi-Rached & Rose, 2010; Rose & Abi-Rached, 2013). The second translational fallacy is the neurotechnological myth that what can be observed by the technology is what is real about human neurobiology, and thus is at the foundations of human experiencing. If we are to continue the pursuit and incorporation of neuroscientific insight, it must be in a manner that makes explicit the philosophical basis of its view of human intersubjectivity, and that is open to the uncertainty and ambiguities contained in the inquiry. While this might provide less satisfying psychoeducative interventions from an explanatory perspective, it will act as a reminder to promote the more agentic aspects of the model described above. The agentic subjectivity of the person is located not in a deterministic enactment of their neurobiology, but rather the real-world exposures, experiments and meaning-making, which shape and reshape our human consciousness and reality.

Third, to differing extents the dominant models are overly structured to changing the perceptive and experiential world of the individual, decontextualising them in practice (if not theoretically) from their interpersonal world and rendering them an objective subject to be worked upon under the neuropsychotherapeutic gaze. Even within TF-CBT, the inclusion of interventions for parental or attachment figures (through psychoeducation and conjoint sessions) is to reinforce the changing responses and meaning-making of the child or young person. There is an inherent paradox in creating models that practise atomised interventions in the traumatised person's life. The more we focus on the individual and their responses, the more we risk losing sight of the interpersonal nature of the traumatic experiences they have had or are having.

The applied Danish philosopher Allan Køster (2017) is critical of mentalisation theory, as he sees it unintentionally replicating a Cartesian mind–body dualism. In conceptualising a social imagination and learning to mentalise about the other, Køster notes the emphasis that is placed on bridging (with imagination) the interiority of one person's mind with that of the other. As with the other dominant neuropsychotherapies and different forms of CBT, there is a tension within MBT over where the interpersonal experience and meaning-making are located. A Cartesian mind formulated as being located in the interiority of the brain perpetuates an incoherence in psychotherapeutic practice. By atomising the human mind in theory or through psychotherapeutic intervention, we are only ever encouraging a partial description of the basis of human relating – something exaggerated in locationist accounts of human emotionality.

In my view, meaning-making and traumatic responses are simultaneously generated by the person, and between the persons involved, in an interpersonal field (following, for example, Fuchs & De Jaegher, 2009). The importance of intersubjective meaning-making is recognised in the central role psychologists and psychotherapists take in working with clients to explore and change the understanding and perceptions of their selves, others and the worlds in which they exist. In this view, it might even be the case that intentionality is both something located in the individual and at the same time co-constructed between the two persons. In the subsequent chapters of this book, I aim to describe in more detail an alternative, more intertwined conceptualisation of intersubjective experiencing, and the consequences it has for supporting people who have experienced interpersonal trauma. As the reader will come to see, existentialism focuses on knowledge through participation (which is not unlike my experience as an ethnographer), whereas empirical neuroscience seeks to understand the objects of our knowledge as an objective structure of existence – one without participation – that stands apart from human construction.

Having outlined three of the core limitations of contemporary trauma-focused psychotherapies, I now turn to consider the possible useful contributions that these models make to our understanding of interpersonal trauma. As an existentialist, I have a foundational belief that all human interventions disclose something about the structure of human existence. While I may not always agree with the epistemological frameworks, or the forms of interventions advocated, there are important contributions within contemporary psychotraumatology (like the earlier theories explored) that can aid us in the development of a more existential understanding of interpersonal trauma and traumatic experiencing.

There are four contributions and disclosures that I include in what follows. First, contemporary psychotraumatology reminds us that our previously embodied experiences of the world are wrapped up in our perceptive and experiential realities in the present. Despite the dualistic theorisation, CBT, MBT and sensorimotor psychotherapies bring our attention to the somatic resonance of so-called psychic wounds, and provide a structured space for clients to focus on and make sense of these. Second, all the above orientations place a significant importance on the framing narrative of meaning surrounding memories of, and responses to, experiences in the past and present. While there is clear value in focusing on meaning-making, it remains unsettling (to the point of repetition) that it is unacknowledged within many of the epistemological stances of contemporary trauma-focused psychotherapies that meaning-making is essentially a political act. Thus, the therapist has an ethical responsibility for the frames and changes that are being co-created with the client about their traumatic experience, their memories, perspectives and the narrative about them.

Third, the models describe in different ways the reality of perceptive and epistemic experiences of danger, threat and relational trust that may be misaligned with the current state of experiencing. Fourth, while seeming to focus on returning to a state of normalcy, most of the models of human experience are fluidic and changeable. As such, the models usefully draw our attention to the potential and possibility for change in different domains of human experiencing (cognitive, somatic, sensorimotor, interpersonal etc.). Relating this back to my reflections on the early psychotraumatology, there is a continuation and strengthening of the agentic being and active intentionality of the person to find change in meaning, acting and responding in their lives. Contemporary psychotraumatology conveys a person who (albeit neurobiologically and neurocognitively) adapts to survive their environment. In the longer term, these adaptations do not serve the person (either because the threatening person or environment is not present), and as such these neuro-alterations no longer serve the person but become repetitions or re-enactments of the past. It is the presence of now maladapted thoughts, sensations, emotions and interpersonal relationships in the present context that are taken into the neurobiopsychosocial gaze and rendered as legitimate sites for intervention. These are expressed in the clinical literature as diagnoses and symptomology.

Finally, there is an important disclosure in contemporary psychotraumatology, which was also present within the paradoxes and tensions emerging from the early psychotraumatology. This disclosure is about the centrality of confrontations with reality in our traumatic experiencing. Whereas the early psychotraumatology itself had a varied relationship with being confronted with the reality of traumatic experiences, contemporary psychotraumatology uses the reality of the experience as a feature within the forms of interventions offered. If we take the use of both imaginal exposure and in vivo mastery within TF-CBT, there is a clear intention to work with the real experience of the traumatic situation or relationships, and to find a temporal orientation in the present rather than an absorption in the memory or sensorial responses of the past event(s).

While all the potential contributions of contemporary psychotraumatologies hold value in approaching an existential understanding of traumatic experiencing, in the next chapter I will use the notion of *confrontations with reality* as a central tenet of my proposed approach. Neuroscience, psychiatry and psychology only take us so far in our understanding of what traumatic experiencing is, and in the remainder of the book I will heed the astute advice of the mentalisation theorist Jon Allen. Allen (2005: xvii) writes: 'We must go beyond psychology and psychiatry to understand trauma fully [...] we need help from philosophy, because trauma confronts us with existential concerns that far exceed the reach of science and medicine'. In Part II of this book, I will turn to explore what the existential features of interpersonal trauma might be, and what this tell us about the structure of human experiencing.

Notes

1 'Neurobiopsychosocial responses' is a somewhat clumsy contemporary term, which repurposes the adoption of biopsychosocial models of health and illness within medicine, psychiatry (see Engel, 1977), and latterly Anglo-American public health and social policy.
2 MacLean's model and ideas were widely popularised with the speculative publication of Carl Sagan's *The Dragons of Eden* (1977).
3 For a more detailed discussion of the synthesised description of the operations of the triune brain, see Minton et al. (2006), and similar approaches by Perry et al. (1995), Rothschild (2000) and van der Kolk (2014).
4 The concept of the 'window of tolerance' in many ways builds upon earlier psychophysiological models of the homeostasis of the human body as an organism (c.f. Cannon, 1963 [1932].
5 See Feldman Barrett (2017b) for a critique of the locationist reductive accounts of, for example, the overemphasis on the amygdala in relation to fear experiences and responses.
6 Readers who are themselves trained or practised in CBT modalities might find my description here frustrating. Inevitably there is limited space to describe the converging and diverging waves within contemporary models of CBT. I hope this limited description provides enough generality to cover most bases of CBT and incentivises those who find frustration with this limited articulation to respond to what is written here and/or undertake more exploration in the rich and interweaving CBT waves.
7 See Cohen, Mannarino and Murray (2011) for alterations in relation to enduring experiences of trauma, including differentiation between real proximate danger and generalised trauma reminders.
8 Readers from a sociological or social psychology background are unlikely to find anything substantively original in my additional point. I am simply bringing to MBT wider observations from the likes of Erving Goffman (1963, 1967, 1986 [1974]) and Harold Garfinkel (1967).

Part II

An existential understanding of interpersonal trauma

5 Existential understandings of human suffering and trauma

In Part I of this book I provided the reader with a broad overview of early and contemporary psychotraumatology. Within this, I have sought to bring attention to paradoxes, tensions and insights that might provide ground for existential understandings of interpersonal trauma. What follows in this part is a synthesis and collage of existing existential thought, and my own proposals for how we might draw on these ideas to better understand traumatic experiencing. In proposing a new model, I am revisiting, revising and repurposing existential themes in order to find new movement through them. This new movement will bring, I hope, a queerer sense of what confronts us at the boundaries of human experiencing.

For existentialists, this chapter will feel like a weaving between the homes and haunts of familiar friends, seeing their works, considering their contributions and reflecting on their offerings and movements from new perspectives. For those coming from the psychological sciences, or with a background in empiricism, the language use, philosophical and theoretical explorations and practical explanations might feel alien, unknown or unsettling. The invitation is to bring the familiar and unfamiliar alike into your reading of this and subsequent chapters. Moreover, any sense of disorientation that may ensue will be of value when we come to deepening our understanding of what is being disclosed about the structure of human existence through the experience of interpersonal trauma.

Existential approaches to psychology and psychotherapy

I will introduce some of the common themes across existential psychology and psychotherapy to provide context for the reader. While existentialism is a philosophical movement most associated with the works and worlds of the French existentialist movement, pioneered by the likes of Jean-Paul Sartre and Simone de Beauvoir, there is no one existentialism or existential school of psychology or psychotherapy (following Cooper, 2017). Many existentialists wrote their work simultaneously and unaware initially of other writers' inquiries (i.e. Eugène Minkowski and Frankl). Some writers and practitioners chose the label 'existentialist' themselves (i.e. James Bugental and Emmy van Deurzen), while others have had it placed on their work in retrospect (i.e. Friedrich Nietzsche and Søren Kierkegaard), and yet others went to great lengths to avoid being called existentialist at all (i.e. Martin

DOI: 10.4324/9781003181675-8

Heidegger). So, when we talk of existentialism, it is better to understand it as a plurality of perspectives (existentialisms), all with different focuses and approaches to exploring human existence.

In a comprehensive study, Edgar Agrela Correia and colleagues (2018) identified four main branches of existential psychology and psychotherapy (see also Cooper, 2017; Norcross, 1987). These include: (a) existential-phenomenological approaches, which tend to focus on non-directively and descriptively exploring the person's experience of their world (influenced by van Deurzen, 2012 (thematic); and Spinelli, 2015 (descriptive)); (b) Daseinsanalysis, which emerges out of European philosophy, and focuses on people's experiences of shared existential structures (influenced by Binswanger, 1963; Boss, 1963; Holzhey-Kunz, 2014); (c) existential-humanistic approaches, which focus on people's experience of the present moment, and use this to interpretatively explore relationships with existential givens, such as death, isolation and meaninglessness (influenced by Bugental, 1965; May, 1958; Yalom, 1980); and (d) logotherapy and existential analysis, which are directive and technique-based approaches focusing on people's value, meaning and purpose in life (influenced by Frankl, 1967; Längle, 2020).

Existential philosophers and practitioners do share a common philosophical ground. Sartre (2007 [1946]: 20) famously wrote that 'existence precedes essence'. He continues that a person 'first exists: [they] materialise in the world, encounter [themselves], and only afterward define [themselves]' (ibid.: 22). Existentialism is thus concerned with the totality of the person's existence – the ways in which we are free (within contexts and limitations) to have choice over the life we live, the meaning we make of it and how we can take responsibility for our existence. Existentialism seeks to open up the world of the person in the present moment, as they experience themselves, others and the world around them (following Spinelli, 2015). In this way, existentialists are not interested in searching for essences of the person, or reducing them to parts of their existence. Another way of expressing this is that existentialists tend to see human existence as a form of emergence or becoming. *Who* we are as people emerges from the fact *that* we are.

Correia and colleagues (2018: 135) found that the three most commonly cited practices across the different forms of existential psychologies and psychotherapies are (a) phenomenological inquiry, (b) addressing existential assumptions and (c) relational practices. A broad description of these three commonly cited practices is given in brief in what follows, as subsequent sections of this chapter will give more substantive exploration and detail.

Phenomenological inquiry emerges out of the writings of the philosopher Edmund Husserl (2012 [1931]). While existential psychologists and psychotherapists have altered and adapted Husserl's initial phenomenological methods, broadly phenomenological inquiry is used to open up the lived world of the client, their assumptions about themselves, others and the world around them (following van Deurzen & Adams, 2016). In practice, phenomenological inquiry involves the bracketing (*epoché*) of our usual assumptions about the world of the client. Existential psychotherapists use open questions to encourage the client to describe and explore their lived experiences and meanings. In doing this, there is a horizontalisation of the content a client brings to the therapeutic relationship (following Spinelli, 2005). In the context of trauma, we seek not to verticalise the relevance of traumatic experiences above the other phenomenological experiences and worldview of the client.

Existential psychologists and psychotherapists further seek to address, and attend to, clients' *confrontations with existential concerns*. This might involve the exploration of philosophical propositions about the structure of human experiencing and existence, and how it is revealed to the person in their own lived experience; for example, an existential anxiety arising out of the realisation of our finitude (death), and how we find meaning in relation to this (for differing accounts, see May, 2015 [1950]; Frankl, 1988).

Finally, many existential practitioners use the immediacy of the *psychotherapeutic relationship* to enable the client to understand their existential situation. For the more relationally orientated existentialists, the purpose of the psychotherapeutic relationship is to establish a whole world of experiencing within the therapy world. This is a co-created world between client and psychotherapist, which can be compared and contrasted with other worlds in which they exist beyond the therapy room. Through experiencing relational intimacy within the therapy world, the client discovers their capacity to agentically co-create their world and to explore different ways of being in relation to themselves and others in their life (following Bugental, 1965; Spinelli, 2005; Yalom, 1980; see also Mearns & Cooper, 2018).

On human suffering

I will next turn back to our inquiry into an existential understanding of interpersonal trauma, by first considering the ways that human suffering has been regarded by existential writers and practitioners. Existential philosophers and psychotherapists have commonly conceptualised the human condition as being in continual relation to states of suffering. The absurdist philosopher and novelist Albert Camus (2005 [1942]) eloquently describes how suffering is a foundational state of our existence. In his retelling of the myth of Sisyphus, he suggests that we must find an absurdist attitude, meaning and even happiness within the endless task of rolling a stone up a mountain. In the myth there is a moment where Sisyphus stands atop the mountain watching the stone roll back down, knowing he must follow it and begin the endeavour of rolling it once again to the summit. Camus suggests that within the never-ending pursuit of Sisyphus, we too can find an absurdist attitude that both celebrates the laborious effort involved in pushing the stone up a mountain, and the moments of peace we may find in 'each atom of that stone, each mineral flake of that night-filled mountain' as we gaze from its summit (ibid.: 119).

Absurdism need not be the only attitude we find emerging out of human suffering. The psychiatrist Irvin Yalom (1980) writes that human suffering more specifically arises out of the *givens* of our human existence. The existential givens are the foundational human experiences and limitations that we have no choice but to be confronted by and will have to face as part of the structure of our existence. For Yalom, the four existential givens are death, freedom, isolation and meaninglessness. He suggests that all of the human givens can give rise to suffering, and emphasises our ability to choose our attitude in relation to our suffering. Yalom's writings (Yalom, 2011 [2008]; Yalom & Yalom, 2021) describe, for example, the ways in which we can confront our finitude with a personal and positive attitude towards death. A personal attitude might enable us to turn towards our own death and find a way of dying meaningfully and with purpose. As such, the emphasis is placed on the attitude that one takes towards the foundations and limitations of human existence. It is this attitude that shapes both our experiences of the existential givens, and the meanings we make out of our experience of them.

Another absurdist philosopher, Arthur Schopenhauer (2004 [1850]), suggests that desires – be they physical, sexual, emotional, relational, aesthetic – cause suffering as we are never able to materialise the desired reality into a lived experience. As such, he advocates a negation of desire and acceptance of our primordial state of suffering. The simultaneous negation and acceptance would enable us to find a way of living a meaningful and purposeful life. Schopenhauer's ideas have strong commonalities with wider contemporary psychotherapeutic frameworks, including Paul Gilbert's (2013) compassion-focused therapy. His model focuses on cultivating a kinder and more compassionate sensitivity to the suffering or distress of ourselves and/or others. Through this, he hopes to bring about greater empathetic awareness and insight into the intentionality of the world around us. Gilbert aims for people to find a motivational attitude, which would enable them to find the courage to turn towards, and find empathy and compassion in, our common suffering.

Both Schopenhauer and Gilbert draw heavily on well-established Eastern philosophical traditions. For example, according to some Buddhist teachings there are four foundational noble truths.[1] The first is that we experience suffering (*dukkha*). The second is that the cause of our suffering is desire (*tanhā*), and this desire can come in the forms of delusion, greed, craving and hatred. The third is that we can end this suffering by liberating ourselves from attachment (*upādāna*) to material objects, aesthetics, our worldview, the rituals we live by, sensual experiences and by setting aside a state of rebirth through extinguishing the causes of our suffering (*nirvana*). Finally, the fourth is an eightfold path to becoming spiritually noble (*magga*). Within this model, the facticity of human suffering must be accepted in order to then counter its causes (through non-attachment) and find meaning (through the purposeful action of living a more spiritual life).

The Danish philosopher Kierkegaard (2008 [1849]: 21, 23) proposes that we are all living in a state of 'despair' (it has a 'generality'), whether or not we are conscious of it. He suggests that despair represents a 'sickness unto death', in that we are unable to 'consume' or 'be rid of' it, nor 'become nothing' by means of escaping it (ibid.: 15–17). Kierkegaard (ibid.: 15–16, 20) asserts that despair in relation to suffering disarms us with an eternal hopelessness where we can neither hope for death nor life, and thus must 'live the experience of dying [that is despair]'. In his formulation, only a leap of faith will alleviate our despair.

Some existentialists have been critical of Kierkegaard's dismissal of hope as a valuable attitude towards our suffering. Elsewhere, I have reappraised Kierkegaard's work (Bush [Boaz], 2018a), and proposed that hope can be incorporated into a valuable psychotherapeutic attitude (following May, 1953; Tillich, 2000 [1952]), which I term *(de)spero*. In this psychotherapeutic attitude, people use their oscillations between despair and hope to find meaning and purpose in relation to their suffering. Similarly, the mentalisation theorist Jon Allen (2005: 238) sees the attitude of 'hope' as a meaningful 'existential stance' in relation to an experience of a traumatic event or situation. The attitude of hope, in the description of Allen, is 'an active process of meaning making' (ibid.). For Allen, existential trauma is the impact on meaning of the reality of an experience. Traumatic experiences 'shatter' our assumptions about the meaningfulness of our lives and the world, and as such this 'undermines the existential foundations of hope'. As traumatic attachments erode a person's mentalising capacities, the emphasis is on the person to refine hope in themselves, others and the world around them (ibid.: 290). Allen sees mentalisation-based interventions as building security, safety and meaning for the person, and fundamentally the hope required to sustain epistemic trust in relations with the world and others.

The existential psychologist Rollo May (1972) takes up in part an alternative existential stance of will-to-power. In doing so, May suggests that we must embrace the potentiality of our power (even in the form of constructive aggression and violence) through suffering and life challenges, in order to grow and develop.[2] A more well-known articulation of this is contained in the German philosopher Nietzsche's (1969 [1883]) writings. He describes (through the voice of Zarathustra) the different forms of suffering we must endure in the transformation of our human spirit. In his description, Nietzsche uses a zoomorphic metaphor to explain the transformation of the spirit. Unlike those lost to the herd, the camel (the person) takes on burdens, and this brings awe and respect for our strength and accumulation of knowledge. However, now a heavy spirit in the desert, we must undergo a metamorphosis into a lion, finding our own meaning, capturing our freedom over the desert through asserting 'I will' and battling the current lord of the desert, a dragon called 'thou shalt'. Having overcome this quest and fight with thou shalt, the spirit becomes that of a child, a new beginning, unburned by what came before, no longer needing to assert its will in contra position to thou shalt and approaching the world with wonderment and a sense of play. Nietzsche sees this transformation of spirit as happening many times over in a person's life, and this transformation enables them to endure their suffering, connect to their agentic power and find meaning in their lives.

Human suffering and the will-to-meaning

Existentialists who have had direct experiences of genocide suggest that finding an attitude towards, and meaning within, their suffering gives them purpose and courage to continuing living even in the most extreme situations and environments (c.f. Bettelheim, 1979; Eger, 2018). Both the essayist Primo Levi (2013 [1958/

1963]) and the psychiatrist Frankl (1967, 1988) describe differing attitudes of their peers inside the concentration camps of the Nazi regime. Levi and Frankl identify how finding meaning and purpose (even in the smallest of daily activities or in the acts of kindness of others) enabled them to survive in this environment. Frankl (2004 [1959]) goes on to put the 'will-to-meaning' at the heart of this own logotherapeutic approach to existential psychotherapy. Logotherapy encourages clients to confront the actualities of their life and find meaning or change within it. As Frankl writes (ibid.: 75), 'everything can be taken away from a [person] but one thing: the last of the human freedoms – to choose one's attitude in any given circumstances, to choose one's own way'. To realise our capacity to choose an attitude towards our suffering is, in itself, an expression of human potential and existential meaning.

More commonly, Frankl's logotherapy is described as focusing on our will-to-meaning, because of the significant emphasis he places on our human capacity to find meaning in our lives. Frankl distinguishes between three sets of values through which a person might find meaning and purpose in their lives and in their suffering (Frankl, 1986 [1946]: xix–xx; see also 2020 [1946]). The first set of 'creative' values emerge from our action in the world, our ability to find meaning in the tasks and life projects we create for ourselves or that necessitate our involvement in them (Frankl, 1986 [1946]: 43). In contrast, the second set are 'experiential' values that emerge from our 'receptivity to the world' (ibid.: 43–44). This receptivity can be realised in, for example, our surrounding or embracing of the goodness, truth or beauty of the world around us (even the projects of others like music, art or theatre), and through experiencing the richness and fullness of another human being. Finally, the third set of values only emerges when the person's suffering is 'unavoidable and inescapable' (ibid.: xx). 'Attitudinal' values are realised in our finding a way to face our suffering and make meaning out of it (ibid.: 43–44).

From the perspective of agentic movement in relation to suffering, we can also describe these three value sets as finding meaning (a) through acting from our own being, (b) by experiencing the world and others within it and (c) by how we adapt to the unavoidable limitations to our human experiencing and possibilities (ibid.: 68). As such, our subjectivity and sense of purpose in life are bound up in the ways we make meaning in relation to our suffering, and live by our meaning, rather than determined by the actuality of a situation or act that gives rise to the suffering (ibid.: 65–68). Importantly for Frankl (ibid., 1988, 2004 [1959]), the ability to realise all of these value sets is founded on the need for the person to take active responsibility for finding meaning in their life. Even the receptivity described within the creative values is also an active movement and approach; receptivity in this sense is an active form of agentic being.

The existential psychologist and philosopher Joel Vos (2018) extends Frankl's triadic framework of creative, experiential and attitudinal values. Vos draws on more substantive and recent evidence to propose the 'meaning quintet' (ibid.: 65–68). The meaning quintet is comprised of five categories of meaning that people can find in their life, and in their suffering. Although specifically designed to relate to human suffering, the meaning quintet is equally applicable to inquiries into human suffering as, like Frankl, Vos sees suffering and meaning as foundational aspects of human existence. Vos suggests that meaning types are interweaving, and proposes that people move through and between types and subtypes as their experiences of suffering change and grow in context and/or time.

The first category of Vos's meaning quartet is a materialist-hedonic domain, valuing material goods, success and pleasurable physical experiences. The second is self-orientated, valuing the capabilities, capacities and resilience of ourselves and the authentic forms of self-acceptance, self-expression and self-efficacy we can practise in our lives. The third is socially orientated, valuing our connections with others, and our belonging to specific communities and expressions of altruistic generosity. Fourth, Vos describes 'larger types' of meaning, which might be better categorised as meta forms of meaning. These meta forms of meaning value a sense of purpose, justice, ethics and engagement in belief and practices that transcend a focus on the self or others, including connecting to experiences of temporality (our orientation in time), spirituality or religion. We could also add here meaning through ecological awareness, and valuing environmental, conservation and preservation beliefs and practices.

Finally and fifthly, Vos describes a set of existential-philosophical meanings, which seem more abstract and are focused on the value of our life and existence. The existential-philosophical meaning can be implicit in the other categories of meaning, or interact with them in society or context-specific ways that frame personal meaning-making. Existential-philosophical values, according to Vos, include the value we find in being alive, taking responsibility for our lives and finding freedom within it – even in situations and conditions where we are limited or have to endure suffering. Additionally, valuing our experimentation and perceptive uniqueness or our connection to others in the world through relationships can be a source of existential-philosophical meaning.

For me, Frankl's triadic framework and Vos's quintet can coexist alongside each other. Frankl is clearly seeking to describe our movement as an agentic being; for him the value and form of meaning are located in movement through time and space. Recall that for Frankl meaning in suffering emerges in *action to, experiencing through, adaptation within*. In contrast, Vos's quintet is a more phenomenological-analytical description of categories of values and meanings. It provides us with a richer articulation of the varied forms of meaning that might arise in relation to suffering, and yet the agentic movement is less obvious at first reading.

We might think of Vos's frameworks as turning within our suffering. Some people turn towards the things of the world, seeking meaning and value in materiality and pleasure. Others might turn towards themselves and find solace in who they are in relation to their suffering. Yet others turn towards others, finding comfort in the connection, generosity and belonging they can experience and offer. Some may turn to create a direction or ethic for their life (possibly guided by the turning of others), and others might find value in contemplating or embracing life itself and the foundations of our existence. The final forms of turning implicit in Vos's work is that of spinning. For Vos (ibid.: 83), traumatic experiencing can disrupt or shatter our meaning and value in life. In such situations, I propose we can enter a state of spinning; that is, continually turning from meaning to meaning, seeking to find a form of meaning and set of values that will ground us and connect us to ourselves, others and the world around us. With the application of turning and spinning to Vos's typology, we can more easily incorporate the explicit ideas of agentic movement within Frankl's work, and add Vos's richer variety of phenomenological-analytical categorisations.

Alfried Längle (2003a) collaborated closely with Frankl, and drew upon logotherapy to create his own modality of Existential Analysis. Längle (2008: 3), in a similar vein to Frankl and Vos, defines existential suffering as 'the felt [subjective] destruction of something dear and/or vital'; put more simply, he articulates this as a 'feeling of loss or impairment to one's existence'. In order to understand the impact of suffering on one's existence, it is first important to have a sense of the existential analytic perspective of our human existence. Längle (ibid.: 4) sees human existence as being based on four fundamental realities: (a) the world, its limitations and conditions; (b) our life and life force; (c) our identity and relationship to others; and (d) the demands and horizons of our life situation.

For Längle, suffering endangers, threatens, disrupts or destroys our relationship with the fundamental structures of our existence. Through suffering we experience blockages in the meaning we make out of our life and the reality of our existence. This might result in us being unable to confront the reality of our existence and turn away from suffering. In relation to the four fundamental realities of existence (ibid.: 4–8), we might (a) experience our suffering as overwhelming and feel unable to overcome the world or find new conditions within it. Alternatively, we might (b) form a preference to not relate, act or experience the world, or (c) resort to self-alienation, avoidance and loneliness by not engaging with ourselves or with others in our lives. Finally, (d) we may feel unable to respond to the world or be actively engaged with it, meaning we lose our relation with the potentiality of our future and experience life as an existential vacuum – without meaning or purpose.

For me, there is an uncomfortable generality of suffering within this articulation of Längle's work. Although the generality of suffering is distributed through, and between, the four fundamental realities of human existence, there is an equalisation of forms of suffering. This implicitly suggests that suffering simply discloses different underlying foundational realties of human existence (ibid.: 6). As such, suffering as a breach or endangerment to meaning in existence, is subjectively horizontalised across experiences of rape, threat to life, bereavement, experiences of shame or guilt and losing a sense of direction in one's life. On the one hand, Längle's horizontalisation of suffering is important as it does not create a hierarchy in the forms of suffering that different people experience. The horizontalisation draws our attention instead to the possible commonalities between different human existences and losses of meaning. On the other hand, subsuming interpersonal trauma (i.e. rape and threat to life) into the generality of human experiences of suffering, potentially undermines the specific disclosures that these forms of experiencing might provide us with about the structure of human existence.

Within Längle's existential analysis, there is an emphasis on the courage it takes for the person to confront the reality of their suffering and therefore the foundations of our existence (ibid.: 7). He proposes that we must find the courage to endure and make meaning out of the reality of suffering. The use of the word 'endurance' (using von Kirchbach's translation) is philosophically relevant in my inquiry. Endurance describes a movement through experiential time – the word etymologically containing the experiential state of suffering as a movement through the duration of time. As we saw in in the work of Frankl and Vos, meaning in relation to suffering is existentially conceived by Längle as movement through time. Thus, suffering is part of a movement related to a confrontation with the reality of our human existence.

Those readers from a meaning-orientated psychological or psychotherapeutic background might be wondering why I am overemphasising movement in the work of Frankl, Vos and Längle. If this is the case, I would ask that you keep this question within view as you continue to read the remainder of this chapter. At this point, let us simply note that agentic movement and meaning might have a fundamental and deep relationship with one another.

For Längle, like Vos and Frankl, making meaning out of suffering is an agentic and active stance. The active motivational stance comes from our responses to the fundamentals of existence, as denotes our participation in our lived reality, rather than a more passive view of waiting for meaning to arise from suffering or avoiding the confrontation of the reality of suffering (see Längle, 2003a, for a useful overview of the existential-motivational perspective). That said, avoidance can also be seen as an active movement away from the confrontation. The stance in Längle's existential analysis is active-motivational because suffering can only be incorporated into our understanding and meaning of our suffering and our responses to it. In incorporating suffering actively into our meaning, we are better able to stay with the confrontation of the foundations of existence, withstand (endure) it and thus realise the potentiality of our futurity. As Längle describes it, 'the act of committing or responding to the situation itself enables a person to find an activity that opens the door to creative and meaningful possibilities and actions. These in turn open the door to the future' (ibid.: 8; see also 2003a, 2003b).

Echoing Frankl's (1986 [1946]: 43–44) attitudinal values, Längle (2008: 9) focuses on the existential concerns of *how* we suffer and *for whom* we suffer – *that* we suffer already being part of the ontological structure of human existence. These two concerns of the ways in which we respond to our suffering, and how we relate to ourselves and others in relation to our suffering, can provide significant existential meaning in the attitudinal values we adopt to respond to the suffering. These could include a wide range of attitudinal responses from privately reflecting on our bravery in facing our suffering, through to actively protecting others from additional suffering. He also draws our attention to what he terms ontological meaning (equivalent to Vos's larger types of meaning). Ontological meaning 'derives from the totality of all that exists and represents the meaning that underlies all beings' (ibid.). It focuses on metaphysical acts of faith in the totality of our existence and offers us the prospect of hope and liberation (or transformation) from (or within) our suffering.

Whether focusing on the will-to-meaning or will-to-power, existentialist writers are unified in their proposal that human suffering is a foundational experience embedded within, or emerging from, the confrontation of the reality of human existence. Moreover, they all agree that a person can find purpose, meaning, power and growth in their life by turning towards their suffering and finding new ways of relating to the foundations of human existence. As Frankl (1986 [1946]: 109) wrote: 'we mature in suffering, grow because of it – it makes us richer and stronger'. This is the paradox of human suffering; while human suffering is inevitable, existentialists see it as necessary for both the destruction of existing meanings and ways of living, and for the possibility of human growth or development. To be clear, the paradoxical feature of suffering is not seen within existentialism as a legitimisation of acts of suffering, nor does it negate the ethical considerations of the actions that bring about human suffering. Frankl and Levi saw no legitimacy or justice in their incarceration and torture. So while suffering is seen to be foundational in the structure of human experience, it does not ethically translate into a justification of enacting suffering upon another.

On trauma and human suffering

So, this leaves us with the question as to whether existentialists broadly consider all human experiencing as a form of suffering, or whether there are specific experiences that we might describe as being existentially traumatic and distinct from the generality of suffering. The Danish existential sociologist and psychologist Bo Jacobsen (2007: 65) attempts to answer this by differentiating between an existential 'crisis' and a 'trauma'. He sees trauma as being something that is 'inflicted' *on the soul* (I infer that he means human consciousness or an authentic form of being) from the outside, whereas an existential crisis is a shock *to the soul itself* (ibid.). Jacobsen writes that interpersonal trauma might result in a crisis, but an existential crisis need not be precipitated by a trauma (ibid.: 65–66). This in itself is not a contentious position to take. Existential philosophy, psychology, literature and essaying are filled with existential crises and realisations that arise out of a sudden awareness of, or new perspective on, the way we are living our lives. That said, significant and foundational existential works focus on crises, which arise out of very specific and tangible contingencies, limitations and traumas in our life – the reader need only glance back to the previous section in this chapter to be reminded of Levi's, Frankl's and Längle's work.

Jacobsen's use of the terms 'on' and 'to' are disclosive, in that they signal the movement of the existential shock to the person. For Jacobsen, trauma emerges and moves from the outside, and crisis arises and moves from the inside (within). The use of internal and external crisis replicates a more dualistic legacy of the interiority and exteriority of human experiencing, and enables him to locate different impacts of the crises on the body, mind or soul respectively. In the previous chapters we saw how both early and contemporary psychotraumatology sought to find ways of transcending the interiority and exteriority of the person in relation to trauma. An example of this would be through the focus on the person's subjective experiences of the (so-called) external event or situation. Paradoxically, and hiding in plain sight (within the 'on' and 'to'), Jacobsen offers us the same transcendence. In suggesting that interpersonal trauma can be *both* an external shock *and* an existential crisis we have a resolution – it is the person (as an experiential and reflexive being) who transforms the external shock into an existential crisis. Where I depart substantively from Jacobsen, is that I maintain the initial traumatic experience (the 'on') *is* a confrontation with the reality of human existence (the 'to'), whether or not the person transforms this consciously or reflexively into an existential crisis.

There are parallels between the descriptions of existential crises by Jacobsen, and the work of the Daseinsanalyst Alice Holzhey-Kunz (2016), whom I mentioned in the Introduction. Both seek to elevate vertically a special form of confrontation with the structure of human existence, which is beyond the specific experiential realities of interpersonal trauma. By way of reminder, Holzhey-Kunz differentiates between two forms of trauma: 'ontic' and 'ontological'. Ontic refers to traumas arising from the concrete limitations of our life, whereas ontological trauma is an 'unshielded exposure' to the human condition (ibid.: 17–18). The distinction between ontic and ontological builds upon the work of the German philosopher Heidegger (2010 [1953]). For Holzhey-Kunz (2016: 17–21), ontic trauma emerges from the experience of an event or situation, whereas ontological trauma arises from a 'special sensitivity' to the structure of human existence. There is a rough equivalence here with Jacobsen's conceptualisation of trauma and crisis.

In the Introduction, I questioned the need to verticalise experiences of more concrete interpersonal traumas, and a more philosophical, ontological trauma, not least because clinical and phenomenological accounts of so-called ontic trauma frequently include descriptions of confrontations with the reality of human existence at an ontological level. The phenomenological overlap between descriptions of interpersonal trauma and ontological trauma are also echoed in Jacobsen's formulation of existential crises. Jacobsen's (2007: 69) description of the characteristics of a state of crisis include a breaking down of our sense of time and space, strong and oscillating feelings and intense mental activity. These three characteristics are featured (albeit in alternative articulations) within the writings of the majority of the early and contemporary psychotraumatologists, as are further phenomenological descriptions he provides throughout the text, such as 'sudden disruption of the normal life activity and continuous flow of time' or 'loss of meaning and world view' (ibid.: 72, 74).

Based on a somewhat brief engagement with the psychoanalytical and cognitive behavioural therapy (CBT) literature and practice, Jacobsen is critical of the usefulness of understanding psychological trauma within existentialist psychology. His aversion to CBT leads him to suggest that therapeutically confronting people with the experience of their trauma or crisis runs the risk of 'violating and breaking down' the autonomy of the person (ibid.: 66). Similarly, he dismisses what he sees to be a causally deterministic psychoanalytic notion that earlier childhood traumatic experiences shape adult reactions to existential crises (ibid.: 67). In theory and practice (as the earlier chapters of this book demonstrate), both the CBT and psychoanalytic positions are more complex and nuanced than Jacobsen allows for in his brief description. They too struggle with the tensions of non- and retro-causality, as well as delve into the ways people's worldview and relationality are experienced and disrupted in the present moment, as well as in the past.

Finally, Jacobsen appraises diagnostic approaches to post-traumatic stress disorder (PTSD)-focused therapies (ibid.: 67–68). I am in full support of his caution over the medicalisation and pathologising of everyday life, and concerns that PTSD diagnoses may become a new threshold for access to therapeutic support. However, to dismiss the traumatic experience at the heart of the PTSD diagnosis as *just* an artefact of a socio-medicalised pathologising label is to philosophically lose sight of the incorporation of the traumatic experience into the being of the person. PTSD as a diagnosis holds value clinically and for individuals as it offers an explanatory narrative for unarticulated and disorientating disruptions in a person's worldview. In summary, Jacobsen's rebuttal to these approaches turns away from the valuable insights CBT and psychoanalytic traditions might hold about the nature of traumatic experiencing, and the structure of human existence.

So, the reader may well be wondering, why then is there a philosophical or psychotherapeutic need to distinguish something special, and above the realities of traumatic experiencing? The reason for the distinction is to protect the notion that some humans have a form of awakened ontological sense of the world and our place within it, and the disclosures this awareness brings about human existence. If we put to one side Jacobsen's dismissal of traumatic experiencing as being something distinct (and less ontologically significant) from crises, there is value in his formulation as it draws our attention to some of the ontological features we might want to consider in our inquiry into traumatic experiencing: of temporal-spatial movement, of a shock to the existing worldview of the person, of the need to find meaning in relation to crises. That said, the everyday legacy of Jacobsen's use of the term 'crisis', is that many leading contemporary existential psychologists and psychotherapists interchangeably use the terms 'crisis' and 'trauma' as if they were describing the same experiential phenomena or disclosing common structures of human existence. Jacobsen's writing, like Holzhey-Kunz's, would not support this interchangeability, and yet in the desire to be part of a movement or market for trauma-focused 'treatment', some existential psychologists and psychotherapists use the interchangeability with existential crises as a way into providing professional training or services to clients.

Heideggerian ontology

A smaller group of existential psychologists and psychotherapists have more explicitly described interpersonal trauma as a specific phenomenon, without subsuming it into the generality of human suffering. Like Jacobsen and Holzhey-Kunz, many of these existentialists have used the ideas and writings of the post-Cartesian

German philosopher Heidegger to inform their theory and practice.[3] Heidegger's philosophy is a dense treatise on the structure of human existence, which is widely influential in contemporary British, European, some American and increasingly international schools of existential psychology and psychotherapy. In what follows, I provide a brief overview of some of the key Heideggerian ideas as presented in his more widely referenced tome *Being and Time*. This brief introduction is far from a comprehensive treatment of his work and is provided here to contextualise the language use and later discussion for readers.

In *Being and Time*, Heidegger (2010 [1953]) describes a specific ontological mode of being, which he termed *Dasein* (being-there). Dasein is a being that is conscious of its own being and therefore implicated in its own existence. This, for Heidegger, is the ontological difference between the human Being (Dasein) and the being of other creatures and things in the world. In exploring and phenomenologically inquiring about Dasein's existence, Heidegger aims to identify the shared givens and structures of existence, which are disclosed (*Erschlossenheit*) through our being (ibid.: 129).

The givens of existence include our thrownness (*Geworfenheit*) into our existence and into a body, social context and world that are not of our own choosing (ibid.: 131–132). The facticity and thrownness of Dasein disclose that our existence is bound up in the world in which we are situated (ibid.: 56–57). This situatedness includes the specific historical moment we find ourselves thrown into, and the facticity of both being related to and bound up in this specific moment in time (*Geschichtlichkeit*).

Dasein is seen by Heidegger to be a being-in-the-world (*In-der-Welt-sein*), and projects (*Entwurf*) itself towards our possibilities and understanding of the world in relation to these disclosed or hidden possibilities (ibid.: 140–141). The world opens up to Dasein through our attunement (*Befindlichkeit*), which is pre-ontologically experienced through the everyday phenomenon of mood (*Stimmung*) (ibid.: 130–136). The ownmost possibility of Dasein is the existential given of our finitude and nothingness. Dasein becomes a being-towards-death (*Sein-zum-Tode*) in confronting, and authentically (*Eigentlichkeit*) opening up, to existential anxiety (*Angst*).

Through embracing our existential anxiety, Dasein can follow the call of conscience (*Gewissensruff*) and move through any uncanniness (*Unheimlichkeit*) or existential guilt (*Schuld*) it might experience. In responding to the call of consciousness, a clearing (*Lichtung*) appears, allowing for the unconcealment of truth (*Aletheia*) and greater understanding (*Vershehen*). Only through facing the existential anxiety and following the call of consciousness can Dasein authentically realise its being-towards-death and possibility (*Vorlaufen/Sein-zum-Tode*). With greater understanding about its existence, Dasein can make a stronger commitment to care (or concern) for its being and that of others (*Sorge/Fürsorge*). Rather than ontological disclosure arising from experience, Dasein can, through concern for its existence, use an anticipatory resoluteness (*Vorlaufende Entschlossenheit*) as an active form of disclosure to face and understand the shared givens of existence. Anticipatory resoluteness creates Dasein's openness to movement (*Augenblick*) towards authenticity (*Eigentlichkeit*) and personal understanding of its own existence.

Finally, Heidegger distinguishes between an ontological and ontic mode of existence. The ontological mode is denoted by our awareness and confrontation with the existential givens, and through authentically turning towards the care of Dasein. This is seen by Heidegger as being in contrast to our ontic concerns, which are manifested in specific expressions or ways of being in the world. In this way Dasein's authenticity is an opening up to our experience of existence. Whereas inauthenticity (*uneigentlich*) is a mode of forgottenness (*Vergessenheit*), falling (*Verfallen*), absorption (*Aufgehen*), or a turning way from our being. We turn away from our being-in-the-world, as we cannot bear the existential anxiety, guilt or uncanniness involved in confronting and embracing the existential givens.

Heidegger's philosophy provides us with many important ontological questions about the nature of human existence and potentially for understanding experiences of trauma. Heideggerian-influenced phenomenology and existentialism have been instrumental in investigating post-Cartesian (beyond the mind–body dualism) explorations of lived experiences, and what they might disclose about the structures of human existence. Frequently, academics in the British and European schools of existentialism insist on embracing and accepting the dominance of Heideggerian-based theory and practice. For me, using the work of Heidegger is fraught with tensions about the person he was, as well as the recognition he sought and the contribution he wanted to make to the world he lived in.

Heidegger was a leading academic during the start of the Second World War. He was clamouring for philosophical notoriety and status within the German National Socialist German Workers Party (Nazi Party), and higher positions at the University of Freiburg. His proxy legitimisation of the Nazi regime and uncompromising reluctance and then refusal to account for his participation in the movement and seeking of recognition and praise by senior Nazi officials are reprehensible.

As I have written before in an open letter entitled 'Haunted by Heidegger', perhaps one can

> understand phenomena, or a mode of existence, by it eluding us in our own lived experience […] Heidegger's quest for an ontology of Being, through Dasein's authenticity, is so compelling, because it describes almost everything he was not in the reality of his own life. Perhaps this was the personal impetus for his philosophical project, to (cynically) mask or (compassionately) understand his own inauthenticity and duplicity.
>
> (Bush [Boaz], 2020a: 7–8)

Beyond this philosophical question, for me there is an ethical question about the appropriateness of using Heidegger's ideas in my own work on interpersonal trauma. Heidegger was a prominent philosopher who was entangled in a project of fascist and genocidal nationalism (c.f. Di Cesare, 2018; Farin & Malpas, 2018; Heidegger, 2016 [2014], 2017a [2014], 2017b [2014]; Mitchell & Trawny, 2017). There is an absurdity in using his work to inform an approach to interpersonal trauma, when his ideas are saturated in the blood, sweat and tears of his own inauthenticity, and his avoidance of the realities of his participation in his existence and historical thrownness. To this day, the Heidegger controversy continues to be as fractious as the protracted controversial discussions that divided the British Psychoanalytical Society between the Freudian, Kleinian and independent traditions in 1942–1944 (see King & Steiner, 1991).

My invitation for existential psychiatrists, psychologists and psychotherapists is to release yourself from the bind of Heidegger. We must accept that Heidegger will remain a spectre in our own writings and profession; however, we must also give ourselves permission to describe the structure of human experience in a way that moves beyond the concepts and language he used. To all readers, if you see commonalities, convergences or conflicts with Heidegger's ideas in this book, you are welcome to embrace them and make of them what you will. Above, I have briefly outlined the Heideggerian ontology and raised a concern about the appropriateness of including his work in the field of psychotraumatology. I now turn to an exploration of the useful applications of his ideas in the work of contemporary existential-phenomenological psychologists and psychotherapists.

Existential-phenomenological understandings of trauma (Heideggerian)

The existential psychologist Chloe Paidoussis-Mitchell (2012) draws on Heideggerian philosophy and existentialism more broadly to provide us with a description of what happens at the confrontation of traumatic bereavement. In her phenomenological study, Paidoussis-Mitchell found that participants experienced an embodied reaction to a traumatic death, which 'jolted' them out of their ontic mode of being. The jolt brought them into an ontological awakening and a simultaneous loss of meaning. The ontological awakening and a simultaneous loss of meaning relate to the person being confronted with existential givens – such as the randomness of life, our finitude and our existential isolation. In the face of these existential givens, Paidoussis-Mitchell notes how her participants experienced a will-to-meaning (not unlike that described by Frankl, Längle and Vos), and a form of spiritual awakening. This spiritual awakening was not necessarily religious, but rather corresponded to the values people found to live by in the course of the traumatic bereavement.

Like Jacobsen and Holzhey-Kunz, Paidoussis-Mitchell too sees there being a threshold that is crossed through the confrontations with the reality of human experiencing (ibid.: 35, 40) – from ontic to ontological awareness. Put another way, she identifies a movement from the realities of the specific experience (in this case a traumatic bereavement) to the realities of human existence (the given of death, finitude and will-to-meaning). The movement is a *jolt*, which signals a violent shake throwing a person through the confrontation into the ontological mode. Paidoussis-Mitchell maintains that what makes traumatic bereavement different from everyday experiences of bereavement is this thrown awareness into the ontological mode (ibid.: 41).

Paidoussis-Mitchell extends the formulation of confrontations with the onto-logical mode of existence in a joint paper with the existential psychologist Susan Iacovou (Iacovou & Paidoussis-Mitchell, 2017). The authors explore British vet-erans' experiences of active service in the Falklands War. Iacovou and Paidoussis-Mitchell describe how active service 'forced' the servicemen 'to come face to face with existential realities' and the existential givens (ibid.: 390). This confronta-tion left them open to their existential situation, resulting in changes to them and to the ways they related to others. Changes included reprioritisations in the vet-erans' lives and a greater value being placed by them on relationality with others (ibid.: 390–391).

The veterans' changed worldviews, values and meanings led to a sense of estrangement and isolation from friends and family, who had not shared in their traumatic experience nor their confrontations with existential givens. A sense of alienation from others resulted in some of the veterans withdrawing fur-ther and feeling more isolated. Some reported ending up in a 'dark place' or re-experiencing their traumatic experiences through flashbacks, nightmares or engaging in behaviours that would threaten or endanger them or those in their lives (ibid.: 392). The authors identified that at a later point, a subsequent life trauma, or a series of stressful life events, would precipitate a form of break-down, which paradoxically opened up the possibility for greater emotionality and relationality in the veterans' lives (ibid.: 293–294). Iacovou and Paidoussis-Mitchell note that the existential confrontation, and growthful change of the person and their priorities, is frequently excluded from diagnostic and some clinical psycho-logical formulations. Likewise, the new ways of being (including emotionally and relationally) and finding of new meanings fall out of much of the PTSD-focused clinical literature.

Clinical psychologists Luke Arnold and Allayna Pinkston build on the work of Paidoussis-Mitchell and others in an attempt to bridge existential and psychi-atric (*DSM-5* PTSD) formulations of traumatic stress and dissociation (Arnold & Pinkston, 2014). The authors suggest that traumatic events and situations share a common existential encounter with finitude and our vulnerability to being hurt by an Other in the world (ibid.: 97). In the Heideggerian view of Arnold and Pinkston, we do not re-experience traumatisation in the present, but rather recon-struct the past experience (in anticipation of a painful future response) in the present moment (ibid.: 98). In this way, traumatic re-experiencing is a potential generalisation of the ontic (i.e. the rape of a young girl by a particular man with brown hair) into the ontological (other situations where men with brown hair are present and proximate). That said, at the same time, the person's awareness of the uniqueness of their own traumatic experience enables them to meaningfully dif-ferentiate their own experience from that of the generalised other. This discloses the existential paradox of being both bound up in relation to others and simultan-eously uniquely alone in our own experience: we are 'being(s)-in-the-world who are simultaneously alienated from and yet painfully close to Others who cannot know our pain as we do' (ibid.: 97).

For Arnold and Pinkston, our phenomenological expressions of our confrontation with the traumatising potential or actuality of the Other, are frequently pathologised by others, and especially in the PTSD diagnosis. They suggest that we might better understand traumatic-stress phenomena as an understandable response to the person's loss of trust, safety and relationality with others in the world (ibid.: 98–99). For example, the experience of dissociation is seen by the authors as an existential movement to gain a felt sense of spatiality – by which they presumably mean distance, as all movement is a form of spatiality – from the self, traumatic event and/or memory of the experience (ibid.). Dissociation is seen to be an attempt to create space from the confrontation of reality.

The authors note how our attempts to make space (or create distance) from the traumatic memory or experience through dissociation is taken up by the Other as a sign of madness and psychopathy, whereas for us it is an understandable and necessary existential movement to survive the reality of existence. The person who dissociates is 'decidedly *being-dys-integrated* or *dys-connected* in the world', and this is a 'protective way of being', which enables their movement through the traumatic experience of memory (ibid.: 100, emphasis added). Dissociative movement is therefore an understandable and yet (according to the authors) a false movement, as it also removes the person's possibility of recognising the newness of the present situation, and further the agentic potential in engaging in new ways with Others in the world. Of course, their analysis relies on the notion that the person no longer experiences a traumatic situation or that the traumatic relationships do not endure into the present.

Similarly, Arnold and Pinkston reframe hypervigilance as a *hyper-attunement* (using Heidegger's meaning) to the actuality of the traumatising potential of Others, and the precarity of the relational world we live in (ibid.: 99). This is seen to be an exhausting mode of Being, as in the attempt to avoid the further pain and traumatisation, the person is turning away from the horrific realisation of the traumatic potential of Others in the world, and our being-towards-death. In a critique of Frankl, the authors suggest that a meaningful attitudinal response to this horror might be to prematurely eschew it. As an alternative, Arnold and Pinkston advocate for the Heideggerian embracing of being-towards-death, which enables us to turn towards both the potentiality of our death (finitude) and living in the present moment. Rather than a loss of meaning, Arnold and Pinkston contend that meaning is lived out in one's being-in-the-world, and that as such, through the experience of trauma we are able to learn to live unresolved and open to the possibilities of unknowing and uncertainty.

Drawing on cognitive-emotional models of psychology, Arnold and Pinkston propose their 'existential trauma therapy' for traumatic stress and dissociation. Their psychotherapeutic response incorporates three interrelated elements of (a) activation, (b) validation and (c) integration (ibid.: 101). Rather than a psychotherapeutically led activation, the clinician uses a phenomenological process of descriptive clarification to open up traumatic experiences as and when the client feels able to reveal and disclose them. In contrast to the traditional cognitive-emotional stance of avoiding the reinforcement of the traumatic experience, Arnold and Pinkston propose that we actively validate the client's experience of the traumatic situation or relationships. In an important critique of the cognitive-emotional approach, the authors note that 'the therapist who systematically eliminates emotional primacy of the traumatic memory by selecting only certain less-activating associations invalidates the mattering of the experience' (ibid.: 101).

For me, there is wisdom in their advocating for staying with the client's felt reality of the traumatic experience, as it avoids an invalidation of their lived reality and the actuality of the situation or event. In a radical validation of the traumatic experience, the existential psychologist or psychotherapist works with the client to face the reality of their pain and find meaning in relation to it, and ontologically in relation to the facticity of their existence. In this way, the focus is on an integration of the person's experience, rather than on extinguishing the client's pain. The existential practitioner focuses on clarifying a person's being-in-the-world instead of adopting the cognitive-emotional approach of counter- or reconditioning the client to feel, and respond in, a different way to the traumatic event.

Integration of the traumatic experience is a by-result of focusing on the client's being-in-the-world, and thus integration is best described as 'both a movement and a recognition of that which has already moved with the passage of time' (ibid.). Existentially, the movement of the trauma into the past mode of being opens up a phenomenological inquiry and clarification about how the person used their agency to survive in the past, and the experiences of loss, guilt and regret related to previous ways of living. Rather than integration being a therapeutic goal in and of itself, integration is therefore emergent within the new ways the client finds to relate to their experience of trauma, and the world in the present (ibid.: 102). This draws on the Heideggerian agentic potential of Dasein to be its ownmost and thus choose itself. Arnold and Pinkston suggest that meaning is disclosed through the ways in which a person uniquely takes up the traumatic situation they have experienced, and therefore taking up new ways of existing in relation to it is an agentic expression of choice, meaning and potentiality (ibid.: 97–98).

Phenomenological-contextual understandings of trauma (neo-Heideggerian)

The phenomenological-contextual psychoanalyst Robert Stolorow provides us with an important contemporary bridge between psychoanalytic and existential approaches to psychotraumatology. His work provides a useful insight into traumatic experiencing in developmental contexts. Stolorow's work draws heavily on the ideas of Winnicott, the self-psychologist Heinz Kohut and latterly from Heidegger.[4]

By way of context, Kohut initially saw so-called psychic trauma as associated with the intensity (over- or understimulation of the experience), although over time he moved away from this conceptualisation to focus on the relational features of traumatic relationships (disappointments) between child and caregiver (Kohut, 1971). In Kohut's (1984) self-psychology, the child relies on the caregiver to be a self-object. The self-object is the child's experience of the other as a narcissistic extension of the self, rather than a separate human being. The child requires available and empathetic attunement of the self-object to develop a coherent and stable sense of self over time. The unavailability of empathetic self-objects in childhood leads to a traumatised experience of the relationship and thus the self in relation to others.

Stolorow, along with his colleague George Atwood (Stolorow & Atwood, 2002 [1992]), continue Kohut's inquiry in describing the intersubjective foundations of interpersonal and developmental trauma. They see human experience as being fundamentally intersubjective, which describes '*any* psychological field formed by interacting worlds of experience' that have a '*reciprocal mutual influence*' (ibid.: 3, original emphasis). Unlike other forms of developmental psychology, and the early Freudians, Stolorow and Atwood see the potential for traumatisation existing within this intersubjective field, and thus the possibility of traumatisation is an intersubjective given – in that we are intersubjectively embedded.

According to Stolorow and Atwood, we enter new situations and relationships with organising principles, which are pre-existing organisations of our sense of self, others and the world that are established from the intersubjective experience of child–caregiver (ibid.: 24). In contrast to many of the object-relation theorists, the authors suggest that the child develops a sense of the real world and reality through the validating attunement of their experiences by the caregiver(s), and these include the preverbal and sensorimotor attunements of the caregiver(s) (ibid.: 27). The validating attunement of the caregiver creates an intersubjective interaffectivity, which is the 'mutual regulation of affective experience within a developmental system' between child and caregiver(s) (ibid.: 31; see also Stolorow, 2007: 3). This positions interaffectivity as the primacy mode of human existence, and at the heart of intersubjective experiencing (Stolorow, 2011c: 19)

When the child encounters a malattuned response to their experiential reality by the caregiver(s), the intolerable affect (emotional state) is repressed into the unconscious (echoing the likes of Fairbairn). For Stolorow and Atwood (2002 [1992]: 31), the repression of these affective states into the unconscious is a defence of the person against retraumatisation and to maintain the required relationship with the caregiver. In a more nuanced description of the intersubjective unconscious, the authors see the repression of the intolerable affect of malattunement as residing in three interrelated forms of unconsciousness: (a) the pre-reflective unconscious, where unconsciously organising principles shape and thematise people's experiences; (b) the dynamic unconscious, where experiences that cannot be articulated are repressed, as expressing them would threaten the required intersubjective relationships; and (c) the unvalidated unconscious, where experiences cannot be articulated as they were met initially by an invalidating response (ibid.: 33). In the case of both the dynamic and the unvalidated unconscious, the child's experiential world is sacrificed to maintain an intersubjective relationship with the caregiver.

Stolorow and Atwood build on Winnicott's (1991 [1964], 2006 [1965]) notion of *indwelling*, or the subjective experience of having and experiencing our self, others and the world through our body. By way of reminder, Winnicott saw the realisation of our embodied self as being developed contextually through the inter-subjective experience of our self in relation to others and the world around us. Stolorow and Atwood (2002 [1992]: 46) suggest that sensorimotor malattunement by a caregiver and latterly another disrupts or 'deforms' the person's own attunement and sense of indwelling or embodiment. The authors identify two broad categories of subjective experiences of mind–body separation. The first results from an initial inability to achieve a sense of somatic indwelling or embodi-ment, and the second is an active misidentification with one's own body to pro-tect against threat or danger associated with continuing an embodied experience (ibid.: 47). Again, these are developed contextually and intersubjectively through the malattunement, the perceived or actual threat of the other and in the first instance the caregiver(s).

Subjective experiences of mind–body separation can be exacerbated by an invalidating caregiver response, which prevents the child from symbolically articulating their feelings as they lack the intersubjective attunement to iden-tify and describe their emotional state. Alternatively, in situations where the affective response of the child is experienced as intolerable or injurious to the caregiver, the caregiver ignores, blocks or further invalidates the child's affective experience (ibid.: 43). Both these exacerbations result in a reversion back to som-atic modes of experiencing and expression (as described in many of the early psychotraumatological cases).

Somatic modes of affective experiencing and expression are described by Stolorow and Atwood as 'concretisations', which are the 'configuration of sub-jective experience' through sensorimotor symbols to maintain the organising principles (ibid.: 45). Somatic concretisations include (a) conversion, where a bodily substitute symbolises the conflictual experience in order to maintain the intersubjective relationship, as (for example) cognising and verbalising the conflict or distress would threaten a required bond or tie with the other; (b) psychosomatic illness or expression, with the difference being that in conversion the expressions of affect (and their intersubjective context) are symbolised, whereas in psycho-somatic expressions these expressions are pre-symbolic; and (c) hypochondrial states, which are formed through anxiety-ridden fantasies about the body. In these states, the person expresses the anxiety of threat to self and life through symbolic-ally locating the concern in failing 'concrete anatomical symbols' (ibid.).

In addition to disrupting our sense of indwelling, intersubjective malattunement can result in a dislocation or confusion of the traumatic experience, and the reason for the caregiver's malattuned response. Stolorow and Atwood suggest that chil-dren readily conclude that they themselves, or their affective response, are in some way responsible for the malattunement of the caregiver. In these cases, the child assumes responsibility for the malattunement and mistreatment by the other, and actively invalidate their own painful affectivity (ibid.: 54; 62–63). The invalida-tion of painful affect enables the person to continue relating to the malattuned caregiver who fails to validate their traumatic experience. Elsewhere, Stolorow describes this as the person concluding that they are inherently bad, which leads to a severe constriction in their 'horizons of emotional experiencing' within relational contexts – as they are deemed to be frightening or dangerous to the person (Stolorow, 2007: 4; see also Stolorow, Atwood & Orange, 2002, for a deeper discussion).

This echoes the work of Fairbairn (1994 [1943a]: 64–65), who suggested that a traumatic situation occurs when the child concludes that they have in some way caused the sense of 'badness' they are experiencing in the malattuned response of the caregiver. Fairbairn similarly proposes that in situations where the caregiver has a high degree of 'badness' (is neglectful and/or abusive) towards the child, the child takes on 'the burden of badness' in order to make their external and internalised ideal objects good (ibid.: 65). As a consequence, the child adopts a 'moral' form of badness, in acting in ways that would be described by the caregiver and others as bad. For the child, moral badness is an important defence as it moves us on from the intolerable situation of being 'unconditionally' bad (i.e. 'bad from a libidinal standpoint' of object-relating), to becoming 'conditionally' bad where the things we do are defined as bad (ibid.: 66). Fairbairn suggests that the more the child 'leans towards' their internalised bad objects, the more conditionally (morally) bad they become.

The child comes to realise that it is 'preferable' to be conditionally bad (do bad things) in relation to good objects (in a good world), than to be unconditionally bad (a libidinally bad person) in relation to bad objects (in a bad world). As Fairbairn wrote: 'It would be better to be a sinner in a world ruled by a God than live in a world ruled by the Devil' (ibid.: 67). As such, the moral defence presents the child with the 'possibilities of conditional (moral) goodness and badness', and thus hope for 'the possibilities of repentance and forgiveness' from the caregiver (Fairbairn, 1994 [1951]: 165).

Returning to Stolorow and Atwood (2002 [1992]: 52), interpersonal trauma is conceived by the authors as painful and unbearable affect resulting from intersubjective contexts, *and* the breakdown of the child–caregiver 'system of mutual regulation'. Interaffective experiences become traumatic when there is a lack of attuned responsiveness by an other within the contextual environment (ibid.: 52–53). Cumulative trauma is thus the inadequate and malattuned response to the child's 'painful affect' once the required protective role of the caregiver has been breached (ibid.: 54).

Having experienced malattunement to their painful and unbearable affect, the person enters new intersubjective contexts with their conscious and unconscious responses to these previous malattunements within the field of this new situation. Stolorow and Atwood argue that it is the current (new) intersubjective context that will co-determine which of the pre-existing organising principles will come into operation in the present moment. A stronger emphasis is placed on the current intersubjective context, as it is this that co-determines the boundaries between the person's conscious and unconscious experiencing and affective response to interpersonal situations (ibid.: 31).

In some situations, the previous incorporations of malattunement and adaptive responses into a person's organising principles will unconsciously sensitise them, (mis)interpreting subsequent (new) experiences as 'actual or impending repetition of the original trauma' (ibid.: 55–56, 63). This is because the experience of interpersonal trauma results in an 'experiential chasm' between the traumatised person and the other (Stolorow, 2007: 14). For Stolorow (ibid.: 19, 41), traumatic experiences shatter everyday absolutisms about the world being safe, stable and predictable, and leave us with a sense of existential singularity, isolation and feeling of solitude. Existentially, trauma 'shatters the illusions of everyday life that evade and cover up the finitude, contingency, and embeddedness of our existence and the indefiniteness of its certain extinction' (Stolorow, 2019a: 74–76). Building on Winnicott, Stolorow and Atwood (2002 [1992]: 57) suggest that the person's interpretation of the new situation or person(s) being potentially malattuned and traumatic, is valid as it is an understandable transference of the intersubjective trauma and lack of attuned response to their previous experiences of painful affect and to the shattering of these everyday illusions of our reality.

Existentially, the experience of trauma is further 'ontologically revelatory' as it discloses a feature of 'authentic existence' (Stolorow, 2011c: 33). Interpersonal trauma confronts us with existential anxiety, as relationally and contextually the experience threatens the possibility of our futurity and brings us into direct relation with the reality of our finitude and possibility of our death (Stolorow, 2007: 37–39). The threat to our futurity and confrontation with our finitude disrupts our lived experience of time. Stolorow (ibid.: 20; see also 2011a) suggests that in the confrontation of trauma, time is experienced all at once, with trauma freezing certain experiences (and the person's horizons of experiencing) as the eternal present. For some people, this results in dissociation, which in Stolorow's Heideggerian frame is seen as a specific traumatic temporality, where the person experiences their existence as being out of the personal and historical flow of time (Stolorow, 2007: 20; 2011c: 54–55).

While Stolorow considered some traumatic states (i.e. dissociation) to be a movement away from the authentic experience of being-towards-death, he proposes that traumatic experiencing can also be a call of consciousness. In a Heideggerian frame, this call of consciousness requires us to embrace our anticipatory resoluteness and choose to be ready for existential anxiety, and thus be authentic in turning towards our possibility and futurity (Stolorow, 2007: 42–45; 2011c: 41–45). As such, the psychotherapeutic focus is placed on addressing malattuned responses to painful affect through the validating responsiveness of the psychologist or psychotherapist (Stolorow & Atwood, 2002 [1992]: 49). In this way, therapy becomes a co-determined interrelationship, and through an attuned response, the psychologist or psychotherapist and client can work together to both build new organising principles and contextually expand the person's experiential repertoire (ibid.: 25). Moreover, co-determined psychotherapeutic relationships enable the person to experience an attuned response to the existential reality of our 'unbearable embeddedness of being' (Stolorow, 2007: 16).

Through the psychotherapeutic relationship, the person can realise their ontological mode of existing by being-in-the-world through care towards the self and
others. Care, as we have seen in the work of Heidegger, enables the person to
incorporate and accept their facility (thrownness), their intersubjective-contextual
embeddedness, the realisation of possibilities and being-towards-death. Moving
away from Heidegger's notion of the existential aloneness of death, Stolorow
(2011c: 67–68) retains the intersubjective stance, suggesting that death and finitude are always relational and thus we can find commonality and kinship in
confronting existential givens.

In a beautiful turn of phrase, Stolorow (2011c: 64; 2007: 49) suggests that
the client can personally and therapeutically find love and kinship-in-finitude,
and an 'existential kinship-in-the-same-darkness'. This emerges from finding
commonality, human understanding and attunement in the world with those
who know 'the same darkness' of interpersonal trauma (ibid.: 19, 49). Latterly,
Stolorow (2019a: 76) has adopted a more active form of therapeutic relationality,
which he terms 'emotional dwelling'. Rather than focusing on therapeutic
empathy, in emotional dwelling 'one leans into the other's emotional pain and
participates in it, perhaps with the aid of one's own analogous experiences of
pain' (ibid.). For Stolorow, this is a more honest form of relating as it enables
both the client and psychotherapist to stay with the traumatised emotional states
of the client, rather than seeking to turn away from the 'unbearable', 'unendurable' or 'unsayable' realities of the traumatic experience (ibid.). In a post-
Heideggerian movement, Stolorow (2019a: 76; 2019b: 100) acknowledges the
need to embrace our own existential vulnerability and find ways of tolerating
and drawing on it (even in the face of our own unbearable pain) to emotionally
dwell in the unendurable pain of others. Stolorow and Atwood (2019c: 116–
117) describe emotional dwelling as 'walking the tightrope' within the psychotherapeutic relationship. The aim of indwelling is not to merely understand
the traumatic experience of the other in their frame of reference; the psychotherapist intends to co-participate in a confrontation of the traumatic world of
the client, and through a dialogical intersubjective system expand the horizons
of emotional experiencing and understanding, so that the client can articulate,
bear and endure these experiences for themselves.

The temptation, according to Stolorow and Atwood (2019b), is to turn away
from confronting the reality of our traumatic experience and its disclosure of our
finitude. According to the authors we re-illusion ourselves about the nature of our
reality, through metaphysical illusions of, for example, the solidness, coherence,
continuity and knowability of our existence and sense of self (ibid.: 88; Stolorow
and Atwood, 2019a: 91–96; see also Stolorow, 2019b: 102–103). Through delving
into this form of *kinship-in-the-same-darkness*, the psychotherapist and client can stay
with the reality of traumatic experiences and co-transform traumatised states into
'sacred' understandings and engagements that are bearable and nameable for
the person (Stolorow, 2019a: 76–77). Further, in this mode of finding kinship-
in-the-same-darkness, Stolorow addresses the absence of the mood of shame in
Heidegger's work. Stolorow (2011c: 107–108; building on 2019a: 76–77) proposes

that shame discloses inauthentic or unowned existing, and thus intersubjective attunement and emotional dwelling within the psychotherapeutic relationship, and disrupts the relational assumption that the person is deficient or defective in the eye of the other. For me, Stolorow's (and Atwood's) articulation of emotional dwelling is a beautiful synthesis of the existential and contextually intersubjective perspectives they have cultivated over the decades of their practices and collaborations.

Worlds of traumatic experiencing (social phenomenology)

Stolorow's notion of kinship-in-the-same-darkness echoes in some ways the writings of the philosopher and phenomenological sociologist Alfred Schütz. Schütz's (1967 [1932]) social phenomenology elaborates on the work of Husserl to provide a more detailed description of the shared structures of intersubjective experiencing. In brief, Schütz adapts Husserl's earlier ideas of the life-world (*Lebenswelt*), to describe our taken for granted (or common-sense) experiences of reality. He contends that our life-world is intersubjectivity co-created through social action, and through social actions our experiences become subjectively ascribed as meaningful within intersubjective fields.

Schütz's social phenomenology of the life-world has a deeper spatial-temporal dimension in his explorations of the proximity a social actor has to others in the social world. Drawing on the work of the French philosopher Henri Bergson (1889 [1927]; 1941), Schütz (1967 [1932]: 45–96) proposes that our primordial experience of the complex world around us is through a lived stream of consciousness. We live within the meaning-endowing acts of existence we and others enact through time (*duration*). We only become aware of our acts of existence and their possibility of meaning when we turn towards our lived stream of consciousness (see also Schütz & Luckmann, 1973: 52–55). This is most easily done when the social acts we engage in recede into the past and thus provide us with a distance from the acts in order to move towards them and reflect upon them. According to Schütz (1967 [1932]), when we reflect upon social acts, they are lifted out of the duration of our lived experience of the stream of consciousness. Turning towards, reflecting upon and examining our acts in the world gives these moments of active experience a sense of discrete or concrete phenomenological significance (ibid.). The act of turning towards (*Zuwendung*) the experience brings meaning (*Sinn*) to the otherwise undifferentiated, primordial stream of consciousness of existence.

Through turning towards our action in the world, we can ascribe meaning to social acts both in retrospect and prospectively in future anticipation. As social action is the focus of Schütz's phenomenology, the movement of action through duration provides the intersubjective ground for the acquisition of meaning (ibid.: 97–138). A person projects forward the completion of an intention of a social act. The intentional goal of the act is brought into being by the anticipation of the action itself, and the past meaning of the action. The projective action becomes a context of meaning (*Sinnzusammenhang*), in which any movement, moment or social articulation of the intended goal or action (through duration) becomes significant for the person (see also Schütz & Luckmann, 1973: 129–130, 213–216). By way of illustration, clients who have experienced sexual trauma will sometimes describe in detail the ways in which the anticipation (or initiation of sex) and the intended goal (or intersubjectively assumed goal) of the action (i.e. acts of penetration or the experience of pleasure) is brought into the present initiative moment of action. The past experience of a sexual act (i.e. previous penetration or sensorial pleasure/absence of pleasure in non-consensual sex) becomes a context of meaning for the present moment of action, and the person's anticipation and perception of the intended goal of the action. The prospective anticipation creates significance in the present moment, which both raises the present moment out of the stream of consciousness and endows it with significance in relation to the past and present meaning of the act.

As with Stolorow and Atwood's phenomenological-contextual understanding, Schütz (1967 [1932]: 97–138) suggests we can gain an intentional perceptive understanding of other people's subjective world. The intentional perspective of the other further intersubjectively co-creates our own understanding and meaning of our experiences. Continuing the illustration above, the perceived intention of the other is intersubjectively relevant for the person. Perceiving the other's intention as being, for example, to penetrate without consent, without the intention of pleasure, to only satisfy their own need, to purposefully ignore signs of physical or emotional discomfort, will be drawn into the meaning-making and significance of the act for the person in the present moment.

For Schütz (ibid.: 29–31, 139–214), the direct proximity to the other adds to our understanding of intentionality. He writes that we have a generalised concept of the lived experience of the other through our individual and collective actions in the world. We also sense the simultaneity of the person's stream of consciousness alongside our own in the world. In some experiences, the other is so distant and unknowable that we rely on cultural classifications and typifications about the kind of person they might be. One might note here some similarity with the ideas of the mentalisation theorists, and our attempts to mentalise about the intentional states of an unknown another. When the other is proximate and/or known to us, we exist in a state of present *synchronicity*. This synchronicity is a foundational state of intersubjective experience, where we share a common sense of reality and existence through a co-existing stream of consciousness. We might not share the same phenomenological experience of the world, but through our perceptions of the other we can gain some understanding of their intentionality.

According to Schütz (ibid.: 29–31, 139–214), those people we can directly experience in the world constitute our Umwelt or immediate social environment. In our Umwelt we are surrounded by consociates – people alongside whom we are associated, partnered or fellowed. Within the Umwelt, we have the possibility of generating a thou-orientation towards the other, where the person is related to as a known other. Through being face to face (literally and emotionally), this thou-orientation can transform into a we-relationship, where the simultaneity of our durations flow synchronically, and the intentionality of the other becomes more immediately inferred (see also Schütz & Luckmann, 1973: 73–78). For me,

Stolorow and Atwood's description of kinship-in-the-same-darkness, is a deeper form of relationality within the we-relationship of the Umwelt.

In contrast, those people who lie outside of our Umwelt to differing extents remain distant others. In the *Mitwelt*, we can establish they-relationships at a distance with our contemporaries. Whereas contemporaries can become, through proximity, our consociates, most remain at a distance and share a contemporaneous stream of consciousness with intentionality that remains unknown and unknowable to us. Beyond contemporaneous streams of consciousness, we can relate to the social world of our predecessors (*Vorwelt*) and of our successors (*Folgewelt*). Like intentionality and relationally in the *Mitwelt*, the *Vorwelt* and *Folgewelt* are only quasi-simultaneous flows of consciousness and intentionality. As these others remain indirect types of persons to us, thus we rely on shared common-sense (contextual) typifications and constructions of who these kinds of people are (ibid.: 79–92).

In including Schütz's conceptualisation of the different social worlds, I am less taken with his specific typology and more with the significance of his proposition that our experience of intentionality of the other relates to the proximity of their flow of consciousness and the meaning-endowing acts of existence that they turn towards in their own lived duration. We might see in clients living with survivor's guilt the turning towards connection to the *Vorwelt* in an attempt to establish the appearance of a proximate simultaneity to their flow of consciousness. Alternatively, other clients who have been betrayed and rejected by others in their *Mitwelt*, might project all hope for proximate simultaneity into their future possible relationship within their *Folgewelt*. These fragmentations of intersubjective relationality and shared contexts of meaning are understandable responses to traumatic experiencing in the past and present. Further, they represent attempts to alter the realities of the flow of consciousness and the distance between people to realise an anticipated act with the goal of social connection.

Schütz's contribution here is useful to understanding the alternative experiences people involved in the same traumatic confrontation can have of the social enactments. I have worked with clients who share the meaning and significance of acts of physical neglect and violence with the family member who enacted them. The family member has reportedly responded with surprise that these acts were experienced as anything other than normative and an insignificant aspect of (for example) parenting. When confronted by the malattunement of the parent, the person is simultaneously confronted by the intentionality of their act (it is permissible and normative in their existence), and the lack of reflexivity upon it (the seeming absence of turning towards the act to make it meaningful or significant). Some clients, who have pursued their horror at the confrontation of the difference in contexts of meaning and significance, have been met by further retraumatisation in the parent asserting that the client's intentional goal is to cause them pain by punishing them for normative behaviour in their social world.

The intentional worlds of ourselves and others has been a central concern both within phenomenology and existentialism. Further, questions relating to intentional life-worlds of others play a significant role in psychotherapeutic relationships. Many clients will enquire about the intentionality of the other – both through known communication or speculated about through the embodied physical or cognitive expressions of the other. In the next section, I will turn to consider how existential-humanistic and logotherapeutic practitioners have incorporated ideas about our experiences of life-worlds into their formations about interpersonal trauma.

Existential-humanistic understandings of trauma (shattered worldviews)

An alternative existential psychological perspective on the impacts of interpersonal trauma on people's world-designs (*Weltentwuerfe*) can be found in the work of Ludwig Binswanger, the Swiss co-founder of *Daseinsanalyse* (see Binswanger, 1958 [1946], 1963, 1986 [1930], for more detailed explorations). He sought to describe an alternative to psychiatric diagnostic classification of people's dilemmas. Rather than taking a psychopathological view of human experiencing, Binswanger contended that the phenomena observed in psychiatric classifications could better be described and understood through phenomenologically opening up the world of the client. Through his phenomenological-anthropological approach, he inquired specifically about the client's world-design and how this was co-created through the contextual situatedness of their lived experience and the world they were thrown into.

For Binswanger, problems in experiencing and living emerged from the lived experience of a person's world-design. In a turn away from Heidegger, Binswanger critiques the idea of the individualised authentic self and reformulates that this can only be realised in relation with the other(s) in the world (Binswanger, 1986 [1930]). In a similar repositioning of the original Husserlian phenomenology of intentionality to Schütz, Binswanger suggests that the person agentically acquires a lived knowledge of the world through experience, through the relational and perceptive experience of the other and the world in which they are situated. This is strengthened by the person's meaning-making through the creation of their world-design and enactments in the world in accordance to it. For Binswanger, world-designs are always agentically co-created through our movement and perceptions in the world. This is akin to Stolorow and Atwood's idea that organising principles are relationally and intersubjectively co-created.

According to Binswanger, so-called psychopathology emerges from the qualities of a specific world-design (i.e. emptiness and limitedness), the enactment of world-designs in relation to others (i.e where the lived reality of the person is not congruent to the world around them), and the disillusionment of a world-design through the experiential and perceptive confrontation of other('s) world-designs or the reality of a situation. The extent to which a person's world-design is seen to deviate from a clinical or collective sense of the normal determines whether or not it is deemed as problematic or psychopathological (following Binswanger, 1958 [1946]).

From the work of Frankl, through Paidoussis-Mitchell and Iacovou, to Stolorow, the disruption and changed worldview or world-design of the person seems to be a common and core phenomenological feature of traumatic experiencing. Vos (2018: 83) extends Binswanger's inquiry by noting that in the context of traumatic events,

> the traumatic aspects of these events may not be the events themselves, but the shattering of our fundamental assumptions. We are confronted in an undeniable way with reality. The more directly physical the events are felt, the more individuals are unable to deny reality.

Vos is drawing our attention here to the relationship between confronting the reality of a traumatic situation, the shattering of our existing worldviews and the possible intensification of the confrontation with reality when it involves an undeniable physicality.[5]

Although Vos is not speaking here of interpersonal trauma, the confrontational physicality of the traumatic realities would equally apply. We could take, for example, the frequently cited examples of injury to the mouth, genitals, anus or more broadly bruising to the body that result from forcible and non-consensual sexual assault. More viscerally, the physicality of the confrontation might be intensified not only by the presence of bodily fluids, but also subsequently any identification and treatment of sexually transmitted infection acquired through the traumatic encounter. In light of Stolorow and Atwood's contributions to the interaffectivity of traumatic experiences, we might add to Vos's observation that the intensification of the confrontation with reality might also involve undeniable emotionality. In any case, Vos's assertion reminds us of the existential importance of phenomenologically opening up both the worldviews of our clients *and* the ways in which confrontations with the realities of traumatic experiences have disrupted or shattered our understandings of who we are, who others are, and also how we realate to the world around us.

Stanley Krippner, Daniel Pitchford and Jeannine Davies (2012: 11) take up the traumatic disruption of a person's worldview within the tradition of humanistic-existential psychology. They suggest that the traumatic disruption of a person's worldview occurs both in their personal life narrative and, existentially, in what they understand the world to be and their place within it. The authors go further in proposing that an experience is only traumatic when it *both confronts and shatters the existing personal myths we have about the nature of reality and human existence.* Our personal myths (or ontological beliefs) are the stories, rules, ideas or ways of living that we use to understand and maintain our worldview (ibid.: 31). Other theorists have varyingly termed these the myths, metaphors (Lakoff & Johnson, 2003 [1980]) or scripts (Steiner, 1990) that we live by.

With a personal myth or worldview disrupted or shattered, there is little meaning and understanding available to the person to make sense of the experiences they have had and to incorporate this lived event or situation into a continuous experience of their self over time. Krippner and colleagues (2012: 15) write that humanistic-existential psychology and psychotherapy are well placed to address both the confrontation and shattering of personal myths, as the focus of the orientation is on human meaning-making, values and creativity (see also Krippner & Pitchford, 2018). The authors psychotherapeutically advocate for a primary focus on understanding who the client is now the world, and use this inquiry as the basis of understanding the ways in which the client 'grapple[s] with the basic nature and meaning of their experiences' (Krippner et al., 2012: 116). Through this, the client is able to re-examine and confront the reality of what they have experienced, and with psychotherapeutic support incorporate the meaning of this experience into their personal worldview.

Krippner and colleagues (2012) illustrate the fraught tensions involved in incorporating a traumatic experience into a personal worldview when it runs contra to the contextual and power system surrounding the person. They give the example of a young woman who is gang-raped by a group of her fellow students. The cultural context of the college, and her wider peer group, wanted to reframe the experience within a more palatable dominant narrative of it being a consensual 'orgy' that she later regretted. The young woman in question was under pressure to incorporate this contextual meaning into her understanding of the experience and her personal worldview. The contextual pressure ran in direct contradiction to her own experience of the event as a non-consensual sexual assault. The authors' humanistic-existential psychotherapeutic intention enabled an honest conversation about the nature of the cultural system in which competing meanings of the event were located. This allowed for confronting the cultural realities of the college system in the United States of America, and in particular permissiveness in the context of sporting prowess and sports industry.

Adopting a humanistic-existential approach enables the psychotherapist to be alongside the client in making sense of the realities of the contextual system; more specifically, how the college marketisation and reputation were at odds with the client's real experience of the college environment and the permissive culture of sexual assault within it (ibid.: 117). The psychotherapeutic stance enables the client to confront both the experience of the rape and the reality of the unjust system in which rape was seen as permissible or excusable. Examining the reality of the context, within the present moment, may open up additional confrontations about the nature of our social reality. This is an important factor in supporting the client to find ways of re-establishing a coherent worldview in relation to their experience of the traumatic event or situation. In agreement with the aforementioned Heideggerian models, the shared exploration of the experiential and contextual factors of the traumatic situation discloses commonalities and differences in the worldviews of the client and psychotherapist. Krippner and colleagues (ibid.: 118) note that the commonalities and differences in worldview can be a way of supporting the client to build trust, hold difference and strengthen their own coherent worldview.

Pitchford (2009) adopted the humanistic-existential approach in his work with veterans who had confronted the possibility of death, non-being and nothingness resulting from active service. Drawing on the work of Kierkegaard (2008 [1849]) and May (2015 [1950]), Pitchford suggests that anxiety is a state of experiencing our possibility of existing, and being active agents in our own life. While working at the Department of Veterans Affairs, Pitchford developed a humanistic-existential psychotherapeutic group approach (modelled on Yalom, 1980; and Yalom & Leszcz, 2005), focusing on providing safety, trust, reconnection and freedom for veterans. The groups were time-limited to ten weeks, with each week being structured around a specific existential theme, including isolation and loneliness. After each ten-week cycle of group work, the group membership would change, with some veterans continuing and new members being incorporated. Each session of the group had two therapists present, so that one could provide additional individual support if a group member became overwhelmed during a session.

Pitchford (2009) uses the groups to encourage self-disclosure and to explore commonality and shared experiences (drawing on Herman, 2015 [1992]), and to role play new possibilities, meaning and ways of being and relating to others. Through group encounters and relationships, the veterans cultivated their awareness of the impacts of their traumatic experiences on their lives. Further, they had the freedom to feel their possibilities for growth and change, and encounter the struggles and difficulties in enacting these changes. Through this, the veterans were able to address and resolve the disruption of their life narratives and existential understandings of the world and their relationships within it.

In a similar vein, the social psychologist Ronnie Janoff-Bulman (1992) writes that trauma shatters our fundamental assumptions about the world, which underpin our worldview. The three core assumptions she identifies are that (a) the world is benevolent, (b) the world is meaningful and (c) we have self-worth (ibid.: 3–17). Embracing these fundamental assumptions enables us to generalise that we are safe and secure in the world, we can trust others and that in some way we are invulnerable to the dangers and threats that the world poses (ibid.: 18–21). The fundamental assumptions are generalisable exceptions we have of the world formed over time from childhood; however, they are also illusionary as they do not represent the reality of the world and the possibilities of exposure to danger, threat and trauma. While maintaining these illusions might be useful in navigating our world, they are maladaptive if we do not reality-test them to situate ourselves in the context in which we find ourselves (ibid.: 21–24). In simultaneously maintaining and reality-testing our illusions, we are able to understand our limitations and those of our context.

Most people do not examine these fundamental assumptions and the nature of their life experiences, meaning that small reality-tests suffice in situating the assumptions within the context of their lives. In contrast, experiences of interpersonal trauma fundamentally shatter these assumptions (ibid.: 51). Janoff-Bulman suggests that an event or situation is traumatic if it is appraised by the person as shattering the illusion of their fundamental assumptions. More specifically, she proposes that an event or situation being 'out of the ordinary' or being 'directly experienced as threats to survival and self-preservation' is what makes the experience potentially traumatic (ibid.: 53–58). Personal experience of the event or situation is powerfully disconfirming of the fundamental assumptions, as the evidential data is grounded in the reality of the person's experience (ibid.: 54). Furthermore, the threat to survival and self-preservation discloses the fragility of our human existence and the possibility of our death and annihilation (ibid.: 56–61). This existential confrontation, for Janoff-Bulman, is a core part of what makes an event traumatic in the shattering of our fundamental assumptions.

The cultural anthropologist Ernest Becker (2012 [1973] : 178) goes further in suggesting that most people engage in a 'serious constriction of the world and of [themselves], in a "refusal of reality"'. For Becker, the experiences and behaviours labelled as 'neurotic' by clinicians is in fact an erosion of the 'clumsy lies about reality' that people tell themselves to avoid being confronted with existential givens, such as finitude and death. He continues:

> Some people have more trouble with their lies than others. The world is too much with them, and the techniques that they have developed for holding it at bay and cutting it down to size finally begin to choke the person [themselves].
> (Ibid.)

Becker sees the erosion of these lies about reality to be a 'failure to be consoled by shared illusions' about the nature of the world and relationships with others (ibid.: 197). Following Becker and Janoff-Bulman, in the experience of trauma the horizons of a personal or shared illusion are shattered and thus we paradoxically become open to both new forms of illusionment and meaning.

In order to incorporate the traumatic experience into their worldview and life, people have to find ways of refinding benevolence, meaning and self-worth in the world. Janoff-Bulman (1992: 117) writes that this allows the person to 'arrive at a new, nonthreatening assumptive world, one that acknowledges and integrates their negative [traumatic] experiences and prior illusions'. Paradoxically, the only way this can be done is by creatively rediscovering the possibility of the very assumptions that have been shattered by trauma, which might include self-blame, survivor's guilt and relativising the experience through comparison with other or possible other experiences (ibid.: 118–132). The notion of reintegrating traumatic experiences into the fundamental assumptions bears a close resemblance to the early psychotraumatological work of Janet (1901). Janet also saw a need for a mental synthesis of new (lived) ideas into old ones, in order to move beyond the disaggregated or dissociated ideas about ourselves, others and the world that have become fixed through the emotional shock of traumatic experiences.

Returning to Janoff-Bulman's conception, shattered assumptions can be rebuilt and integrated into new illusions through (drawing on Frankl) (a) suffering for a purpose (Janoff-Bulman, 1992: 133–135); (b) learning lessons about oneself and life, or reconsidering what is important to us (ibid.: 136–138); (c) attitudes we take towards others, including seeing our suffering as a form of altruism (ibid.: 138–139); and (d) finding choice 'even in the face of uncontrollable, unavoidable and negative outcomes' (ibid.: 140). In rebuilding our shattered assumptions through the discovery of choice, Janoff-Bulman (ibid.) proposes that existentially choice can be realised through our 'interpretations and reinterpretations, appraisals and reappraisals, evaluations and revaluations made of the traumatic experience and one's pain and suffering'. While we may not be free from the reality of the traumatic experience, we can agentically choose the ways we integrate this into our sense of self, others and the world we live in. As such, for Janoff-Bulman (1989; 1992: 175; Janoff-Bulman & Berg, 2013 [1998]), both illusionment and disillusionment offer a creative potential for the person to find new ways of existing in relation to the reality of the world and new meaning within it.

The German-Swiss existential psychiatrist Karl Jaspers (2003 [1954]) offers a similar appraisal of illusionment and disillusionment, through his description of a limit, border or *boundary situation* (*Grenzsituation*).[6] Jaspers suggests that we cannot 'evade or change' a boundary situation; rather, we must acknowledge and confront it (ibid., 1948, 1956, 1995 [1971]). Traumatic experiences would be an example of Jaspers's boundary situation, in that the acts themselves disrupt or shatter the lived worldview of the person and bring them into a stark confrontation with the realities of human relating. For me, the notion of a limit, border, frontier or boundary within the experienced traumatic situation is crucial. Phenomenologically, interpersonal trauma is described as threats and incursions of people's boundaries. Whether they be of bodily integrity or understandings of human relationships, the form of human relating takes us beyond the limit of what is expected, known, understood, meaningful, safe and so on. As such, we could understand a feature of 'traumatic' experiencing as being the movement beyond a known mode of existing.

Building on this further, Jaspers (1948, 1956, 1995 [1971]) provides us with a description of the phenomenon of illusionment and disillusionment (*Enttäuschung*). I have previously applied this description to exploring the ways in which clients are confronted by the reality of a situation, leading to a disillusionment with the reality they had known and a sobering up to the reality that lies before them (Bush [Boaz], 2018c; see also Merleau-Ponty, 1968 [1964]: 40–42). The confrontation with reality results in *Ernüchterung* – that is, a sobering up to the reality of their situation. For me (following Jaspers), it is the entangled experience of both *Enttäuschung* and *Ernüchterung* that enables the person to find altered or new modes of existing in the moment (initially as adaptations to the confrontation), and over time (through the discovery and expansion of new modes of experience).

Returning to Janoff-Bulman (1992), it is through the confrontation with the reality of our traumatic experience that the potential for re-illusionment is possible. Janoff-Bulman echoes the ideas of Bowlby (1973) and the early attachment theorists in proposing that in incorporating reality-tested ideas about the nature of the world (and others) into our new foundational assumptions (and the illusions we use to maintain them), we can prepare ourselves for further adversity and suffering in the future, without also experiencing the shattering of assumptions.

Finally, Janoff-Bulman describes how our attempts to re-establish the fundamental assumptions of our self-worth, and the world being benevolent and meaningful, can be undermined by the existence of the other. These challenges arise from prevailing societal and relational discomfort arising from stigma around mentioning the form of traumatic experience, through to explicit blame in locating responsibility for the traumatic event onto the traumatised person (Janoff-Bulman, 1992: 147–157). Further, the shattering of assumptions also breaches the foundations of social relationships. People therefore have to find ways of navigating their relationships as partners, children, parents, lovers, friends or colleagues, while attempting to integrate and rebuild their foundational assumptions. The need to both maintain social relatedness and rebuild our foundational assumptions can result in significant withdrawal, avoidance of relational intimacy and difficulties in communication (ibid.: 157–161).

Logotherapeutic and existential-analytical understandings of trauma

The French philosopher and existential-psychoanalyst Georges-Elia Sarfati builds on Janoff-Bulman's ideas by bringing in Frankl's notion of *noögenic neurosis* and applying this to the case of traumatic experiencing. Sarfati (2016) proposes that while people experience the specific traumatic phenomenological impact described in post-traumatic stress, they too are confronted with the tragic triad of finitude, guilt and suffering. It is this confrontation with the tragic triad that leads to an existential vacuum, which is expressed as an existential crisis in our perceptions of the world (worldview) and of meaning in one's life (ibid.: 240). For Sarfati, the traumatic disruption of the existential (noö-)dynamics leads to a simultaneous loss of assumptions about the nature of our world (building on Janoff-Bulman) and 'the collapse of subjective values' that make our life project valuable and meaningful to us (ibid.).

For Sarfati, post-traumatic recovery or growth can only be said to occur when the person finds a way to both overcome the impacts of the psychosocial post-traumatic stress and resume their existential life project (ibid.: 242). This is seen to be achieved in two distinct phases of logotherapeutic response. This first focuses on recovering the *common sense meanings* a person has about themselves and their world, akin to Janoff-Bulman's incorporation of the trauma into the illusions we live by. The psychotherapist provides psychoeducation about the impact of trauma on the person's sense of self and world, focusing more specifically on psychosomatic and psychosocial disruptions. This intervention operates at a level of common and shared meaning, aiming to restructure the person's fundamental beliefs about the nature of their world (post-trauma) and address phenomenologically their confrontation with the structures of their life-world.

Second, the person moves towards reconstructing and restructuring their personal meaning on a noögenic level in order to resume their specific existential life project. In contrast to the first phase, the logotherapist provides noetic education about the nature of our existence and the importance of value and meaning in our lives. In this way, the intervention attends to the existential dynamics, supporting the person to reconstruct their life project and phenomenologically explore the possible personal meaning that relates to this project. The second phase aims to enable the person to existentially affirm their life, with meaning for themselves.

For Sarfati (ibid.: 242–243), the two phases do have an implicit hierarchical relationship, with the first psychotherapeutic phase being foundational for the second logotherapeutic one. Once the two phases are completed, there is then potential for a coming together of the forms of psychotherapeutic and noetic education, to allow for the realisation of the universality of the tragic triad, and the personal experience of trauma and life project within this existential given. From my own clinical work, I remain sceptical about any separateness of these two phases, noting how in reality clients move within and between symptomological and existential concerns. Phenomenologically, there is more to be gained for the client by looking at the interrelationships between disruptions in personal and common-sense meanings, than separating them out as distinct disruptions. Our personal life projects are contextually situated, and thus the so-called common-sense meaning is dynamically implicated in any noetic dilemma.

Alternatively, Längle offers us an existential-analytical perspective on the shattering of worldviews through traumatic experiencing. Within his formulation of existential analysis, experiences of trauma lead to changes both in our structural (existential) anchoring of the experience, and our ability to process the experience as part of our existence (Längle, 2007: 111). Längle proposes that uniquely in the experience of trauma, all four basic conditions of existence are *equally* affected by this change. The experience of trauma results in disruption to our existing comprehension of (a) what the world is, and its limitations and conditions (leading to shock); (b) our own life and life force (leading to pain); (c) our identity and relationship to others (leading to feelings of loss); and (d) the demands and horizons of our life situation (leading to contextual incomprehensibility) (ibid.: 111, 114; 2008: 3–4). At the extremity, the impact of traumatic experiencing, and the resulting incomprehensibility of our existential anchoring, can lead to a fixation within all four basic motivations related to the conditions of existence (Längle, 2007: 111). These fixations manifest in the basic motivations of (a) hostile or suspicious attitudes towards the world, (b) feelings of emptiness, (c) social withdrawal and (d) feelings of hopelessness and equivalency of all activity.

Längle goes on to consider the impacts of trauma on the person's ability to process information about the trauma and new situations in their life. He writes that the traumatic disruption of personal processing of existence leads to a 'protracted process paralysis' (ibid.: 111, 113). In this protracted paralysis of processing, images, thoughts and memories of the traumatic experience return to the person, leading to an eventual emotional numbness and anhedonia. In terms of action, the person becomes reactive and avoidant, with any attempt at active engagement in the world resulting in nervousness, irritation or overexcitation.

The traumatic impact of personal existential processing leads to further felt alterations across the four basic conditions for existence (ibid.: 114). First, the person loses the feeling that they can have a real and agentic existence in the world. Second, our ability to internalise the experience for ourselves and make it meaningful is disrupted. This can lead to a personal lack of awareness or realisation of the significance of the traumatic experience, leaving it unincorporated and experienced as alien to the self. Third, the experience lacks personal and emotional resonance, which overwhelms our connection to existential values that provide meaning to 'how' we suffer, and 'for whom' we suffer (ibid.; also see 2008: 9). Within this lack of personal resonance is a collapsing of our experience of time, bringing the traumatic experience(s) repeatedly into our experience of the present moment, which further disrupts the resonance of new situations. Finally, the impacts of personal existential processing result in no meaningful horizon of experiencing, closing down the possibilities of future growth and development beyond the impact of the traumatic experience (Längle, 2007: 114).

Drawing heavily on the work of Freyd (1994, 1996), Längle (2007: 114) proposes that the deepest impact of trauma is the shattering of, or shock to (*Erschütterung*), our basic trust in something greater, which can hold us and absorb our human experience of the traumatic situation(s). Trauma acts as a disillusioning betrayal of the personal existential foundations required for us to find meaning, motivation and action in the world. The de-anchoring of our existential foundations necessitates a healing presence of the other (ibid.: 114–115). According to Längle, the focus of this presence is through dialogue to address the client's avoidance behaviour and non-contextualised experience of the traumatic situation(s) at the time and in the present (through associative memories). The aim of the dialogue is to rebuild the client's capacity for self-dialogue and thus to re-anchor them in their existence and to integrate what they have experienced into their sense of self, others and the world around them.

In existential-analytic practice, the psychologist or psychotherapist works on the specific foundations of existence that have been de-anchored (ibid.: 115). In re-anchoring our four foundational and existential references: to the world, life, our self and meaning. To re-establish our *reference to the world* (*Weltbezug*), the psychotherapeutic dialogue focuses on the client's experience and core assumptions (*Weltbild*) of reality. Further, we explore the existential givens related to this. This is similar to the approach taken by Janoff-Bulman, although Längle does not consider this a process of re-illusionment but rather a re-establishment of meaningful contact with reality. Moving on to the *reference to life* (*Lebensbezug*), attention is brought within the dialogue to the active co-creation of the psychotherapeutic relationship. The client is able to test the relational boundaries of trust and safety. Over time, this allows for the confronting of the feelings relating to the traumatic experience, with the emphatic response of the psychotherapist.

In contrast, *reference to the self* (*Selbstbezug*) is psychotherapeutically achieved through encouraging the client to explore their own freedom and self-organisation. This is brought about through the use of Längle's method of *personal existential analysis* (*Personalen Existenzanalyse*), which includes description of the traumatic situation; elaboration of the subjective situational meanings; integration of the perceived value, challenge or meaning and one's sense of self; and commitment to inner motivation for active involvement in the world (for more detail, see Längle, 1993, 2003b).[7] Finally, for Längle (2007: 115), the *reference to contextual-meaning* (*Kontextbezugs/Sinnbezug*) can be restored through dialogues that open up the possible existential meaning of the traumatic situation(s). Within this there is a focus on accepting that which cannot be understood to be part of an overarching reality (*übergreifende Realität*), which is disclosed by the unknowable to us (ibid.). Längle's advocation of the existential-analytic method aims to lead to restorative changes that enable people to both re-establish their anchoring in the foundations of our existence and restore our ability to process the overwhelming experience of the trauma.

Existential psychotraumatology or modal existentialism

In the previous sections of this chapter, I have examined some of the possible existential perspectives relating to interpersonal trauma. As with all books, this is an incomplete presentation, with many more existential practitioners generating models and practices that I have been unable to include given the time available for me to write this book. Yet more existential offerings are being gently held for forthcoming chapters, so those reading in a linear fashion should not conclude that the inquiry ends at this moment of the book – I continue to weave within and between a wider range of existential ideas as my own proposed model is explored.

Before moving on to introduce my approach to understanding interpersonal trauma, it feels important to draw the reader's attention to four core existential premises that I have identified as emerging from across the literature and models reviewed thus far. These four core existential premises relate to the commonalities across interpersonal traumatic experiencing and include the following:

(a) interpersonal trauma involves an experience that results in confrontations with reality.

(b) these confrontations are existential movements in relation to reality (i.e. awareness, recognition, disillusionment).

(c) these existential movements resulting from a confrontation include agentic movements in relation to the self, others and the world around us (i.e. a jolt, disruption, shattering, a turning away from or towards).

(d) these existential movements are contextually and intersubjectively situated and co-created over time and space.

My proposition is that these four core existential premises provide us with a ground for the formulation of an existentialist psychotraumatology, one that is more attuned to a person's confrontation with reality and existential responses to this.

The existential psychotherapist Hans Cohn (1997: 16) poignantly noted that there has always been a tension within and between existentialism and (existential phenomenology), with existentialists wanting to attend to ontological concerns and phenomenologists being accused of being lost in the ontic concerns of a situation. For me, a phenomenology aiming to recreate an empiricism of the empirical sciences falls short. Likewise, an existentialism that seeks to ascertain the structure of our existence without a ground in the ontic is a metaphysical myth or abstraction of human existence. In this book, I am proposing that the ontic and the ontological are inseparable, and that perhaps even that the distinction between the two is problematic and unnecessary in contemporary existentialism and psychotraumatology. The so-called ontic is our contextual-embeddedness in the experiential reality of existence; the ontological is our agentic participation (through our so-called ontic experience) in the structure of existence. The specific ways we are in the world are intersubjectively incorporative of an *onto–ontic entanglement*.

Thus, the only way of exploring traumatic experiences that incorporates both the confrontation with the reality of the experience(s), and the existential and intersubjective movements of the person in relation to it is through a focus on what is available to both the person and the psychotherapist: the agentic expressions and articulations of confrontation and movement. I call these agentic expressions and articulations of confrontation and movement: *modes of existence*. What I am formulating here is a *modal existentialism*, one that is not concerned *that* we exist (this being an existential given), but rather with *why*, *how* and *for whom* we exist. In this sense, modal existentialism is concerned with a person's modes of existence in the confrontation with reality and how these can be *generatively elaborated* through time and space.[8]

The phrase 'generatively elaborated' discloses here the idea that our modes of existence (the way we agentically, individually and collectively express and articulate confrontations with reality) generatively elaborate (another agentic-structural movement) the realisable structures of human existence, and the world around us. This means that the structural reality of existence is generative (changed and ever changing through our agentic movements) and can only be known through the inquiry and examination of modes of existence, which phenomenologically are expressions of this generative movement. Moreover, this means that the confrontation with reality within any modal expression of existence is contextually bound to the moment in the generative-structural movement of existence. The so-called ontological mode of existence is nothing more than an attempt to abstract our awareness of generative movement and modal expressions of existence.

In summary, what we call traumatic experiencing could more usefully be thought of, and described phenomenologically, in terms of existential movements. That is, movements towards a confrontation with both the reality of a traumatic situation(s), and the generative foundations of our human existence. Further, interpersonal trauma defined in this way is not just movement towards and within the confrontation, but also movements beyond and in the wake of the confrontation(s). It is important to note here that in the case of interpersonal trauma, the confrontation is not necessarily chosen, nor does it necessarily arise from spontaneity or opportunity. This gives the modes of movement and the forms of confrontation specific qualities. These specific qualities are the subject of inquiry in this book.

Existential features of traumatic experiencing

In what follows I give an overview of the modal existentialist model of traumatic experience. This is based on a descriptive synthesis of the four core existential premises emerging from the existing literature base and my own phenomenological inquiries into traumatic experiencing. More detail on the features of traumatic experiencing are given in the subsequent chapters of this book. The overview provided here can act as a reference point for those taking a non-linear approach to reading this book, or as a guide for those joining me on the weaving path of my discussion.

Modal existentialism sees traumatic experiencing as having the following phenomenological features, qualities and movements:

a. Traumatic experiencing involves encountering the reality of a situation[9] that:
   i. goes beyond a limit or boundary of the person's known mode of existing;
   ii. directly or indirectly involves an actual and/or perceived act(s) or inducement of harm, and/or threat to life, and/or breach of our current mode of existence and/or our continuity of being.[10]
b. The experience of approaching, and going beyond, this modal limit or boundary is experienced by the person as a crossing place between worlds, and modes of existence.
c. In confronting this boundary, we are also confronting the intersubjective reality of our situation. This is a queering of our reality as we have known it.
d. Through the confrontation with reality, we are 'called' to change our lived modality (through movement) and the world (as we know it now) to an (as of yet) altered or unknown or un(dis)covered mode of existence.
e. The 'call' to change our lived modality leaves us standing at the precipice of disillusionment or re-illusionment, additionally being confronted with:
   i. disillusionment with the world and our relations within it, by crossing this limit or boundary, and subsequently sobering up through (dis)covering new modes of existing; *and/or*
   ii. the incorporation of this newly confronted reality into our re-illusionment about the world, and our relations within it.
f. Our disillusioned or re-illusioned mode of existing represents an awakening of our primordial impulse to philosophise within an intersubjective context, and to find the kind person of we want to become.
g. Our primordial impulse to philosophise is a modal call to find our way back to relating to ourselves, others and the world around us, through the use of new movements and changed modes of existence.
h. Being confronted with our previous modes of existing, our current modality and our potential to move between and within modes of existing is a queering of existence. This queering of existence brings us close to the realisation

of the liminality, ambiguity, horror and terror of the structure of human existence.

i.   New modes of existence incorporate the intersubjective and embodied knowledge and experience of having crossed the boundary of a confrontation with reality, and the modal re-experiencing of this confrontation(s) in new ways in the moments and through the movements of our existence.

j.   Modal elaboration incorporates reflexive awareness of our modes of existing, and the (re)(dis)covery of generative freedom, choice and responsibility for older and newer modal movements and expressions.

Theoretical clarifications

Reflecting back on these emerging features, it feels that in some way traumatic experiencing is phenomenologically more specific than generalised philosophical or psychopathological conceptions of human suffering. Existentially, interpersonal trauma does not have the same meaning as might be used currently in clinical or lay spaces. It is not a referent for the situation(s), the ongoing impact on the person, nor the meaning ascribed to the situation(s). It is not shorthand for a diagnosis (i.e. PTSD), nor for suffering and distress, although these might arise within or between modes of existing. In a *modal existentialist* framing, trauma can be described as *an interpersonal confrontation with reality, and the incorporation of this confrontation into an existing or emergent mode of existing, through the disillusionment or re-illusionment of an existing mode.* Trauma endures to the extent to which the new mode of existing is primarily emergent from the confrontation, and the modal responses arising from it.

In my formulation, we can see the importance of the intensity of the confrontation with reality, and the existential movements one makes to find modes of existing in relation to the confrontation. I am not saying here that existential confrontations with reality are exclusive to traumatic experiencing. I am open to, for example, Holzhey-Kunz's (2014, 2016) and Bugental's (1965)[11] proposals that the confrontation can emerge from a sensitivity to existential concerns. It is more that interpersonal trauma discloses a generative modal structure of human relating, more specifically through both the confrontation with reality in its immediacy (in the moment or aftermath of the event) and through the insidious creeping towards the confrontation (as can be the case in childhood neglect, harassment, or domestic abuse). Finally, confrontation with reality is movement of experience, allowing for repetitious and circularised exposures to the reality of a situation.

As presented above, mode(s) simply means existing in a particular way in relation to reality. The mode of existing incorporates the lived experience of the situation, the impact on the person, their relationships with others, and the meaning, values and worldview they incorporated into it. For Heideggerians, mode might equate to the specific way in which Dasein is being-in-the-world(-with-others). In this sense authenticity and inauthenticity would be modal, and how authenticity and inauthenticity are manifest and disclosed in our specific acts of being-in-the-world(-with-others), is our mode of existing.

The mode of existing incorporates the embodied experience of the situation, the impact on the person, their relationships with others, and the meaning, values and worldview they incorporated into it. Modes of existence are an amalgam of conscious and non-conscious states of existing, which emerge from the specific lives and embodied, intersubjective contextuality of the person who is traumatised. The term 'mode' in this sense is resonant with the existential notion that existence precedes essence, and more specifically, it places an emphasis on emergence as a mood and movement of becoming. Moreover, following a more Nietzschean (1914) reading, the notion of being might be better understand as a mode of becoming.

Having outlined a modal existentialist model of traumatic experience, I will turn in the following chapters to explore the features, qualities and movements of traumatic experiencing from different existential dimensions. First exploring how we experience the movements of confrontations with reality, I will then go on to explore the ways in which we incorporate these movements into our embodiment, identities, relationships with others and the world around us.

Notes

1 For more information, see UNHCR (2012) and the Buddhist Society (2020).
2 Rollo May is sometimes more readily classified within the will-to-meaning branch of existential philosophies and psychologies. My reading of his works is that he also offers significant insights into the agentic and dynamic nature of power in relation to meaning. I would refer readers to his lesser-referenced work, and contribution, in *Power and Innocence* for further exploration (May, 1972).
3 In reality, few academics and practitioners engage with the totality and complexity of Heidegger's work. His writings remain largely inaccessible to many, and the resurrection and reapplication of arcane German terms can at times be disorientating for the reader. I have had to read his renowned work *Being and Time* (2010 [1953]) and the *Zollikon Seminars* (2001) multiple times over the years to understand his philosophical intentions, proposals and areas of ambiguity. From my personal conversations, I know that many leading psychologists and psychotherapeutic scholars continue to debate, and be confused by, some of the more abstract aspects of his writings and the relevance of their application to contemporary psychotraumatology.

  I am honest here about my own struggles with reading Heidegger, as many existential writers and practitioners see being fully literate in Heideggerian theory as a badge of honour and a foundational requirement for existential psychological or psychotherapeutic practice – with the notable exception of contemporary logotherapy and Länglean existential analysis. I am not one of those existentialists, and the invitation in this book is to hold his work lightly, as just one contribution to existential thought and practice.
4 Stolorow's theory and practice predates his exposure and interest in the philosophy of Heidegger. In many ways, Stolorow's contextual-intersubjective formulation of psychoanalysis provides a more robust foundation for his existentialism and the later turn to Heideggerianism. While there is significant continuity between Stolorow's earlier and later formulations of trauma, after the Heideggerian turn he replaces much of his own terminology with some of the conceptual phrasing and language use mobilised by Heidegger (and/or his translators).

In my exploration of Stolorow's work, I interweave the non- and Heideggerian ideas, as this does not substantively disrupt the core tenets of Stolorow's propositions. Further, I do this because I see significant value in his pre- and non-Heideggerian work, and because (for me) the unification of Stolorow's own non- and pre-Heideggerian existentialism with the post-Heideggerian turn offers more insight than reading or presenting them as separate theoretical moments or models in Stolorow's works.

5 For the moment, let us put to one side Vos's notion of the undeniability of physical confrontations of reality, as in later chapters I explore personal denial of reality as a mode of existing and experiencing.

6 While I have drawn on reflections of Schütz and Luckmann's (1989 [1983]) boundary crossing in everyday life, my own formulation does not incorporate their description of these situations.

7 Those practitioners working with eye-movement desensitisation and reprocessing (EMDR) can consult the work of Rudolf Leuenberger (2008), who draws on Längle's first fundamental motivations (the real ability and capacity of the subject) to existentially describe the contributions that EMDR could make (see Shapiro, 2018). Leuenberger suggests that EMDR is a procedural and methodological intervention, which enables people (albeit through the use of verticalised and highly structured protocols) to face the reality of their traumatic experience, endure the confrontation and accept the existential givens they are confronted with. As such, they are able to incorporate them into their first fundamental motivations for existing.

8 I am borrowing the terms 'elaboration' and 'generative' from Margaret Archer's (1995) version of *critical realism*; however, the meaning is different in my work.

9 By 'situation', I do not mean a moment in time. The use of 'situation' here follows Jaspers, so in this context it could be enduring experiences or relationships from another or others.

10 Initially, I included the word 'intention', which seemed to work for interpersonal trauma; however, when considering single incident forms of trauma, it did not work, unless a form of fatalism or spiritual intentionalism was projected onto it – such survivorship from natural events, major incidents or accidents. Notwithstanding this observation, the primary focus of the exploration in this book remains on interpersonal trauma.

11 Although I have reflected upon the work of Bugental (1965: 288–289, 293) and his formulation of the confrontation of existential anxiety to inform my own thinking, the reader will note that my use of the idea significantly diverges from his existential-analytic framing of the reality of existential isolation from the other.

Bugental writes (ibid.: 289) that 'the confrontation of the basic givens of our being means an unflinching acceptance into full and feelingful awareness of one's limitedness and vulnerability, of one's unrelenting responsibility, of the external silence of the world in the face of our most desperate pleas, and of the ultimately unbridgeable chasm that separates each from the other. It is the rare person, if any exists, who can truly accept all this into their being'.

6 Existential understandings of traumatic embodiment and identity

Trauma is not just a psychological confrontation with the reality of a situation, but an existential movement of the totality of the human person through space and time. In this chapter, I will explore the features and qualities of the existential movement of traumatic confrontations through the dimensions of our embodiment, lived experience of time and space and the way we experience our sense of self and identity.

Traumatic embodiment

Within a phenomenological frame, Husserl (2012 [1931]) suggests that primarily we experience ourselves, other people and the world around us through the movement, perceptions and actions of our lived body (*Leib*). In the early and contemporary psychotraumatologies, we saw the centrality of the person's relationships with, and movements of, their body in their experience of traumatic situations and relationships. In the case of interpersonal traumas, the movements between, and within, human bodies are of the utmost interest. Inquiry into the human body, and its relationships with other bodies, can begin to disclose the lived existential movements of confrontations with traumatic reality. As May states (1972: 76):

> Experience puts the accent on action, living out something, or feeling it […] By experiencing something, we let its meaning permeate through us on all levels: feeling, acting, thinking, [reflecting on] and, ultimately, deciding […] one experiences as a totality.

The existential-phenomenologist Maurice Merleau-Ponty (2012 [1945]: 147) provides the ground for a deeper understanding of our embodied confrontations. He writes that our bodies are our 'general means of having a world'. By this he means there is an entangled relationship between the reality of our body and the world around us. We inhabit 'the world by our body' (Merleau-Ponty, 1968 [1964]: 28), and in this sense our embodiment cannot be abstracted in reality from our perceptive experiences of the world around us. As a post-Cartesian phenomenologist, he is drawing our attention to the 'coexistence' of our 'sensorial and

DOI: 10.4324/9781003181675-9

corporeal exploration' and our 'mental inspection' (i.e. reflections and thoughts) within the perceptions and experiences we have of the world around us (ibid.: 31, 38). As such, there is a complex intertwining reality between what is described as 'our anchorage in the world' through our body, and the generative influence of our embodied acts on the world around us (ibid.: 147; see also 2012 [1945]: 84).

We only understand our world through our 'embodied' experience, or rather, as Merleau-Ponty (2012 [1945]: 91) describes it, the 'movement of existence'. For me, Merleau-Ponty's focus on the *movement* of embodiment is important, as it discloses the generative structure of our existence. It incorporates the fluids, thoughts and substances that flow through, around, into and out of us; the coexisting bodies, objects, non-human animals, cultural artefacts and networks of significance that interact, and co-shape, our embodiment and understanding with the world around us and the experiences we have. Our embodiment in this sense is simultaneously the personal 'mine' that the existential philosopher Gabriel Marcel (1949, 1950, 1952 [1927]) refers to, *and* the lived experience of our interweaving movement through personal and collective time and space. Here, we can begin to better understand that what is approaching and *moving* through a boundary situation of trauma is not just a worldview, but an embodied and relationally situated person. Further, in this sense there is no distinction between the traumatic situation or relationship, or the traumatised embodiment of the person. The traumatised and traumatising bodies are already given as a body in action, and thus an embodied situational movement. Attempts to make categorical distinctions between the traumatic situation (as a social artefact of an adverse childhood experience (ACE) or diagnostic category of post-traumatic stress disorder (PTSD)) and the embodiments of the persons acting and experiencing is an abstraction of reality (elaborating on Sartre, 2003 [1943]: 367).

Merleau-Ponty (drawing on Bergson) writes of an ontology of the 'flesh', in which he continues to explore the intersubjective and generative features of our embodiment (see also Sartre, 2003 [1943]: 336–337). Merleau-Ponty (1968 [1964]): 18–49) notes that 'there is only an elaborated world [...] the intertwining of my life with other lives, of my body with [other bodies and in] the interaction of my perceptional field with that of the others'. He terms this intertwining embodiment of ourselves and others as *intercorporeality* (see also Tanaka, 2013, 2015). A more expansive understanding of our embodiment is also resonant with the eco-phenomenological accounts of human consciousness. For example, David Abram (2011: 254) echoes Merleau-Ponty's description of interweaving embodied movements in his observation that 'only by entering into relation with others [human and non-human] do we effect our own integration and coherence [...] Each being that we perceive enacts a subtle integration within us'.

Merleau-Ponty (1968 [1964]: 141–144, 168, 172) terms this more expansive view of intercorporeality with non-human animals and the world around us, our *interanimality*. In the confrontation of the reality of institutional and/or familial maltreatment (neglect and abuse), some of my clients have enquired: 'Am I a human like other people are humans?', 'How is the way they treated me any worse than a battered dog?', 'Am I just a pigeon to be kicked away?', 'Maybe a rat has a better life than me', 'Maybe I'm more like a cockroach than a person, humans don't survive these conditions'. While some eco-psychologists might philosophically be uncomfortable with clients' zoomorphic descriptions, for me these questions disclose a modal uncertainty about interanimality. The person's experience of dehumanisation through the confrontation of interpersonal trauma also opens up valid philosophical questions about the dominance of anthropocentrism within many human cultures (especially within the Anglo-American context). It further brings attention to the ontological closeness between the interanimality of human and non-human beings. This echoes socio-historical psychological narratives, across cultures, about the animalistic nature of madness and traumatisation. To explain away the reality of our human capacity and potential to enact harm, violence and pain towards another, we describe traumatic experiencing as animalistic, as if it is not of the human world but a regressive devolution of our humanity (following Foucault, 2009 [1961], 2003 [1963]).

Thomas Fuchs and Sabine C. Koch (2014) draw out more explicitly the notion of *interaffectivity* as an additional feature of Merleau-Ponty's *intercorporeality*. For the authors, intercorporeality incorporates an intertwinement of two or more embodied affectivities. Each person within an intersubjective system is continuously modifying the other person's affective and bodily resonance. Readers will note the striking similarities between this description of intercorporeality and the phenomenological-contextualism of Stolorow and Atwood (2002 [1992]). In this way, intersubjective affectivity is a primordial state of existential movement (e - *motion*). We speak of the way in which we are moved by the emotionality of others, and how our emotional world moves us. This is because interaffectivity is situated in movements both within, and between, intercorporeal bodies. Interaffectivity discloses the paradoxical personal-collective feature of traumatic experiencing. The intersubjective quality of personal trauma means that interaffective experience is, too, a co-construction of intercorporeal movement – shared and circulating within, and between, bodies. These interaffective experiences are infused with wider social constructions and power dynamics of the affectivity of social kinds of bodies (i.e. female, migrant, lesbian, gay, bisexual, transgender, queer or questioning and others (LGBTQ+), children's etc.), which are flowing through our intercorporeality (following Ahmed, 2004).

Fuchs and Koch's interaffective addition to Merleau-Ponty's formulation is useful in understanding interaffective complexity reported in some abusive and emotionally coercive relationships, and how this form of emotional relating can be sustained and endured over time. This form of traumatic interaffectivity has been well documented (albeit using alternative language) in the wider psychotraumatological literature and presented cases (c.f. McCrory & Viding, 2015; Rothschild, 2000). In the case of child sexual abuse or sexual violence, studies have noted the ways in which people experience, for example, genital, other somatic or cognitive arousals in relation to the experience of sexual trauma (c.f. Herman, 2015 [1992]). The intercorporeality in these cases discloses a perceptive ambiguity of consent within a traumatic encounter, and subsequent confusions in meanings and significance of embodied responses that seem to belie the harm and distress being experienced by the person. The seemingly paradoxical psychological responses also disclose the interanimality of our existence, whether we see this as an existential phenomenon or as being stimulated by biochemical responses seen in the possible alternations in levels of noradrenaline or endogenous opioids, such as endorphins.

This can be compounded by the visceral nature of sexual violence, where there is ambiguity over the intercorporeality and intracorporeality (following Merleau-Ponty, 1968 [1964]: 261) of bodily fluids and emissions; where the person cannot determine whether the saliva, semen, blood, tears, lubricant, scent, pheromones, sweat etc. is theirs, of the other or something that is itself a product of the interanimality of the encounter (see also Laing, 1971 [1961]: 140–141). This is an example of what Merleau-Ponty terms the *reversibility* of our intercorporeality.[1] He illustrates reversibility in his description of touch as 'landscapes interweav[ing]': 'I can feel myself touched as well and at the same time as touching' (Merleau-Ponty, 1968 [1964]: 142). Reversibility here adds to the ambiguities of traumatic embodiment, and its resonance in the body as an interweaving of the intercorporeal reality. The movement through a confrontation of our intercorporeal reality in interpersonal trauma can result in a *reversible entanglement*. The reversible entanglement of our intercorporeality and intracorporeality can be seen in the questions my clients have frequently brought to the psychotherapy room in the wake of interpersonal trauma. Common questions include: 'Why did my body respond like that?', 'Am I responsible for what they did?', 'Did I enjoy it like [they] insisted I did?' Reversible entanglement further problematises more cognitive attempts to distance the traumatising other within concretised notions of (for example) stranger attacks. By virtue of our intercorporeality, the traumatising other becomes *known* to us intercorporeally through the co-experiencing of the attack. The reversible entanglement of the attack creates further complexity in distinguishing the known from the unknown, and what is of each of us, and co-created through the enactment of the attack.

Merleau-Ponty extends his description of intercorporeality by bringing our attention to both its visible and invisible dimensions. He suggests (ibid.: 144) that 'this flesh that one sees and touches is not all there is to flesh, nor this massive corporeity all there is to the body'. For him, intercorporeality extends beyond the visible into the invisible domains of myth, archetype, culture, meaning, significance and attitudes. His analysis echoes the more sociological writings of Bruno Latour (2005; Latour & Woolgar, 1979), Pierre Bourdieu (2003 [1979]) and Michel Foucault (1979, 1990 [1984], 2003 [1999]) who also describe the ways in which our embodiment is inscribed by the cultural mechanisms of any given society.

If we apply this back to the case of sexual trauma, we can see how the ambiguities and reversibility of movement within traumatic confrontations incorporate the invisible framings of such a movement's existence. Merleau-Ponty (1968 [1964]: 48) describes the invisible framings of an intercorporeal encounter as the inter-world (*l'entremonde*). This inter-world includes the 'elaborated' meanings and significance of the encounter between the persons involved, and the relationships and situations within wider elaborated contexts. For example, until relatively recently in some countries rape within heterosexual marriage was considered permissive as a conjugal and connubial right rather than an illegal offence. Further, in some cultures a wife's refusal of sexual interaction could be used by a husband as a legitimate case of the defence of rape within an application for divorce. This equally could apply to the well-documented secrecy and shame surrounding signs or knowledge of physical or sexual abuse, where families or communities seek to maintain a reputation or status, and control the disclosures of trauma (following Herman, 2015 [1992]).

Temporal-spatiality of traumatic embodiment

Having explored what traumatic embodiment within the confrontation of reality might be, I now turn to the spatial and temporal dimensions. Merleau-Ponty (2010 [2001]: 44) conceives of a *body schema*, which is a communicable (verbal and non-verbal) synthesis of 'all possible activities' and the possible 'bodily state' of the person. This body schema is an organisation of the body's 'relationship to its surroundings' and brings together as a system our embodied perception and position in our environment. This creates a system that can be communicated to other bodies, and through intercorporeality there is communication, signification and interpretations by each person as to their own, and others', body schemas (ibid.: 247, 437). Elsewhere (ibid.: 437), he more usefully describes this system as a synthesis, which mirrors the phenomenological nature of 'perception [as] a synthesis of all possible perceptions'. What is important about the synthesis is that it recognises the active movement of our bodies though space, in that the synthesis 'is actualised by the [agentic] power that I possess to move myself' (ibid.).

When applying this specifically to traumatic embodiment, we can see that the experience of crossing a traumatic boundary situation gives rise to spatial alterations in the body schema – both as it is communicated to ourselves, and others, through our intercorporeality. Here we can make an explicit link to the neuroceptive alterations described in contemporary psychotraumatology. We can also consider how this relates to the significant literature base on unexplained somatic phenomena following interpersonal trauma (be it psychogenic seizures or chronic pain), and Stolorow and Atwood's (2002 [1992]: 45) description of concretised somatic modes of experiencing.

More specifically, Merleau-Ponty (2012 [1945]: 84) adds that 'regions of silence are thus marked out in the totality of my body'. This silencing of elements of the body schema can be seen in clinical accounts of sexual anorexia, anhedonia or other forms of sexual or genital sensation alterations that can happen following experiences of sexual abuse and/or sexual violence (c.f Mackey et al., 1991; Oei et al., 1990; Rellini & Meston, 2011). Similarly, drawing on Merleau-Ponty's (2012 [1945]: 78–91) discussion of phantom limbs, we can see how unexplained somatic symptoms could be understandable syntheses of traumatic experiencing in the body schema. In this way the body schema, and its communicative changes, are indicative of *moving* through the traumatic boundary situation, and signify or disclose the ways in which relationships in our intercorporeality have been disillusioned or re-illusioned as modes of existence.

It is important here to restate that the body schema is also a lived attitude towards our position in the intertwining with others, and thus includes our actualities, potentialities and possibilities of movement through space. This can be seen in the well-documented and observed behaviours of those who have experienced interpersonal trauma; for example, in the case of hugging and physical proximity following child sexual abuse, where a child freezes and does not reciprocate when being hugged, having previously been tactile before the change in their body schema. The child communicates the need for distance and the discomfort with human touch and embrace, and through intercorporeality this is either heeded or unacknowledged by the other (see also Merleau-Ponty, 2010 [2001]: 437).

To illustrate this further, with colleagues I have drawn on case material to describe how young people can have somatic responses to situations that are seemingly unrelated to the situation they are facing (Brennan et al., 2019). With an understanding of the way in which these responses are elaborated through the intercorporeality of a traumatic experience, we can better see the embodied significance of these representing ways the young person survived in a traumatic environment (see also Zyromski et al., 2018). The somatic phenomena we noted ranged from shaking, holding their breath in an attempt to prevent others sensing that they perceive a threat, through to actively using aggression in order to create greater distance from an adult who is too proximate to them. This echoes the cases cited by Herman (2015 [1992]) in the presentations of somatic modal responses to trauma enduring years after the event.

The intercorporeality of traumatic experiencing brings into sharper relief the polarities of proximity and distance from perceived threats to our existing and emerging modes of existence within our environment. For example, Ogden and Fisher (Ogden, 2015; Ogden & Fisher, 2015) suggest there are explicit and implicit embodied responses to physical touch, which they define as a 'somatic sense of boundaries', where, for example, someone does not reciprocate a hug, avoids someone standing behind them or physically leans back or turns away from a kiss on a cheek (c.f. Dunleavy & Kubo Slowik, 2012). Here again, the active somatic response is protective for the person, in that their body schema has retained knowledge of the traumatic experiencing and creates new modes of relating to others. However, it paradoxically can create the conditions for increased isolation and a loss of opportunities to discover more positive forms of intimacy between people.

This is also why the negotiation of space has become such a prominent feature of contemporary body, somatic (see Marlock et al., 2015; Pesso, 1972), play, drama (c.f. Gil & Dias, 2014), dance and movement therapies (Cristobal, 2018). There are significant debates continuing over the use of touch within the therapeutic encounter and how clients can experiment with proximity and distance (and a sense of relational safety) within the therapy room and beyond. This allows for a safer space to re-enact and experiment with disillusioned and re-illusioned modes of existing that have emerged from confronting the reality of crossing the traumatic boundary situation (see Perry with Szalavitz, 2011, 2017).

The enduring changes in 'bodily resonance' (to borrow the term from Fuchs & Koch, 2014) demonstrate the ways in which both the embodied experience of crossing the boundary situation, and the disillusioned or re-illusioned modal responses, are incorporated into the movement of our body through time and space. In a similar vein, Frankl (1967: 88) suggests that 'everything in the past is saved from being transitory. Therein it is irrevocably stored rather the irrecoverably lost'.

Merleau-Ponty (2010 [2001]: 131–132) describes this incorporation as 'sedimentation'. Ernesto Spinelli (2005, 2015) reuses this term to explain the ways in which lived experiences and worldviews become sedimented. He notes that our present lived experiences of the world, and others in it, are built upon previous embodied lived experiences, and further that we can transcend this sedimentation through new experiences (de-sediment). That said, when we face moments of crisis or difficulty in the present moment, it can kick up sediment (as modes of existing) from the past. This also provides an existential equivalency to the intrusion symptoms and alterations in arousal and reactivity of PTSD set out in the clinical literature (c.f. APA, 2013), including flashbacks and heightened startled reactions. In this way, we might also think of re-illusionment as an attempt to (re)cover – that is, to re-cover-up the sedimentation of traumatic experiencing and the confrontation with reality – and disillusionment as an attempt to (re)(dis)cover – that is, to dis-cover or discover beyond sedimented and known modes of existing and experiencing.

To imply that spatial and temporal dimensions of traumatic embodiment are separable is problematic, as temporality is always simultaneously spatial movement. Even if we take the example of clock time, we use the movement and positioning of astronomical bodies to determine the time and day in which we are located in the present moment. It is more coherent for us to speak of temporal-spatial embodiment, and in the preceding discussion the reader will have already seen that lived time cannot be abstracted from the interweaving movement of bodies through space. Here, I will more specifically consider the alterations and disruptions in the lived experience of temporal-spatiality emerging from confrontations with reality and crossing the boundaries of traumatic situations (see also Herman, 2015 [1992]; Ratcliffe et al., 2014: 8–10).

From a neurobiopsychosocial perspective there is seen to be a hyperarousal that emerges out of traumatic experiencing. This hyperarousal activates the adrenal system (inducing forms of excitement), which can lead to altered experiences of increased speed and emotionality. Additionally, we can recognise that an alternative response seems to activate the opioid system (inducing forms of euphoria), which too can result in an altered tempo-spatial reality, where our life-world seems to slow down. These neurophysiological responses can work biphasically (meaning at the same time or in succession), so that our felt reality can be experienced as fluctuating paces of temporal-spatial embodiment. We might use the metaphor of a wave to understand the oscillations and extremities that can be experienced within these temporal-spatial modes of embodiment: a calm sea, where the movement and flow of time is so incredibly slow that it seems as if the water were in stasis;

stormy waters, where the wind, rain and currents become a dramatic symphony, co-creating an immediacy of movement towards the progression through time.

The phenomenological psychiatrist and philosopher Thomas Fuchs describes how traumatic experiences can leave us being out of step with the world around us. He calls this *desynchronisation*, where we feel we are in a state of being 'too late' or of being 'too early' in relation to the social processes of our time (Fuchs, 2013: 82–83, 97). Similarly, Stolorow (2003) describes interpersonal trauma as creating a fundamental disruption in being-in-time, and the 'unifying thread of temporality'. Using a more psychoanalytic frame, Stephen Seligman (2016: 119–121) similarly describes a blurring of past and present time into an anticipated 'post-traumatic fixation', and situations where past trauma is experienced as if it were occurring in the present time. Within these lived experiences, futurity has a vacuity – it is denied, lost or abstracted (ibid.: 122–123). This can be seen in the experiencing of flashbacks (c.f. Duke et al., 2008), memory alterations (c.f. van der Kolk, 2005), and dissociation from the present moment (c.f. Lanius, 2015; McNally, 2005: 93).

The phenomenological psychiatrist Minkowski (1970 [1933]) provides ideas to better understand the interrelationships between our experience of time and our embodied movement through time. Drawing heavily on the work of the French philosopher Bergson (1889 [1927]; 1941), Minkowski describes the way in which our consciousness of temporality is experienced as a lived time (*temps vécu*). According to Minkowski (1970 [1933]:18–22; 38–43), within duration (*durée*), we have a primordial vital impetus (*élan vital*). This ensures a flow through the unfolding of time, and thus towards the future. Working in parallel to this is our 'vital contact with reality' and our own personal impetus (*élan personnel*). Within these, we find (or not) our syntony (our resonance) in the world. Further, we construct our sense of continuity, self and spatiality in time. This allows us to conceive of, and situate, our own contribution to the *élan vital* (ibid.: 22; 44–47, 64–70, 73). In this sense, we are primordially in a state of becoming (*le devenir*).

Through these *élans* we encounter our struggles to maintain a sense of continuity and the vital contact with reality. Thus, it is our resonance in the time-world that constitutes our *temps vécu*, and therefore constitutes the perceptions of time and space around us. Traumatic phenomena, from a Minkowskian viewpoint, emerge from fundamental disruptions and distortions in the experience of the *élans*, and in the consequential impact on a person's resonance (syntony) in time-space.

Our agentic being is a core aspect of our personal *élan*, and is part of our core vitality. Minkowski (1958: 83) notes that our action is 'an essential phenomenon of life', in that 'all that lives is active, and all that is active lives'. The temporality of activity and movement can be seen in it containing the 'factor of the future'. Furthermore, 'through its activity the living being carries itself forward, tends towards the future, creates it in front of itself' (ibid.). In this way, Minkowski concludes that 'fundamentally, activity is lived duration connected to the idea of the living being. It is active duration or, better, duration orientated towards the future'. Conversely, he adds that 'all lived duration that tends towards the future can only be active' and founded on movement (ibid.). Therefore, disruptions in our lived time are inevitably reflected in how we act in time-space, and the visibility of our future orientation.

Modal change is not a singular movement from one mode of existing to another. In the temporal-spatiality of disillusionment and re-illusionment there is an interpenetration and intertwining of existing and emergent modes. To borrow again from the later work of Bergson (1941), there is a reciprocal interpenetration of the present into the past, enabling new modes of existence to generatively be experienced and elaborated. In this sense, modes do not have concrete or rigid boundaries, but rather are fluidic and movable in their expressions and articulations (influenced by Luce Irigaray, 1992 [1982]). In a different context, Foucault (2002 [1969]: 193) notes 'the contemporaneity of several transformations does not mean their exact chronological coincidence: each transformation may have its own particular index [modality] of temporal "viscosity"'. Thus, through the viscosity of traumatic confrontations, there is a *generative co-creation of interpenetrative modes*, in which ever-succeeding and intermingling disillusioned and re-illusioned modes emerge.

In a similar vein, I have previously (Bush [Boaz], 2019) drawn on the ideas of the existential-phenomenological philosopher Emmanuel Levinas (2001 [1947]) to propose an existential analysis of fatigue. I suggest that in the phenomenon of fatigue, there is an 'experiential gap' between what clients experience as the present moment, and the lived time they are participating in. I draw attention to the fundamental paradox of being negatively suspended in a form of 'effortful being' and offer a light (to borrow Levinas's articulation) to more positive forms of fatigued being, including finding a ground (coenaesthesis), taking a position and creating a new attitude towards our present. At the centre of this analysis is the need to reorientate clients' spatial-temporal reconstructions to committing to action in the present. My analysis describes the different ways in which people attempt to suspend themselves in order to avoid, slow down, deny or recoil from confronting the reality of a situation. Suspension is paradoxically seen in this regard to be an active mode of existing.

Temporal-spatial fragmentations of agentic potential

The application of Minkowski's ideas to my modal existentialism might seem disorientating for some readers, so I will briefly illustrate with my previously published case of Nathan (Bush [Boaz], 2020c),[2] who also demonstrates the centrality of agentic potential. Nathan's experience is fragmented along temporal-spatial and relational axes. The general features of the fragmentation of his agentic potential are present in many of the clients I have worked with who have had traumatic confrontations in their life. Not all modes of existing locate agentic fragmentations in past-present or past-future agentic fragments; other clients have alternatively placed them within and between wake-dream world fragments, sober-intoxicated world fragments, intellectual-embodied world fragments or intimacy-sexual world fragments. Some non-existential psychologists and psychotherapists might want to term this fragmentation agentic 'splitting', so it can more easily be incorporated into existing conceptual frameworks. We could add to this many other disillusioned or re-illusioned modes of existing, for example, May's (1972: 50, 103) notion of 'pseudo-innocence', where a person avoids confronting their own power in order to remain under an illusion about the world and relationships around them.[3]

Nathan refracted his temporal-spatial experience of being actively agentic, and having meaningful human relationships, in the present in a modal response to the reality of his experiences of childhood neglect. Nathan experiences his social world as distant from him. He describes his movements and conversations in the world as being heavy, clumsy, pointless and lost. This is reflected in his relationship with others, who reportedly do not seem to understand who Nathan 'really is', nor can they 'bring themselves' to form meaningful relationships with him. Each moment in his present feels, at the same time, stretched out and unnecessarily long, fast paced and shallow.

In contrast to his present time, Nathan describes his life in an imagined 1940s, where (in and among the difficulties of wartime Britain) there is a collective sense of purpose and possibility. He has a clear sense of being active in the world: doing a job he enjoys (being an engineer) and where his relationships with others are positive and in the moment. For example, he retells a beautiful and meaningful romantic (imagined) encounter with a female engineer before they both leave the imagined location that they are temporarily living in. He sees himself as happy, active and content in this imagined and alternative time, even if it might have led to an early death through armed conflict.

The description of Nathan's two time-worlds immediately discloses the lack of syntony within his lived time. Further, the descriptions of moments of time seem to indicate his attitudes towards the fragmentation of his *élan personnel*. In Nathan's present time, a moment in time is experienced as out of synchronisation with those around him – his moments as 'heavy, clumsy, and pointless'. Whereas the world around him oscillates between contradictory stretched-out-ness and fast-paced-shallowness. In contrast, in the past time-world, moments are precious and lived time stretches out before him in a meaningful way, with the only given parameters being contingent factors relating to wartime.

Moreover, we can see significant distortions in the resonance of lived time within the parameters of Nathan's past time-world too. Had he lived during this period of time, he could have been called up to active military service, and as such the presence of war would be more proximate and imminent. Further, this past time-world is a fragment in imagined time – there is no substantive account of the conditions of his imagined self growing up in 1920s Britain, in the wake of the First World War. Nor is there the anticipation of feeling out-of-time, as the imagined self ages through the socio-economic and political changes of the subsequent decades. Somewhat paradoxically, the lived time in his imagined past time-world also lacks a fundamental contact, and resonance, with the reality of the time described, and has a telling absence of imagined futurity.

In Nathan's case, we see a refraction in his agentic being. Present time seems to lack the possibility of active and meaningful action, whereas the past time-world is filled with active engagement and personal commitment – to work, love and the imagined time-world around him, though it is important we note that this agentic refraction into the past time-world is a futile form of becoming, given the impossibility of its realisation by Nathan. Importantly, it is lacking in futurity, which leaves it being contained as a fragment in imagined time rather than a lived possibility.

Nathan's experiences clearly show how clients can locate imaged versions of themselves being active in an imagined past-present. The refractions in his agency and relationships with others could only be healed through a real-world confrontation of himself as an agentic being in the present. While, existentially, we can understand his desire to find a meaningful relation to the present, we should not be too quick to dismiss the significance of his past time-world. This imagined-fragment-in-time clearly had meaning for him, and also contained all the ingredients (albeit infinitised) he needed to restore his *élans* and sense of *durée* – and thus holds the modal possibility of new forms of movement.

From an existential perspective, this past time-world fragment makes sense; it mirrors an early situation of childhood neglect where he had to use his own creative adaptations to exist and find agentic meaning in the world. The close-by, but not fully proximate, war echoes the intra-familial neglect and constant threat of aggression in the home. The opportunistic use of small moments of time, in this past time-world, could relate to the moments of respite, relationality and freedom he experienced as a child. We can further understand this past time-world as representing a creative and powerful preservation of his knowledge of a mode of agentic existence and active participation in the world.

The psychotherapeutic focus is on the rediscovery of agentic and intersubjective modes of existing in the present time – and through this, re-establishing Nathan's *élans*. Minkowski (1958: 84–85, 87–90) considers our agentic potential as expansive and as enabling us to contribute to something greater. The possibility of Nathan's rediscovery of this is signalled in the significance of his constructed engineer in a society at war. This is then realised through his bringing of his refracted agentic, and intersubjective self, back into present time through real-world experimentation.

In my psychotherapeutic practice, I refer to people's temporal-spatial fragmentation of agency as a person's *time arc(s)*. In the present moment, some clients' time arcs are constricted, with clients seeking immediacy in the world and in relation with others, as if the expanse of the future possibility did not lie before them. Other clients have almost infinitised time arcs, locating their agentic potential and modal change in an ever-unreachable future moment. Such clients reverse the time fragment seen in the case of Nathan, locating all agentic responsibility in a time they simultaneously hope for, and avoid. Time arcs, as qualities of modes of existing, expand and contract according to the intersubjective context in which the person is experiencing their life. The fragmentation of agentic potential is important in traumatic confrontations with reality, as it preserves a primordial wisdom that we can actively find new modal expressions within, between and beyond our known modes.

Traumatic experiences of disembodiment

The ways in which we move in time-space is another way of describing our modes of existing. Modes have their own forms of movement and connection to the reality of a situation or relationship. In this section I consider the ways in which people's modal responses to a confrontation with reality might incorporate the experience of being distanced from one's intercorporeality. I will aim to more explicitly describe what is known in the clinical literature as the phenomenon of *dissociation* – and sometimes in more specific formulations as *derealisation* and *depersonalisation*. Within a modal existentialism, dissociation could be described as a mode of existing-out-of-time-and-space (building on Bush [Boaz], 2020c).

A useful starting point for my exploration of dissociation[4] is the work of the Scottish existential psychiatrist R. D. Laing. Laing (1972 [1959]: 78) notes that dissociation is a common, temporary state in people who 'find themselves enclosed within a threatening experience from which there is no physical escape'. In some situations the only form of escape is a seeming 'estrangement and derealisation'. By derealisation he means situations where 'the body may go on acting in an outwardly normal way, but inwardly it is felt to be acting on its own, automatically' (ibid.). Further, Laing notes that this may be a 'desired state', which enables people to deal with, and 'disentangle' themselves from, 'the dangers that threaten [their] body' (ibid.: 66–67). This form of depersonalisation (as it is called in the clinical literature) is an understandable mode of existence to emerge from a traumatic situation where we need to attend to our survival and protect our existence from the danger of another.

Laing (ibid.: 67–68) further describes a partial dissociative state (using the example of a client who has experienced a 'stranger' attack and violence) to illustrate the ways in which we experience our sense of self becoming somewhat divorced from the sensations, feelings and physicality of the body. Within this analysis, he notes that our thoughts seem to turn to sense-making (even in the moment). His client describes, first, surprise at the attack and then explores feelings of hopelessness and meaningless. As Laing notes, what is given up is the physical damage to the body, and in this way the dissociative mode provides the client with psychological space away from the full intercorporeality of the attack, and thus enables him to make an interim sense of it and survive it in the present moment.

Continuing the exploration, Laing describes the loss of a sense of personhood that occurs in the experientially *unembodied* self. He suggests that the 'body is felt more as one object among other objects in the world than as the core of the individual's own being' (ibid.: 69). Extending this further, Laing describes how in existing-out-of-space-and-time, clients experience their body as not only 'operating to comply with and placate others, but as being in the actual possession of others' (ibid.: 144). This is clear in narratives of those who have experienced interpersonal violence, and especially where there is coercion and control, including child grooming and child sexual abuse. The person experiences themselves as an object in the world of the other, to be done unto, and with, as the other sees fit (see Sartre, 2003 [1943], for a similar conceptualisation of relationality here too).

Laing notes that to other people relating to the person, it might seem that the agentic potential of the person is lost, or that they are in an unreal or dreamlike state. However, in reality he asserts that they are 'excessively alert' to the world and actively engaged in 'observation, control, and criticism vis-à-vis what the body is experiencing and doing' (Laing, 1972 [1959]: 69, 78).[5] This seems to echo the common client descriptions of being outside of their bodies in the moment of traumatic experiencing, and those who report reoccurring dreams or flashbacks that are experienced as if they were watching a film of the traumatic encounter. Furthermore, it pre-empts more contemporary understandings of biophysiological stimulation and response that can happen even in the most adverse of experiences; for example, where the somatic response is protective in the moment (i.e. a freeze 'sleep' state), but leaves the person with feelings of shame, guilt or confusion about the experience. These unembodied modes of survival could be seen to be akin to Laing's 'denial of being, as a means of preserving being' (Laing, 1976 [1969]: 150). For example, feigning sleep, not crying out for help, or being very still during sexual abuse, violence or rape could induce a sense of numbness or a perceptive distance from the encounter, enabling the person to survive the attack.

Despite the protective features of dissociative responses, Laing (1972 [1959]: 66) claims that even the 'unembodied person' is 'inextricably bound up' with the relationship with their body – that is, being trapped within, or floating away from it. In this way, their embodiment continues to be experienced as a base for contact with other bodies intercorporeally (ibid.: 67). As such, Laing (ibid.: 69) suggests that the 'relationship with [ourself] and [our] body [...] can become very complex'. We can see from Merleau-Ponty's contribution that unembodiment, as a mode of existing, can become incorporated into our body schema, and thus be enacted as a way of responding to both direct traumatic events and also a general mode of relating to the world around us. Paradoxically, even within an unembodied state, bodily perceptions and sensations remain present, or fluctuate in and out of conscious awareness. Many clients report flashbacks to, or in-event experiences of, the visceral nature of the intertwining human bodies involved. This allows for bodily sensations to be creatively and imaginatively transformed by the person into other experiential constructs (i.e. abstractions of thought, intellectual reasoning, problem-solving or meta-observations and spiritual dialogues etc.); however, the fundamental relatedness of intercorporeal traumatic experiencing cannot be negated (see also Lanius, 2015).

Existential features of traumatic identities and relations

I have explored in the above sections our intercorporeal temporal-spatial movements through the confrontations with reality in traumatic experiencing. I sought to describe how this movement can give rise and emergence to elaborations of existing modes, and to new modes of existence, which respond to and incorporate these experiences. I will next delve deeper into the disillusioned or re-illusioned modes of existing that can emerge, and how they awaken our primordial impulse to philosophise. Within this, I will offer a more detailed analysis of the ways in which we find the kind person we want to become, and how we make sense of relationships to others in our life.

As we have seen, traumatic experiencing can fundamentally change our mode of relating to ourselves and others, be it the forms of intimacy, proximity or touch we are able to tolerate and engage in. This is especially the case when interpersonal trauma has involved a violation of safety, trust, mutuality, dignity and bodily integrity (c.f. Herman, 2015 [1992]: 51; Ratcliffe et al., 2014: 3–7). This can result in a form of existential solitude (*Einsamkeit*) (Jaspers, 1948: 299) or singularisation (Stolorow, 2011c), where we feel we are existentially alone, beyond the boundary situation and distanced from meaningful contact with others. This is more than a psychic atomisation; it is a lived, embodied and relationally experienced distance from the reality of our intersubjective proximity to others.

Even when we re-illusion ourselves in order to protect against the confrontation of the reality of a situation, we can hold back, control or not disclose the traumatic experiencing. In some way we believe we are alone in the experience (Herman, 2015 [1992]). This perceived isolation from others can lead to validations or invalidations by others of the mode of existing that has emerged to survive within, between and beyond a traumatic situation (building on Herman, 2015 [1992]; Stolorow & Atwood, 2002 [1992]; van der Kolk, 2014). I will now turn to consider the experiences that can heighten this sense of existential isolation.

It is important to reiterate here that all modes of existing are valid responses to the confrontation with the reality of a traumatic situation. Even those modes containing qualities many of us find problematic (including denial, deception, manipulation, feigned passivity) are valid forms of illusionment and survival in the face of trauma. The concern for existentialists is more about the problems that arise for people when they assume they have a *modal singularity*, which incorporates a more constricted quality of existing. A modal singularity occurs when a person engages in the epistemic fallacy that they only have one mode of existing, that their totality of existence is reducible to this one mode and that this mode of existing is all they are and all they can be in the world.

Existential guilt and regret

I will now turn to consider some of the ways in which a disillusioned or re-illusioned mode of existence interacts with ideas about existential forms of guilt and regret. Frankl (1967: 33, 87; 1988: xi, 51–52) suggested that guilt (along with pain and death) is part of a 'tragic triad' and an experience we all have to confront. May (1953: 110–113) adds that guilt is a fundamental aspect of the human existence, which is 'rooted in our existential structure'. Cohn (1997: 72) takes us further into understanding guilt's existential features by distinguishing between three forms of guilt. The first is an 'unfounded (neurotic) guilt', where a client is generally guilty, without being able to specify an action to which the guilt relates, or is disproportionally guilty about an action that does not warrant a guilt response (ibid.). The second is 'real guilt', which Cohn suggests 'needs to be faced' (ibid.). This relates to guilt arising from a criminal act or purposeful intent to harm another. It is this form of guilt that most closely relates to our common usage of the word. The final form is an 'existential guilt', which he sees as 'an intrinsic aspect of existence itself' (ibid.). It is this latter form that I explore next.

May (1958: 54–55) locates the ontological 'rooting' of *existential guilt* in the 'forfeiting of potentialities' (building on Heidegger's analysis; see also Boss, 1963: 270). More succinctly, Otto Rank (1936: 211, emphasis added) wrote: 'We feel ourselves guilty on account of *the unused life, the unlived life* in us.' Note that Rank refers to 'unused' and 'unlived life'. This draws attention to the negated potentiality in our lives. He is referring to the choice and decisions we did *not* take in the past, and consequently the life experiences we have *not* had, or the imagined lives we had *not* lived. We saw a version of the unlived life in the case of Nathan and his preservation of his agentic potential in an imaginal past-world fragment. Existential guilt, therefore, relates specifically to our modes of existing in the world.

We can understand how people who have crossed the boundary of traumatic situations can lament the relationships they have not pursued, the connections that have avoided and the loss of the dreams and hopes they had for themselves before they experienced the interpersonal trauma. Further, this existential guilt arises from awareness and/or implicit perceptions of a gap between the embodied life we are living and the life we want to be (or think we 'ought to be') living (following May, 1992: 36–38). Some people might feel existential guilt about becoming a person who cannot experience pleasure during sex with someone they love (*anhedonia*), or lament that they find themselves observing their intimacy with their child in a detached and unemotional way, as if they are watching a film they are disinterested in (*dissociation*). The feeling of existential guilt is transformed within traumatic experiencing into what the existential-humanistic psychotherapist Witold Simon (2009) describes as a mourning of the 'person one could have become'. The guilt-ridden mourning for Simon is an existential transition through which the traumatised person has to pass to be present with the person they have become.

I suggest that by taking up new disillusioned or re-illusioned modes of existence, the person is intercorporeally aware (even in a pre-reflexive or non-conscious way) that this arises from, and endures in relation to, the confrontation of the reality of a traumatic situation. Further, disillusioned or re-illusioned modes of existence are, by their nature, a taking up of possible responses to survive and make meaning out of the experiences we have had. Here, we encounter a paradoxical feature of existential guilt. As Chris Scalzo (2010: 87), in line with a Heideggerian perspective, writes: 'In each context, opportunities and limitation are always created and yet we will only ever be able to choose one singular option.' Reflecting on this, Yalom (1980: 277) suggests that 'one is always "guilty" – and guilty to the extent that one has failed to fulfil authentic possibility'. The paradox is that guilt, in its existential form, will be ever present, for in each moment we can only ever choose one singular option (one potential), meaning that by virtue of our existence we will always be 'being-*guilty*' (Heidegger, 2010 [1953]: 279, emphasis added).

Thus, the taking up of new disillusioned or re-illusioned modes of existence enables the person to retain the potentiality of their agentic being, and opens up a future for them, although they might not experience it as such. In the case of survivor's guilt, the above analysis holds; however, the imaginal unlived life of the other is intersubjectively woven into the lived and unlived life of the person. In this sense, the continued existence of the survivor is a continual confrontation of the non-survival and unlived potential of the other within the flow of time-space.

Associated with our existential guilt is the phenomenon of *existential regret*. By this I mean the concern or preoccupation about the time one has lost by continuing to exist in a disillusioned or re-illusioned mode. Building on this, Marijo Lucas (2004 [1959]: 59) suggests that existential regret emerges from existential guilt as 'a profound desire and aching to go back and change a past experience in which one has failed to consciously choose or made a choice which did not follow one's beliefs, values, or growth needs' – an attempt at a *retro-fixative* movement. Herman (2015 [1992]) notes how many people who survive traumatic environments and situations become preoccupied with what they could have done to have changed their role in the situation(s). Further (as we saw in previous chapters), returning to memories and meanings around them is part of the experience of crossing the boundary of interpersonal trauma.

In a Nietzschean analysis, May (1953: 11–13) describes the pressure to conform that is driven by notions of *what one should do* or *how one should be*, in order to fulfil a mantra of social, moral and ethical bodily conformity. Some people may use this as a way of protecting against the threat of further traumatisation or the avoidance of confronting the reality of a situation (through rapid re-illusionment). It is in the pursuit of questions of *should* that people lose sense of *what they want to be*, and *how they want to be* in the world. May (ibid.: 17–18) argues that we are at risk in these moments of losing 'our awareness of ourselves', and therefore become lost in the ambiguities of intercorporeality – akin to what Frankl (1988) terms the 'existential vacuum'.

The realisation that existential guilt and regret emerge from the experience of interpersonal trauma is compounded by the atomised notion of responsibility in some existentialist, psychological and psychotherapeutic thought. As Yalom (1980: 320, original emphasis) writes, 'if one accepts responsibility for one's life situation and makes the decision to change, the implication is that one alone is responsible for the past wreckage of one's life and *could* have changed long ago'. Lucas (2004 [1959]: 60) suggests that this can lead to further anxiety and stress as we must 'confron[t] our inability to go back and reclaim the moment when we had the ability to choose'. He further suggests that for some, existential regret can be overwhelming and result in a paralysis, meaning that people lose hope and perspective on the ability to make new choices in the present moment (ibid.: 66). The contemporary psychotherapy focus on self-compassion and kindness is important here, as we must honour that our disillusioned or re-illusioned modes of existence were creative responses to confronting the reality of the situation.

The creative responses were generatively related to the contextual limitations of a traumatic situation. Modal creativity emerges within intersubjective constraints and limitations, and thus there is still scope for us to expand our horizons into new modes.

Existential writers agree that the key to resolving existential regret is not dwelling on the life that was *not* lived, and on the time spent in a particular mode of existing following the crossing of a boundary situation and confrontation with reality. Rather, they advocate a focus on the meaning that we have given to the life we *have* lived, and the possibilities we have not pursued. As Yalom (1980: 221) reminds us, 'nothing in the world has significance except by virtue of one's own creation'. Frankl (1988: 98), too, suggests that 'meaning is more than being' and characterises existential regret as a 'noögenic neurosis' resulting from 'existential frustration' – a frustration in finding a 'will-to-meaning' and experimenting with new modes of existing (Frankl, 2004 [1959]: 106–107).

Existential shame, embitterment and humiliation

People experience an immense sense of loss of 'worth and dignity of the human being' when confronted with interpersonal trauma (building on Lee, 2005; May, 1953: 70). The result can be feelings of worthlessness and valuelessness about the possibility of any mode of existence, and especially those that seem to be beyond the frame of traumatic experiencing of the confrontations with reality (building on Baldwin, 2017 [1963]: 13–16). This in itself can lead to further humiliation within the incorporeality of the relations between ourselves and others.

These experiences of humiliation and worthlessness are incorporated into disillusioned and re-illusioned modes that involve forms of self-condemnation and self-criticism, which could manifest in hatred for others (May, 1953: 108) and/or self-hatred and self-harming behaviours (Austin, 2016; see also Allen & Oleson, 1999; Downs, 2012; Kaufman & Raphael, 1996). We might call this sense of worthlessness *existential shame*. By this I mean shame that specifically follows on from an awareness of the gap between the mode of existence we are living and want to live (existential guilt), a frustration with the modal life choices that have been made and an inability to go back and pursue alternative possibilities (existential regret). In my formulation, existential shame is a dynamic state emerging within and between the flows of existential guilt and regret. Stolorow (2011b: 286) reminds us that a 'move toward greater authenticity' is often 'accompanied by an emotional shift from being dominated by shame to an embracing of existential guilt'. While I would not use the Heideggerian framing of authenticity in this discussion, his observation still stands if we replace 'greater authenticity' with 'an alternative mode of existing'.

Erving Goffman (1990 [1963]: 57–128) suggests that people[6] can become socially 'spoilt' if they are seen to have a stigmatising characteristic, for example, 'abnormal' behaviours, bodies, illnesses or social statuses. He writes that the 'discredited' are those whose stigma is known by other people (i.e. someone with a visible impairment), as opposed to the 'discreditable', whose stigma is only revealed in certain situations (i.e. through sexual behaviour). People who have experienced interpersonal trauma may fear that their mode of existing (especially if it is re-illusioned) is discreditable (could be revealed to others) or discredited (known by others to be not who they want to be/become). The medical sociologist Graham Scambler (1986; Scambler & Hopkins, 1989) expands Goffman's description by distinguishing between 'felt' stigma and 'enacted' stigma. The former is the stigma that results from the anxiety of managing the discredited mode of existing, and the latter the experiences of stigma in relation to others interacting with our mode of existing. Building on Goffman and Scambler, this would create an existential conflict between the 'actual' experience (disillusionary) of ourselves and the 'virtual' (re-illusionary) modes of experiencing that are stigmatised intercorporeally by the other.

Our own existential shame can give rise to interpersonal dynamics of shame. The presence of the other person is crucial in the Sartrean conception of shame. In Sartre's (2003 [1943]: 276–325, 364) more conflictual basis of interpersonal dynamics, the presence of an other is problematic for the person. In experiencing the presence of the other person, we also sense and experience ourselves as an 'object' in the gaze of the other (ibid.: 103–129, 222). By making me an object in their eyes, the other is rendering me a being-in-itself (*être-en-soi*). That is, a fixed material being without consciousness and whose purpose is derived from its nature. As a result, I fight back, wanting to retain my freedom as a subject that is a being-for-itself (*être-pour-soi*), that is, a conscious human being, who has the freedom to determine their own nature and purpose in relation to nothingness (ibid.: 95–126). This conflictual dynamic within modal existentialism is a movement away from the intersubjective incorporeal reality of human relating. We can understand how, within the context of traumatic confrontations, experiencing the other as an agentic person with realisable potential might be a frightening or daunting prospect.

According to Sartre, in attempting to retain my subjectivity, I seek to make the other an object (and thus a being-in-itself). Paradoxically, at the same time I am too drawn to become a being-in-itself, seeing the grounding in the world the other acquires through my looking at them as if they were an object within it (ibid.: 362–382). The other mirrors my concerns, wanting both to retain their freedom and similarly render me an object in their gaze. Sartre characterises this as a circular process, in which both I and the other are paradoxically enriched by our mutual failure to fully realise either becoming a being-in-itself or being-for-itself for each other (ibid.: 363–364, see also 383–452 for proposed masochistic and sadist attitudes relating to this dynamic).

For Sartre, this circular dynamic gives rise to shame, which is by its 'nature *recognition*. I recognize that *I am* as the Other sees me […] the Other *looks* at me and as such he holds the secret of my being, he knows what I *am*' (ibid.: 246, 385, original emphasis). Being seen through the gaze of the other is confronting as it brings awareness to the gap between the mode of existence we are living and how we want to live our lives. Thus, through the conflictual intersubjective dynamics of shame we are brought back to a more existential shame in who we are becoming. Drawing on a more Bergsonian, Minkowskian and Schützian perspective, we might say that the conflictual dynamics of shame arise from the movements (or dance) between proximity/distance and synchronicity/dsynchronicity of another's lived experience. As Sartre notes: 'Shame is shame of *oneself before the Other*; these two structures are inseparable. But at the same time I need the Other in order to realize fully all the structures of my being' (ibid.: 246, original emphasis).

When our mode of existing becomes stigmatised, conflictual and discredited through the intersubjectivity of ourselves and the other, we can move into a mode of *existential humiliation*. Within the mode of existential humiliation, we see mistrust and a lack of safety at every turn. We are saturated by the dynamic flows of existential guilt, regret and shame, and no modal movement alleviates us from the overwhelming reality of a situation or relationship. Every modal movement and expression is an articulation of humiliated existence. Modes of humiliation face the past with rumination, suspicion and a lack of faith in the possibility of modal movement. People in this mode of existing find comfort in non-resolution of conflict and the denial of the possibility of movement and the generative opening up of new modes of existing. In some modes, humiliation is directed intersubjectively towards the other in the form of *existential embitterment* – that is, a seeming hatred for the modal movement and explorations of the other. The modal movement of the other in the confrontation of reality becomes an affront to the humiliated mode of existing as it discloses the epistemic fallacy of an *existential singularity or fixity* of humiliation. In this way, humiliated modes can never be satiated, as their relational expression is vengeful and attacking. The person claws at themselves and others in an attempt to (re)discover an expansive modal movement; however, in doing so they attempt to render the other into the existentially humiliated mode they embrace (following a more Sartrean reading of intersubjectivity).

In this way, existential humiliation is also an attempt at agentic suspension (building on Bush [Boaz], 2019). The movement of existential humiliation is an attempt to press oneself into the ground in such a way that one is unable to establish a position from which to move. It does not represent a mode of disembodied merging with the ground to feel the movement of the earth or to be held within the animated movement of the world around us. Rather it represents an agentic attempt to bury oneself under the weight of the ground of a confrontation with reality – to allow reality to bear down upon us until all animated reality of ourselves, the other and the world is diminished. In the modes of existential humiliation, it seems as if others are in a position to move over us, as if we were a grounding to move across.

The sense of being under the ground on which other people walk, crawl, roll over makes it harder for us to locate our agentic contribution to the modal expression, and thus take responsibility for it, as we feel subject to the infinitised or known other who moves over us, as they would another ground. The movement away from *existential humiliation* is to feel the hard ground beneath us, find comfort and rest in it, and see that we may too wriggle, crawl, walk, jump, leap and dance over it. In (re)encountering our modal movement, we better understand the relationality of the ground (solid and fluid alike) and the proximity of the other as being co-generative in expanding beyond humiliation as a modal response to the reality of a situation.

On survivalism and survivorism as positive modes

Paradoxically, all the above modal states (existential guilt, regret, shame, embitterment and humiliation) are examples of our awakened primordial impulse to philosophise following the confrontation with reality. In what follows, I explore two ways in which a new mode of existing can incorporate traumatic confrontations into the formulation of modal identifications. Here I use the term 'identity' as the articulated self-sense of the person we have become in our mode of existing (building on Baldwin, 2017 [1963]: 84). This articulation could be realised through the descriptions and narratives we have about our life, the patterns of behaviour we display or the kinds of people we are drawn to spend time with.

Existential guilt, regret, shame, embitterment and humiliation complicate the endeavour of finding modes of existing that enable us to incorporate the experiences of interpersonal trauma into the kind of person we want to become. As the existentialist writer James Baldwin (ibid.: 17) astutely observes: 'People find it very difficult to act on what they know. To act is to be committed, and to be committed is to be in danger. In this case, the danger […] is the loss of their [existing] identity'. The relationship drawn here between self-knowing, action, commitment and identity is important, as it signals the ways in which modal responses can give rise to forms of identity and meaning-making that become sedimented and core movements within the kind of person we become in the world.

Baldwin (2017 [1963]: 43) further draws our attention to the importance of finding an attitude (a mode of existing) that is embedded in the reality of the experiences we have had. He suggests that people who find themselves caught between their distrust of their own experiences and the reality of the situation(s) they have faced become lost in a 'labyrinth of attitudes' (ibid.). The person's labyrinth of attitudes tends to be borrowed and encultured from 'historical and public attitudes', which may not relate to the person, their own experiences or the present they find themselves in. Many existential and sociological writers have described the ways in which people find attitudes, freedom and meaning within constrained situations (Baldwin (2017 [1963]: 13–16, 42; de Beauvoir, 2015 [1948]; Camus (2005 [1942]; Foucault, 1979; Goffman, 1968 [1961], 1990 [1959]; Lupton, 2004), even in conditions where they are subject to others, regimes or situations that would seemingly curtail their agency.

Building upon the notion of finding the freedom and power of movement within limited situations, I have identified within the existing literature two positive forms of traumatised modal identity: *survivalism* and *survivorism*. In these two forms, the mode of existing that has emerged from the confrontation of the reality of the situation is transformed into a propulsion through time-space towards other environments and persons (potentially less harm-inducing) that enable them to continue to realise their power, freedom, agency and find meaning in their life, within limitations.

Survivalism is the modal identity of embracing the confrontation of reality as a fundamental premise of existence. Further, it is an investment in growing and strengthening modes of existence in order to survive in a world of adverse, stressful environments and potentially threat-inducing relationships. This form of existing can be incredibly meaningful for people: be it the human rights activist who works to challenge the harm of institutional injustices, or the child who finds themselves in another violent relationship attempting to change their friend's behaviour towards them. In this way, we can see that rather than re-living or re-enacting the crossing of the boundary situation of trauma, these modes are generatively elaborating experience of confronting a traumatic reality to inform their agentic mode of existence.

Survivorism is a mode of existence where a person's identity is orientated in reciprocal relation to the traumatic situation and the experience of it. The mode of existence focuses on both disclosing (directly or indirectly) their experience of trauma and their ability to move beyond it to connect to the world around them, and using their experience of trauma as a core explanatory mechanism to understand the experiences they have in the present. For me, this conceptualisation is different to an identity founded upon victimisation, where a person attempts to retain the negative position of a traumatised person as reductively a victim in and to all situations.

Both survivalism and survivorism are generative modes of existing, which move beyond victimisation through traumatic confrontations. Echoing the perspective of Frankl, the existential psychologist Edith Eger (2018: 9) proposes that while victimisation is a lived experience within traumatic confrontations, the identification with victimhood is a chosen response. In her autobiographical account of surviving the Nazi concentration camps, Eger writes that victimisation comes from the outside, whereas victimhood is an attitude that emerges from our own personhood. Thus, the identity of victimhood is something we can choose to hold on to (as a modal possibility), or move within and beyond. Modes of victimhood are seen in this way to be negative movements of incorporation of traumatic experiences. They are negative in that these modes of victimhood can be used to paradoxically justify the intersubjective weaponising of the distress and pain of traumatic confrontations. Intersubjective weaponising includes the paradoxical re-enactment of interpersonal trauma as forms of revenge or entitlement to immoral behaviour – and thus perpetuate cyclical movements of violence (see also Gabay et al., 2020, for an alternative personality construct description that I am not aligned to).

In contrast, survivorism is a paradoxical movement of liberation, in that the person incorporates the referent of the event, relationship or situation in order to agentically escape being defined and constricted by the traumatic experience. Expansion emerges from the movement with the referent of the traumatic confrontation, rather than an attempt to suspend one's modes into a singularity. This positive mode of survivorism is popularised in the mental health survivor's movement, in the work of the founders of support organisations (e.g. those aimed at supporting the victims of rape or torture), and the advocates of lived experience informing policy design and institutional reform in the United Kingdom and internationally. Equally, it can be found in people who spend significantly long periods of their life only socialising with other people who have had similar experiences of trauma, or participate in closed groups for survivors of (for example) domestic violence, child sexual abuse or rape. This mode may or may not use formal diagnoses (i.e. of PTSD or complex PTSD) to give legitimacy to people's survivorism and/or use it as a signifier or shorthand in relating to others.

Being positive modes of movement, survivalism and survivorism are generatively also acts of resistance (building on Foucault, 1998 [1976]; 2010 [2004]; Butler, 2011 [1993]). These modes are movements of resistance in that they actively incorporate the confrontation of reality and experience of trauma into a mode of existence that has forms of meaning, purpose, power and freedom. Despite the resistant potential, survivalism and survivorism can become habitual modes of existing. While initially they might be forms of liberation – in representing movements of liberation within, and from, the traumatic situation(s) – the modes do not always provide the ground for new and emergent modes that can flow with and beyond the person's past confrontations with reality. That said, I maintain survivalism and survivorism are positive modes in the sense that they signal a continuation of movement through the confrontation with reality, rather than seek a suspension of agentic potential.

Incorporating confrontations with reality through interpersonal trauma into modes of existing, enables a generative participation in modally changing the social world around us. This echoes the meaning of the word 'use' in Baldwin's (2017 [1963]: 71) notion that accepting 'one's past – one's history – is not the same as drowning in it; it is learning how to use it'. Modal survivalism and survivorism can result in *modal activism*. Modal activism seeks to address the permissive intersubjective contexts and institutional structures, which allow for (or actively promote) the emergence of interpersonal trauma and violence. As with all movements and responses, modal activism has disillusioned and re-illusioned modes.

The extent to which modal activism is re-illusioned depends on the personal tolerance for re-encountering our own personal confrontation with reality, and those who share similar lived traumatic experiences. Disillusioned modal activism risks exhausting movements of overwhelming waves of confrontation with reality, each taking the person deeper into a totalising confrontation with the polarities and extremities of horrific and peaceful movements of existence. *In this sense, the world is a more brutal and more joyous place than we dare let ourselves believe or realise.*

In contrast, at times many of us (myself included) have engaged in a more re-illusioned form of modal activism. We have actively (consciously or nonconsciously) chosen social causes that meaningfully incorporate the reality of our own confrontation with reality, although from the perspective of a less proximate traumatic experience. By advocating alongside others, within a mode of kinship-in-the-same-darkness (following Stolorow, 2019b: 67–77, 102–103), there is a simultaneous sharing in the similar traumatic confrontations with reality, while attempting to maintain a safe distance between our pain and that of the others. As

Stolorow and Atwood (2019c) note in their description of indwelling, in reality the distance between the emotional worlds of our modal activism and the other is an illusion. Our interaffectivity implicates us co-creatively in the world of the other, and thus re-illusioned modal activism encounters continual displacement, confusion and ambiguity over whose pain is being advocated for. At its most extreme polarity, some re-illusioned modal activism becomes a negative movement within generative modal change. This occurs in situations where re-illusioned modal activists engage in radical movements away from their own lived experiences, stating these have no intercorporeal or interaffective relevance for their mode of existing. As such, like those choosing modes of victimisation, the re-illusioned modal activist risks paradoxically advocating for or perpetuating cycles of interpersonal trauma and violence (see also Eger, 2018: 263–264, 280).

Some might read survivalism and survivorism as articulations of 'post-traumatic growth' (c.f. Calhoun & Tedeschi, 2013; Greenberg et al., 2018; Jacobsen, 2006; Tedeschi & Calhoun, 2004; Vachon, Bessette & Goyette, 2016). My concern with the notion of 'post-traumatic' is the value judgement of perceived negative and positive responses to traumatic experiences. For me, I think of all modal movements as human growth. The positive and negative in my usage is about movement through intersubjective time-space, rather than the human or social value of the modality. As Laing (1971 [1961]: 128) astutely notes, an 'existential phenomenology of action is concerned with the movement, the twists and turns of the person as one who puts [themselves], in different ways, more or less, into what [they do]'. Thus, many of the aforementioned modal movements could be encapsulated in this emerging field of so-called post-traumatic growth.

Traumatised kinds of person

Within the above description of modal identities, I am reminded of the work of the philosopher Ian Hacking (2007: 288–289), who describes the 'making' of different 'kinds' of people. Hacking (1999) suggests that in order for a kind of person to become knowable in society, we first must have an embodied language by which we can describe them (Hacking, 1991, 1992). Only through shared descriptions can we have an idea of what the kind of person is. Hacking uses a number of examples to illustrate this, including a discussion of various diagnosed mental health conditions (Hacking, 1995, 1998) and autism (Hacking, 2009).

His clearest articulation of 'kinds' is in his exploration of the 'making of child abuse' (Hacking, 1991, 1992). In this work, he differentiates between objects (behaviours, acts or practices, i.e. of habitual or ritualised child abuse) and the concept, classification or rather idea of 'child abuse', 'child abusers' and 'child abuse victims'. He argues that the concept of these kinds of people has been elaborated from the historical development of the idea of 'child abuse'. Without this core idea of 'child abuse', there would not be these kinds of people in our society. In this, Hacking is not saying that the interpersonal enactments would not exist (i.e. the act of, for example, an adult touching a child's genitalia), but rather they would not be described as 'child abuse' and would not give rise to positional identities relating to it ('abuser', 'victim', 'bystander', 'witness' etc.). I call these positional identities *contra-modal* movements as they are defined in contra-position to another actual or imaginal modal movement.

Because the idea of 'child abuse' does exist in society, it enables individuals and groups of people to remake their experiences in relation to it. Thus, once we have the classification – a language – of 'child abuse', we get the notion that there is a definite type of person related to it (the 'child abuser', for example), and this kind of person becomes reified through our practices, beliefs and structures that we build around them (child protection, safeguarding, vetting procedures etc.) (Hacking, 1999: 27). However, Hacking (ibid.: 10) writes that these ideas do not operate in a vacuum, and that they are made and remade in relation to a matrix in which the idea operates. This could be akin to the inter-world described by Merleau-Ponty, which includes shared and conflicting cultural myths, significations and meanings. For Hacking (similarly to Latour, 2005), this matrix can refer to the social systems, structures and documents (etc.) that are created to interact with the kind of person that has been made (i.e. child protection plans, diagnostic criteria for PTSD etc.).

In relating this back to the earlier discussion of modal identity, we can see how both survivorism and survivalism rely to some extent on the notion that 'kinds' of intercorporeal acts constitute a traumatic experience. Further, the person's incorporation of the kind of person they have been, or are becoming (into movements of modes of existence), enables an elaboration of the kind of traumatised identities that exist within society. For this reason, Hacking (2007) calls these 'interactive kinds' as traumatised kinds are in a continual interaction with the people who occupy those kinds, and as such are informed and elaborated by changes in both collective understanding and enactments of this kind of being. This is in a similar way to how Merleau-Ponty (2012 [1945]) describes movement and change in the intercorporeal inter-world, and incorporates what I mean by *generative* movement.

We can see the generative movement of modal identities in the recent lay reclaiming of clinical diagnoses as a social identity, for example, recent shifts in the making and remaking of autistic kinds of personhood in the Anglo-American context, in which the introduction of neurodiversity as a lay identity has shaped clinical understandings and articulations of autistic personhood (c.f. Baron-Cohen, 2017; Silberman, 2015). A similar generative cycle seems to be emerging in the Anglo-American context, with people increasingly self-diagnosing or identifying as having complex PTSD or so-called borderline personality disorder (BPD). The taking up of diagnostic labels as interactive (generative) kinds produces new knowable forms of personhood within society and thus creates meaningful explanatory mechanisms for the self and other. There are generative tensions involved in the making of interactive kinds, including the simultaneous increasing of feminist critiques of the use of BPD as a diagnostic label (c.f. Nicki, 2001, 2016; Shaw & Proctor, 2005), and lay communities reclaiming it as a positive identifier of modal responses to traumatic experiencing.

Generative tension is understandable within the movements of making and remaking traumatised kinds of people. Through the intersubjective remaking of kinds, the social dispersement of explanatory narratives can become attractive to those who want to make use of the diagnostic identification for the purpose of displacement or deception. As such, within diagnosed and undiagnosed kinds of people, there are some who are drawn into participation in these modes of existing, despite not actively identifying with them beyond the social benefit the status might confer (c.f. Matto, McNiel & Binder, 2021). Paradoxically, these false modal movements are core to the generative movement of kind-making and remaking. The cases of false accusations of violence and public acquittals go on to shape public and personal perceptions and explanatory narratives around the kinds of people who have traumatic experiences, and actions people in relation to these kinds (cf. de Roos & Jones, 2020; Weiser, 2017).

Notes

1 Whenever I reread Merleau-Ponty's description of the *reversibility* of our intercorporeality, I am also reminded of Sartre's (2003 [1943]: 625–663) earlier fascinating exploration of slime, slimy and sliminess. This discussion of the qualities of sliminess contains expressive movements of our intercorporeal reversibility too.
2 I have slightly modified the identifiers and descriptions to retain client anonymity.
3 I am reminded here of a similar observation by Baldwin (2017 [1955]: 178), who eloquently notes that 'people who shut their eyes to reality simply invite their own destruction, and anyone who insists on remaining in a state of innocence long after that innocence is dead turns himself into a monster' (see also, ibid.: 16–17).
4 An alternative analysis based primarily on the work of Heidegger can be found in Arnold and Pinkston (2014). Laing's work resonated with my formulation more, so I have focused the discussion here.
5 This Laingian understanding of dissociative experiences is compatible with other neuro-psychotherapeutic conceptualisations, for example, in the trauma curve explained in Vogt's (2018) somatic-psychological-interactive model.
6 Goffman is writing in a social psychology frame and thus uses a form of self-construction and the notion of a 'presentation of the self' and 'spoilt identity' in his original publications. I have used the terms 'person', 'mode of existence' and 'experienced by' instead to create a coherence with the argument I have built on Merleau-Ponty's notions of embodiments and intercorporeality.

7 Existential ambiguities, liminality and reality-denial in traumatic confrontations

In the previous chapter, I described modal existential understandings of traumatic embodiment and identities. In doing so, I explored examples of the modal movements and modes of existing that emerge out of disillusionment and re-illusionment in confrontations with reality. In this chapter, I will return to the theme of intersubjective ambiguity, which is at the foundation of human existing, and a tension within modes of existing. I will consider the possible impact that ambiguity has on our understanding of traumatic experiencing, and modal movements resulting from confrontations with reality. More specifically, I will propose a way of understanding the existential horror and terror emerging and arising out of traumatic confrontations. This will lead me to describe in more detail what is meant by *reality* in a traumatic confrontation with reality, and further how ambiguity and liminality queers the turns, movements and reality we experience. Finally, I will apply my formulation of confrontation to our intersubjective and contextual reality, suggesting that human and family systems can engage in reality-denial and reality-augmentation in modal attempts to turn away from traumatic confrontations with reality and the foundations of our existence.

Intercorporeal ambiguities

Following Laing (1972 [1959]: 131), there is a fundamental ambiguity within the intercorporeality of our existence. Previously, I explored the notion of touch. Touch, for Merleau-Ponty (2012 [1945]: 95–96; 1968 [1964]: 56, 261), is an ambiguous 'double sensation' in the ambiguity of who is touching, and being touched by whom, in a given encounter. Further, through the intercorporeality of interpersonal trauma, the other becomes 'inscribed' in our embodiment of traumatic experience and subsequent modes of existence, and vice versa we in theirs (Merleau-Ponty, 1968 [1964]: 143). As Laing (1971 [1961]: 81–82, original emphasis) writes, 'each person is always *acting* upon others and *acted upon* by others'. The ambiguity of intercorporeal inscription can be seen, for example, in experiences of rape, sexual violence and sexual abuse, where there can be significant confusion reported by clients about the nature of the situation being faced and the client's own role within it (also following Laing, ibid.: 140–141). Thus,

DOI: 10.4324/9781003181675-10

the givenness of our intercorporeality, and its resulting ambiguities of movement, creates additional complexity in our agentic modes of existing.

An alternative form of ambiguity that arises more specifically from illusionary modes of experience (Laing, ibid.: 108) draws our attention to the etymological commonalities between illusion and collusion (the Latin verb *ludere*, or to play). The ambiguity of playing along with a traumatic encounter can be seen as a form of re-illusionment, possibly a necessary mode in order to survive a threat to life or bodily integrity: a touch, a kiss, a smile, a nod, a look, a whisper in a loving and nourishing relationship that might communicate deep connection, mutuality, respect and growth. In modes of traumatic collusion, these intercorporeal gestures are transformed into non-verbal expressions of a secret bond, and their possible invisibility (both in terms of concealed physicality and significance) creates an active form of re-illusionment.

What is seen as a person being complicit in their traumatisation and sustaining the traumatising relationship with the other over time (collusion), could in this instance be a protective response while the situation endures (following Herman, 2015 [1992]), though we are left with the paradox of the traumatised person becoming active in the endurance of this way of relating. Using a more compassionate framing, we might see this collusion as an understandable mode of survivalism – an attempt by the traumatised person to render the other relationally knowable and safe, given their possible proximity.[1] The illusionary nature of collusion is maintained, for Laing (1971 [1961]: 143), as confronting the reality of one's role in sustaining the conditions that enable the traumatic experience (irrespective of its survivalism) is 'untenable' for the person. From my previous description, we can see how a disillusioned modal response of one's positioning in a traumatic relationship could throw the person back into a state of existential guilt, regret, shame and humiliation, or they could be left with movements of irreality or unembodiment.

Alongside collusion, ambiguity arises in traumatic experiencing through what Laing (ibid.: 82–83) describes as 'complementarity'. This is where the presence of the traumatising other is necessary for a person to intersubjectively continue in a particular mode of existing. Complementarity is where 'the other fulfils or completes self […] One speaks of a gesture, an action, a feeling, a need, a role, an identity, being the complement of a corresponding gesture, action, feeling, need, role, or identity of the other' (ibid.: 98–107). Complementarity gives an insight into those clients whose mode of existence evoke relationships with specific kinds of other(s) in order to maintain a specific traumatic identity (c.f. van der Kolk, 1989). We can see this intercorporeally in people who (following trauma) become attracted to, avoid or are disgusted by another's perceived gender, body shape, scent, body or facial hair (or lack of), height, form of laughter or crying, form of walk, style of dress and so on. As difficult as it might be for us to acknowledge, *when we continue to live in modal relation (even contra-modal) to the traumatising other(s), we are living in a state of complementarity*. The modal identities of 'traumatised' and 'traumatising person' emerge from the crossing of a boundary situation and our confrontation with reality. The modal positions of 'traumatised' and 'traumatising' are 'contradictory and paradoxical' identities as they rely on an intersubjective commitment to complementarity (extending Laing, 1971 [1961]: 87). That said, complementarity may not be of the traumatised person's making or choice (it may be imposed coercively by the other), although by modally living in relation to it, the traumatised person in some way is living in a complementary mode of existence (following ibid.: 98–107).

Existential horror and terror

The spectre of the traumatising person haunts our movements emerging from confrontation with reality.[2] This haunting is reminiscent of the Sartrean notion of a present-absence (Sartre, 2003 [1943]: 32–35, 366). In Sartre's example, he enters a cafe expecting to see his friend Pierre sitting at a particular table, and instead is confronted by the absence of Pierre. Sartre describes Pierre's absence as haunting the cafe, and thus he experiences nothingness in the place of Pierre's presence – that is, the presence-absence of the negation of Pierre's presence. In a similar way, we encounter the presence-absence of the traumatising other haunting our new experiential situations (also following Eger, 2018: 21). Presence-absences are modally incorporated into new relationships, what we might call 'displaced re-illusionment': displaced in that we bring the intercorporeal sedimented memory of the traumatising other (by way of a haunting) into our relationships with non-traumatising others in new situations.

This haunting is further intensified by experiences of invasive sensations, memories or thoughts, or the throwing up of sedimented responses to trauma from the past, which are incorporated into our mode of existing. Haunting can manifest in abstractions within our creative imagination, through unembodied experiences, through the ambiguities of time and place (as in dream, wake, trance and altered states) or through somatic presentations (as in numbness of the body, or an absence of pleasure or excitement). Another way of articulating this haunting of the traumatising other(s) is through a new formulation of *existential horror and terror*.

Levinas (2001 [1947]: 54, 58) notes that horror emerges from the dark (in contrast to the light of knowing), and signals existence with 'no exits'. In traumatic experiencing, the horror *emerges* from the intercorporeal interanimality of the encounter(s) with the other. As Becker (2012 [1973]: 35) notes, there is a simultaneous pleasure and horror that paradoxically can be found in our realisation that 'blood and excrement, sex and guilt' relate to the 'constraints of [our] basic animal condition' and the 'incomprehensible mystery of the body and the world' (ibid.: 35). In our experience of horror, we are thrown into a confrontation with the boundaries of our existence – in whatever way one wants to frame these, be it Frankl's (1988) tragic triad, or Yalom's (1980) givens of human existence.

Our existential horror can be intensified in situations where the traumatising person is 'meant' to fulfil myths and significations of social roles (as Merleau-Ponty acknowledges is part of our inter-world), for example, those of caregiver, grand-parent, lover, teacher, coach, confidant, friend and so on. This is the horror of confronting both the interanimality and incorporeality of the other, and disillusionment: disillusionment of who the other is, or who they modally have become, the reality of their mode of existence and the knowledge that we too share the modal potentiality to move towards becoming this kind of person. A Levinasian reading of horror suggests that horror results from something that exists, in contrast to the more Sartrean spectre of nothingness.

Längle expands on the Levinasian ideas of horror, by exploring what is confronted within the reality of a traumatic experience. He contends that what is experienced in a traumatic situation is not so much fear but acute *existential horror* (*Das Entsetzen*) at the *incomprehensibility* of the reality (*Unfasslichkeit der Realität*) being confronted (Längle, 2007: 110; see also a similar earlier discussion in Längle, 2005). The incomprehensibility of the reality being confronted is equivalent to the 'crushing power of reality' described by Becker (2012 [1973]: 54). Incomprehensibility arises from disillusionment of our previous mode of existing (incorporating our worldview), which is shattered or disrupted by the confrontation. The horror at the incomprehensibility of the reality incorporates a disruption in our self-perception, self-assessment and self-esteem (Längle, 2007: 110–111).

Echoing a more Jasperian reading, Längle describes horror existentially being as an expression of shock (*Erschütterung*) or harrowing (*Erschütternden*) wonderment arising from the incomprehensibility of the depths of existence (*Unfasslichkeit der Abgründigkeit der Existenz*), and our lack of trust and understanding in the face of this incomprehensibility (ibid.: 110). While Längle (ibid.: 114) suggests traumatic confrontations bring the person to a standstill psychologically, physically and relationally, in the modal perspective the person remains in movement. We could note here that the shocking or harrowing wonderment Längle talks about is a movement, this time expressed in German as a vibration emerging from the moment of confrontation with reality. Thus, the horror of the confrontation with reality is something to be incorporated within disillusioned and re-illusioned modes of existing.

Alongside the existential horror of the incomprehensibility of the traumatic reality is our *existential terror*. I describe existential terror as an actual and perceived anticipation of repeated traumatic experiencing the next time we encounter the person(s), or others in the world (see also Herman 2015 [1992]: 33–50, for an alternative framing). Existential terror *arises* from (and to the extent to which we have incorporated) the traumatic experiencing in our body schema and mode of existence. Existential terror is intensified if the person has had multiple or enduring experiences of interpersonal trauma, if they remain in contact with the traumatising person or if the threat of the person terrorising them remains. Paradoxically, Laing (1976 [1969]: 145) infers that we might choose to feel this existential terror (whether consciously or not), by actively continuing to remain in traumatising relationships, and this might even become a survival strategy that some people use to 'experience real alive feelings'.

Reflecting on being incarcerated for his homosexuality, Oscar Wilde (1907 [1897]: 109) tells a friend:

> I know that on the day of my release I will merely be moving from one prison into another, and there are times when the whole world seems to be no larger than my cell and as full of terror for me.

The anticipatory terror remains present and projected forwards for Wilde, as the society to which he returns continues to criminalise his sexuality, and thus invalidates and delegitimises his very existence, irrespective of his modal expression. Thus, the existential terror arises from the prospect of living in a world where he could at any moment be subject to harassment, violence or degradation by state actors, and subject to legal proceedings and/or incarceration for the mere existence of his sexuality. His description of the movement from prison to the outside world, and the shrinking of the 'whole world' into the size of a cell, reminds us of the spatial dimensions of existential terror. Wilde incorporates into his awareness a knowledge that his mode of existing will be both restricted (*the shrinking*) and constrained (*one prison to another*) if he is to find the possibility of forms of free movement in the society in which he lives.

What is described here is something more than other intra-psychic and interpersonal notions of projection, transference or hypervigilance. This is a terrorised mode of existing: *the terror that we will not find a path towards a mode of existing, which would enable us to find courage in the moonlit darkness of the night, and walk proudly in the light of day.* In some ways, being with the horror of the other (i.e. staying with being horrified by the actions of the other) is a more comforting mode, as the locus of the confrontation seemingly emerges from the other and loses sight of the intersubjective intercorporeality of our existence.

Building on this, the incorporation of existential horror and terror into a mode of existing is a temporal-spatial one, in that the emerging (*existential horror*) and arising (*existential terror*) are movements situated within intersubjective lived experience.[3] This explains the ways in which existential horror and terror become sedimented in our modes of existing: through the features of *horrification* and *terrorisation*. These features of horrification and terrorisation are incorporated into the ways we understand ourselves, other people and our relationships with the world around us. To be horrified at the way people treat each other, or to be terrorised by the idea of relating to other people, is also to be existentially horrified and terrorised by our own sedimented experience of trauma, the embodied, relational memory of it and at the same time the ways in which we have disillusioned or re-illusioned ourselves. In short, *our existential horror and terror are at the same time our own, and dispersed through the anticipated prospect of all forms of human relating and modes of existing.*

The movement between our existential horror and terror are what the existential philosopher and psychotherapist van Deurzen (2010: 138) might describe as 'onto-dynamics'. These are the polarities and paradoxes that are at the heart of our existence and disclose 'the values […] towards which we are pulled, or from which we are pushed away' (ibid.). Rather than seeking to dismiss or to resolve the tensions between our values, van Deurzen encourages us to use personal reflection and therapeutic spaces to confront the conflicts, polarities and contradictions continued within them. From this, we can use these tensions to understand our modes of living before our experience of trauma, during it, and our modes of existing that may emerge for the future (building on ibid.: 141). van Deurzen continues that it is the movement within the field between these opposing forces that creates the tension, space and motivation for living. As such, we can understand the oscillation between the extremities of the polarities of existential horror and terror as representing the movement between gaining and losing perspectives and meanings in our lives. Also, it suggests that this movement enables discoveries of new modes of existing.

So here again we see the temporal-spatial dimension of traumatic experiencing. Existential horror and terror remind us that the movement need not be linear in direction, and can oscillate between re-illusionment and disillusionment, and different modes of existing. The existential movement of terror and horror is as shaky as the rage we feel, as frozen as the numbness we contend with, as circular as the spiralling overwhelm of the memories or daydreams we have. In this, there is some semblance here with my own critique of Kierkegaard's (2008 [1849]) description of despair and hope (Bush [Boaz], 2018a), and people's experiences of the COVID-19 pandemic (Bush [Boaz], 2020b). In my paper on despair and hope (Bush [Boaz], 2018a), I suggest that it is the oscillation between hope and despair (and what I call a resulting attitude of *(de)spero*) that enables people to find an expansive awareness, meaning and purpose in their life.

Within the oscillating movement of the onto-dynamics created by existential horror and terror we are caught in a world of tensions. As such, to find an orientation within the tension, we sometimes must have the bravery to confront the reality of the horror of a traumatising other, in order to escape the terrorising anticipation of an infinitised and hypothecated threat towards our existence from them. At other times we must turn from the horror of the other and the reality of their mode of existence, in order to be terrified by the prospect of remaining in full relation to them, and use this to find an alternative mode of relating to them and others.

Dispersement and liminality

To extend my description above, experiences of existential horror and terror seem to be less about the anxieties of death or nothingness (contra terror management theory and anxiety buffer disruption theory,[4] see Arnold & Pinkston, 2014; Laing, 1972 [1959]; Sartre, 2003 [1943]), and more about the experiential reality of existing between modes. In this sense, I believe it is more productive to think of our primordial state as being a modal dispersement, rather than existing in relation to our finitude. I will briefly describe what I mean by modal dispersement; however, I will refrain from a deeper exploration as it is beyond the scope of this book and it will no doubt be the subject of future inquiry.

We could conceive of the foundation of our existence as *primordial dispersement*. That is, we emerge from dispersed matter (a non-personalised, abstracted, yet symbiotic and interactive cosmos) and return to this mode in a state of death and decay – following in the Epicurean proposition. As David Abram (2011: 230) describes, our bodies are a 'sensitive threshold through which the world experiences itself'. Thus, we, and the world in which we are generatively situated, are modally transformed and metamorphosed in the interweaving movements before, during and after the modal states we think of as lived human experience. Death anxiety and existential confrontations with finitude are just one manifestation of existential concerns relating to primordial dispersement. I am not seeking to deny the facticity of our death, nor dismissing the central role that ideas about finitude play in our modes of existing. Rather, I am aiming to contextualise our experiences of death and finitude within a broader foundational existential structure of primordial dispersement

The existential psychiatrist Yalom considered for a moment our primordial dispersement; however, he later turned away from it, finding it a discomforting thought and preferring to focus his attention on the anxiety of death and finitude (see his discussion in Yalom, 2011 [2008]). Despite this, Yalom reflects on death as a form of dispersement in noting that after our death, we leave intercorporeal traces of ourselves (and our actions) in the ongoing present moments of the world. Yalom calls this phenomenon *rippling*, which he describes as

> the fact that each of us creates – often without conscious intent or knowledge – concentric circles of influence that may affect others for years, even generations. That is, the effect we have on other people is in turn passed on to others, much as the ripples in a pond go on and on until they're no longer visible but continue at a nano level.
>
> (Ibid.: 83)

Frankl (2020 [1946]: 52) similarly echoes the sensing of our dispersement beyond the facticity of our death in stating that 'what we "radiate" into the world, [are] the "waves" that emanate from our being, that is what will remain of us when our being itself has long since passed'.

The reason for the inclusion of the idea of primordial dispersement is that traumatic experiencing brings us into close proximity with the reality of our possibility of dispersement. It is for this reason that the experiences of trauma, and the subsequent movements, disclose many forms of being *between* modes of existing. Being *between* modes could also be termed *liminality*.[5] Through traumatic situations we incorporate our experience of liminality into our modes of existing, and the more liminality we encounter in our interanimality, intercorporeality and inter-world, the greater the intensification within our modes of existing. The experience of liminality (existing-between-worlds) is a foundational feature of our movement within and between modes, and without it we seek to singularise our mode into something that seems fixed, concrete, immovable and unmoved by our experiences. Needless to say, liminality bears some resemblance to both the Freudian (1955 [1919]) and

Heideggerian (2010 [1953]) notions of uncanniness (*Unheimlichkeit*). We could see how unexplainable shaking or psychogenic seizures (within the liminality of exist- ential terror and horror) fit well with Freud's (1955 [1919]: 226) description of the uncanniness of the seemingly mechanical animation of the person.[6] That said, the focus I have placed on being between modes of existing as a form of liminal uncanniness is beyond the intended use within Freud's or Heidegger's conceptions.

The radical object-oriented philosopher Timothy Morton (2019) describes a spectral phenomenology, which might incorporate the dispersement and lim- inality of our existence. He writes that 'we coexist *with* and *as* ghosts, specters, zombies, undead beings and other ambiguous [and uncanny] entities [...] nonhumans, including the "nonhuman" aspects of ourselves' (ibid.: 54–55, 61– 67, 72, 90, original emphasis). What he terms our 'symbiotic real' (akin to a worldly intercorporeality) gives rise to an uncertain ontological status, a new onto- logical understanding that blurs the visibility and invisibility of phenomena, which to encounter is both horrific and beautiful to us (ibid.: 66–69; see also Baldwin, 2017 [1963]: 84). The ontological uncertainty of the spectrality of our existence is in itself perceived as ontologically 'dangerous', 'disturbing' and/or 'amazing' by some people (Morton, 2019: 76).

The reality of our composite existence is so monstrous for some, that we re- illusion ourselves to perceives ourselves and our bodies as a singularity, and thus to limit the sensing of our primordial, symbiotic interdependency (dispersement). Foundational re-illusionment in the face of primordial (symbiotic) dispersement aids us in describing re-illusionment as a protective mode of surviving the reality of our existence. A full confrontation with the reality of our dispersement might evoke the existential anxiety of becoming a dispersed being. Rather than this being an aspirational state of nirvana, it could lead to so-called 'psychotic' abstractions of all grounding and meaningful experiencing of a comprehensible reality and modal worldview. Spectral phenomenology offers another dimension in our understandings of how modes of disillusionment and re-illusionment incorporate our confrontations with reality – to the extent to which we can tolerate our prox- imity to the confronting (perhaps affronting) reality.

We can apply my extension of Morton's spectral phenomenology more spe- cifically to inquire about the symbiotic reality of our spectral existence within the movements of interpersonal trauma. The symbiotic reality of interpersonal trauma is disclosed in, for example, the transmission of sexually transmitted infections (STIs) or viruses that can haunt the immunity of our cellularity in the wake of sexual violence or abuse. Further, it can be seen in the aforementioned impacts of trauma on our immunoendocrinological (c.f. Sherin & Nemeroff, 2011) and autonomic nervous systems (c.f. proposals by Porges, 2009, 2011). In a more explicit way, non-human animals can be figural in the spectral haunting of inter- personal trauma. If one considers, for example, the case of torturous, inhumane and degrading treatment, we can see spectral interanimality expressed in sleep deprivation through the use of barking dogs; their saliva mixing with the fear and sweat of a detainee, and the heat the dogs transmit, which is in turn transmitted to the detainee. Likewise, spectral interanimality is disclosed through the stress this places on the ecology of our own human system, the biphasic releases of our endogenous biochemistry, the more hostile environment this creates for our own microbiome, the nausea that ensues as the waves of spectral movement radiate through our mode of existence. In this way, interpersonal trauma sits at the nexus of our intercorporeal interanimality, and brings us into confrontation with our spectrality – *of being between modes of existence and worlds of experience.*

The queer phenomenologist Sara Ahmed (2006a; 2006b) would remind us that existing between worlds as liminal or spectral beings is not negative modality. It can bring joy, discovery, excitement, liberation and close connection with other liminal peoples, non-human animals and environments (echoed in other terms by Stolorow, 2007). Indeed, we can see how liminality, and the experience of existential horror and terror, awakens our primordial impulsion to philosophise, to make meaning out of our incorporeality, liminality and to find the kind of person we want to become – albeit within constricted and limited situations. Following Ahmed (2006a) and Jaspers (2003 [1954]), this can give rise to awe and wonderment at the terrible actualities and horrific possibilities of human existence, imaginations and the fundamental nature of relationships. Paradoxically, we can glimpse here that the horror, terror, fear, awe, wonderment of traumatic experiencing can all give rise to the primordial impulsion to philosophise what Jaspers (2003 [1954]) describes, and thus direct or guide us towards finding the kind of person we want to be and become.

Queer turns and modal movements

Ahmed's (2006a) queer phenomenology offers us a deeper perspective on the movements of disillusionment and re-illusionment emerging from the traumatic confrontation(s) of reality. She suggests that our bodies are not merely objects in the world; rather, we embody a point of view moving through the world, interrelated to other corporeal entities (human and non-human alike). In the language of Ahmed, traumatic experiencing is a disorientation of our embodied movement through the world. Extending her proposition, the paradoxical movement of trauma and the confrontation with reality is its queering potential to shake us out of any given modality we have been existing within and between (ibid.: 19). As a queering liminal experience of being-between-worlds and modalities, our horizons of movement are opened up and expanded (albeit disconcertingly in existential horror and terror) beyond our known experience of the world.

Here we come to understand that at the foundation of modes of existing is the human movement of turning. Our ability to turn in different orientations and across different planes of experiencing enables the generative movement of modes of existence. Turning here is not just a physical movement but an existential one. Existentially, turning opens up new horizons of experiencing and offers the possibility of new modes. As Ahmed notes (ibid.: 15), 'depending on which way one turns, different worlds might even come into view. If such turns are repeated over time, then bodies acquire the very shape of such direction'. Further, she astutely suggests that

> moments [of] disorientation are vital. They are bodily experiences that throw the world up, or throw the body from its ground. Disorientation as a bodily feeling can be unsettling, and it can shatter one's sense of confidence in the ground or one's belief that the ground on which we reside can support the actions that make a life feel livable. Such a feeling of shattering, or of being shattered, might persist and become a crisis. Or the feeling itself might pass as the ground returns or as we return to the ground. The body might be reoriented if the hands reach out and find nothing, and might grasp instead the indeterminacy of the air. The body in losing its support might then be lost, undone, thrown.
>
> (Ibid.: 157)

Following Ahmed (ibid.), and Frantz Fanon (2004 [1961], 2008 [1952]) before her, I propose that disorientation is only problematic if it is seen from a more Westernised notion of the linear directionality of human movement and modes of existing. If we see human movement as being founded on our capacity to move between worlds of experiencing, turning and opening up new horizons of modalities, then disorientation can be seen in a valuable and existential light. Re-illusionment is a (re)turn to (re)orientating into a known mode of existing. Disorientation is a part of the disillusionment we experience in the traumatic confrontation with reality because it turns away from the illusion that we are linear beings. From the modal existentialist perspective, our quality of movement at the foundations of human experiencing is described as turning, spinning, spiralling, rolling and any other descriptor that discloses our capacities and possibilities for (re)(dis)covering new horizons and modes of existing. As Ahmed (2006a: 16) similarly notes, opening up our movement and following the unexpected line 'gives us the chance for a new direction and even a chance to live again [a generative mode of existence]'. In this framing, psychogenic movements are also queering, in that they are a revising of both our sensing of spectral and dispersed existence, and our attempts at turning to new horizons of experiencing modal movement.

Given my reformulation of Ahmed's description of orientation and disorientation, how might modal existentialism understand the relationships between (dis)orientation and (dis)illusionment within the context of a traumatic confrontation with reality? I propose that *orientation* is a movement and (re)turn towards modes that resonated before the traumatic confrontation with reality, and thus re-orientation is a quality of re-illusionment. Re-illusionment is an attempt to re-orientate back to the previous mode of existing, or one that incorporates similar movements and directionality. In contrast, *disorientation* is a movement which emerges out of the disillusionment of a traumatic confrontation with reality. Disorientation incorporates attempts to generatively create new horizons of experiencing and modes of existing, which incorporate the reality that has been confronted through the trauma. Finally, *(dys)orientation* is a movement drawing upon pathologising ideas about traumatic confrontations with reality and attempts to use psychiatric and medical modes of existing to incorporate the experience into an existing or new mode. As indicated in the earlier section on kind-making, this can be an agentic and generative modal identity; however, it relies on contra-positioning and repositioning to retain its movements.

This formulation might seem strange to some, as in psychiatric, psychological and psychotherapeutic literature disorientation is usually characterised as problematic and a sign of existing or emerging psychopathological experience. The paradox in my description of it here is that it is a quality of (dis)covery of new horizons and modes of experiencing. Thus, to find new movements, we have to move through a process of (dis)orientation. Queerly, for some of us this might be an easier movement as the society and cultures we find ourselves in were never orientated to modes of existing that resonated with us or incorporated our modes of existing. For others, the movement will be the lostness, undoing and thrownness Ahmed describes, as there is no known horizon of experiencing or permissive culture around them to provide the ground for movement (see also Fanon, 2004 [1961], 2008 [1952]). This will heighten the queer liminality of their movements and turns.

Using the word 'horizon' here is problematic as it brings to mind a horizontal line. Freeing ourselves from the linearity of a two-dimensional horizon, we can begin to understand the horizons of human experiences. Even taken from the perspective of our planetary location, we move on a moving sphere turning, spinning, rotating, circulating on its relational orbit. If in reading this, the movements and sounds of a Sufi whirling (or turning) dervish comes to mind, you are sensing an embodied representation and expression of what our existential movement might look like.

Finally, the queering qualities of movements and modes of existing bring us to re-examine the seeming singularity of confrontations with reality. Even in the earlier accounts of developmental or cumulative trauma, the generative iteration of the relational encounters is flattened in the pursuit of a descriptive singularity for child sexual abuse, domestic violence, torturous treatment and so on. Ahmed (2006a: 39) asks us to consider the 'ethno-phenomenological' question of:

> How did I or we arrive at the point where it is possible to witness the arrival of the object? How is the arrival a form of witnessing in which 'what arrives' becomes a 'what' only in the event of being apprehended as a 'what'?

In the case of traumatic experiencing, this leads me to ask what is being encountered in the intercorporeal enactment of interpersonal trauma. A singularised and atomised account of the enactment might conclude that it is just the confrontation with traumatic reality of the other in the moment of experience. Taking a more meta-phenomenological stance, might not the confrontation generatively incorporate all previously encountered confrontations in the person's life?

This question might sound abstract, so let us consider a more tangible example. The re-enactment of previous experiences is common in interpersonal cycles of violence, albeit in new and elaborated forms of action. For illustrative purposes, let us take the example of rape, where an adult who has been abused in childhood, sexually attacks another person. It is the attacked person who encounters the arrival of another adult within the traumatic event of a sexual assault, and witnesses their arrival intercorporeally through the proximal-relational act. The attacked adult can phenomenologically apprehend the experience of the sexual assault in the moments of enactment. Whether they comprehend the enactment as the *what* of *sexual assault* depends on the extent to which ethnologically they understand the significance of the experienced act. Further, to apprehend ethnologically the *what* of the *sexually assaulting adult* is to *turn* to a horizon beyond the present foreground of enactment, that is, to see the confrontations with reality that are disclosed in the movement of the adult, which led to their arrival in the encounter.

The background (previous modal movements) leading to the attacking adult's arrival is their incorporation of a mode of existing in relation to their own experiences of child abuse, which involves their own witnessing of the arrival of a sexually assaulting adult. It is unlikely that a child, let alone an adult, can apprehend the arriving 'what' that they are witnessing. The partiality of their apprehension confers an ambiguity as to the phenomenological experience of the arriving other. In this way, personal histories are spectral, in that they are 'behind the arrival of "the what" that surfaces' (ibid.: 44). So, what arrives in a traumatic confrontation with reality is also a liminal spectre of the generative and genealogical embodiment of multiple confrontations with reality. The traumatising person is not merely arriving into our awareness through the enactment, but spectrally interweaving and possibly inter-merging our modally sedimented confrontations with reality.

On confrontations and turning with reality

As I have described, our confrontations with traumatic reality are imbued with existential horror and terror. Existential horror and terror emerge and arise from the opening up of the reality of our existence. They are compounded by the ensuing incomprehension and disorientation, which obscures the totality of reality being confronted. The incomprehensibility and disorientation within confrontations with reality relate in part to our individual or collective human capacity to comprehend the complex movements of all *that is*. We lack the ability to comprehend the confronted reality even when we use our tools of modal expression (technologies, philosophising, social institutions etc.) in attempts to make sense of it. That said, through modes of existing we can incorporate foundational movements that bring us closer to comprehending the reality of existence. In this way, each unique mode of existence and confrontation with reality discloses a specific feature, quality and structure of our existence.

At this point in the book, I do not intend to walk in the philosophical marshland that is an inquiry into the nature of reality. Some readers might be frustrated by my lack of definition of the totality of reality (all *that is*). For me, the lack of definition is an important feature of existential modalism, as it enables us to inquire phenomenologically into the lived and enacted consequences of more constricted, and expansive, horizons of experiencing. As such, I propose that *confrontations with reality* is an existential-phenomenological and descriptive term. It refers to the quality of the feature of reality that is being confronted through an interpersonal experience. Descriptively, we could inquire about the ways in which interpersonal trauma(s) brings about confrontations with dimensions of existence. These dimensions include the following:

- *Personal reality*: the lived, embodied and experienced worldview of the person, realised and enacted through their mode(s) of existing. Personal reality is not an atomised individuality. *Personal*, in this formulation, refers to the agentic movements I make in my mode(s) of existing – even when they emerge in dialogue with a proximate or imagined other(s) or world around me.
- *Intersubjective reality*: the co-created experiences, enactments and meanings of the person in relation to known and/or proximate others through the simultaneity and intercorporeality of their modes of existing.
- *Contextual reality*: the sociocultural and political laws (formal or informal), rules, attitudes, narratives, myths and behaviours that generatively govern, give reference(s) and meaning(s) to our interpersonal enactments, experiences and mode(s) of existing.
- *Dispersed existence*: the incomprehensible, dispersed and generative features, qualities and totalities of all *that is*, which are disclosed through, within and between modes of existing and our tools of modal expression.

The dimensions set out above are purely descriptive. I hesitate to call the above categorisations *dimensions*, as the term communicates some form of verticalisation of reality, and the notion there is separability between dimensions. The dimensions are, like our intercorporeality, intertwined and generatively co-creating and shaping our experience of them as we participate in the dance (modal movements) of reality. Another way of thinking about this is that we all modally glimpse different features and qualities of reality depending on the specific lived confrontation of reality we have, and our modal response(s) to it. The experience of these dimensions by the person varies significantly according to their own situatedness, and is more or less constricted or expanded according to the modal movements and horizons of experience they are about to turn towards/away from.

When we attempt to incorporate confrontations with reality into modes of experiencing, we engage in disillusionary and re-illusionary turns. These turns bring into existence more descriptive experiential-dimensions of reality within, and between, the four dimensions described above. I do not intend here to provide an extensive or exhaustive list of disillusionary and re-illusionary turns to incorporate the confronted reality. By way of illustration, in my earlier discussions I have explored four existential turns that can emerge out of confrontation(s) with reality. The first is the experience of *queer realities*, which is the incorporation of lived spectral, liminal and existential movements and turns within, and between, our modes of existing. The second is *irreality*, where we incorporate the shock or shaking of confrontation(s) of reality into our modes of existing, and all our subsequent experiences of reality are felt to be on shaky foundations. The third is *unreality*, where our modes of existing incorporate the incomprehensibility of the confronted reality through experiencing oneself, others or the world around us as being not of a known reality. The fourth is *surreality* or an *ab-reality*, where we attempt to incorporate the incomprehensibility of our confrontation(s) with reality into our mode(s) of existence, though embracing our impulsion to philosophise about the nature of our reality and the structure of human existence.

What are descriptively considered to be *queer, irreal, unreal, surreal* and *ab-real* experiential-dimensions of reality are contingent on the situatedness of the person (and their mode of existence) within the society, culture and historical period in which they live(d). As such, the extent to which a modal incorporation of confrontations with reality can be intersubjectively described as disillusionary and re-illusionary is contingent on the situatedness of the person. This re-emphasises the importance of working phenomenologically with clients to open up their descriptions of their confrontations with reality, the movements and turns they have made to incorporate (disillusion or re-illusion) themselves in relation to it.

Modes of existence emerge generatively within the relational confrontation with the reality of the other. The intersubjective intercorporeality of our situatedness provides ground for our comprehension of reality, and our disillusionary and re-illusionary turns and movements. Frankl suggests that reality is always relational. He writes that,

> only when one aspect of reality is counterposed to something different does either come into being. Anything real, that is, requires as a precondition the reality of something other than itself. 'To be' equals 'to be different' – that is, 'to be different from something'; relationship is supremely important. Actually, only the relationship 'exists'. We might therefore state it this way: all this has its being only with reference to something else. Differences in states of being, however, can be simultaneous, or can follow one another.
>
> (Frankl, 1986 [1946]: 5n)

For me, Frankl is describing here the dynamics of generative modal movement within interpersonal trauma. The traumatic confrontation expands the horizons of experience to the extent that the relationality with the other becomes the anchor for our experience of reality (to borrow from Längle, 2007). Our initial modal movements of disillusionment and re-illusionment incorporate to differing extents the perceived difference of the modality of the other.

Paradoxically, the modal movements of relational difference also possibly explain why some people experience non-traumatic relationships as re-traumatising confrontations. In a non-traumatic relationship, the person is confronted with another kind of other, one who is different in their mode of existence to the known traumatising kind of person. As such, the paradoxical impact is that the difference between the traumatising and non-traumatising other becomes a new confrontation of the reality of modal possibilities, and thus can reify the modal response of the traumatised person. In some situations, the person can be more distressed by the confrontation with non-traumatising others (*the realisation that other knowable people, and the knowable world, need not be traumatising*), than staying in relation to a traumatising other. For some people, moving into a world with more expansive horizons and modal expression, can be experienced as so real that is feels irreal (*disillusioned*) to the person. This has been the case for clients who have grown up in constricted, coercive and controlled environments (such as closed religious communities or neglectful families).

Reality-denying and reality-augmenting systems

An investigation of cultural trauma and its relationships to human social systems is beyond the scope of this book. That said, it is important to bring our attention to the inter-systemic features of interpersonal trauma. Human systems (i.e. societies, cultures, political movements, institutions, religion, communities and families) and their modal expressions (i.e. technologies, social media memes, land use, public discourse) are created to govern, discipline, recreate and maintain *practices of reality* (expanding on Foucault, 1979, 2009 [1961]). Practices of reality are a plurality of competing hegemonic and countercultural modes of existing that are generatively co-created and articulated through formal (institutionalised) and informal (networked) enactments.

As social actors we agentically participate in the generative movements and collective modalities of human systems. I write 'the plural of modalities', as it is more astute to describe human systems as a dynamic dance of disillusionments and re-illusionments to multiple and simultaneous confrontations of personal, intersubjective, contextual reality, and dispersed existence. Our own attempts to incorporate traumatic confrontations with reality into modes of existing interweave (between, within, against, beyond) this dynamic dance of *reality-denying* and *reality-augmenting* systems. Just like our own confrontations with reality, human systems (and their collective tools of modal expression) generatively engage in competing modes of disillusionment and re-illusionment when confronted by reality. As we personally turn within our confrontations with reality, so too do our human systems turn, spin and generatively roll across the ground of our dispersed existence to (re)(dis)cover new horizons of possible existence, or (re)cover older modes of movement.

As our human systems turn away from the multiple confrontations with reality, it creates permissive (re-illusioned) movements that enable interpersonal trauma to emerge. This can clearly be seen in the example of institutional abuse of children and young people within religious organisations and residential school settings. In the United Kingdom, independent inquiries have demonstrated how institutional movements enabled the covering and (re)covering of child sexual abuse, and the myriad of sociocultural policies, behaviours, practice, power and modes of related that permissively enabled this (Independent Inquiry into Child Sexual Abuse, 2018, 2020a, 2020b, 2020c).

At a systemic level, modes of re-illusionment include substantial modal efforts to cover and re-cover traumatic confrontations and experiences. We need only refer back to earlier chapters of this book to see the consequences of Freud's turn away from the reality of traumatic experiences on subsequent psychoanalytic and psychotherapeutic theory and practice. Miller's (1984 [1981]) investigations describe how traumatising adults in a child's life attempt to reverse the reality of a situation, in order to justify their traumatic enactments. Bowlby (2005 [1988]), Freyd (1996, 1994) and Allen et al. (2008) all note the ways in which a child (through the encouragement of adults) would augment their reality in order to maintain trust and relationality with a caregiver. Winnicott (2018a [1965]), on the other hand, demonstrates how a traumatising adult could expose a child to both the overwhelming reality of a situation and their existence. Herman (with Hirschman, 1981), alongside many feminist scholars, provided detailed accounts of the ways in which families created cultures of silence to avoid and deny traumatic realities and situations. The intersubjective modal responses explored above are all examples of reality-denial and reality-augmentation within an extended family system. The modal expressions of secrecy and coercion are ways of retaining illusions and re-illusioning a system, to turn away from (deny or avoid) or soften (augment) the confrontation with a traumatic reality.

By way of illustration, we can delve further into existential formulations of traumatic confrontations within the idea of family. Through exploring these contributions, we might understand more about systemic disillusionary and re-illusionary turns.[7] The existential psychiatrists Laing and Aaron Esterson (1974 [1964]) propose that in addition to the interpersonal relationships of a family, we all have an internalised 'family'. This internalised 'family' holds in our mind the roles, personalities, physicality, emotionality and relationships between the family members (Laing, 1976 [1969]: 3). The Laingian internalised model of the 'family' is not substantively different to the intersubjective working models of Bowlby (1973) or the organising principles of Stolorow and Atwood (2002 [1992]), and incorporates the modes of mentalising and epistemic trust described by the mentalisation theorists (Luyten & Fonagy, 2019). In modal existentialism, the described internalisation is a generative incorporation of the reality of our intersubjective intercorporeality into a mode of existence.

Laing (1976 [1969]: 13) suggests that a family crisis occurs within a family if any member attempts to remove themselves from this internal idea of the 'family', or their place within it. In his case description, Laing identifies the movements family members make in order to avoid a crisis in the family and the 'family'. The modal experience of a 'family' has a hold over members because it holds significance for their existence. As Laing (1971 [1961]: 136) writes, 'every human being, whether child or adult, seems to require significance, that is, place in another person's world'. When a traumatic situation disrupts a person's modal placement within a family system, the family attempts to defend against this disruption (Laing, 1985 [1965]). Transpersonal defences are where one person 'attempts to regulate the inner life [or modes of existing] of the other in order to preserve his or her own' (Laing, 1976 [1969]: 12).

Transpersonal defences are examples of reality-denial and reality-augmentation within family systems. Defences identified by Laing include 'invalidation', or the denial of people's lived experiences and perceptions. In many of the cases he (Esterson and the team) worked with, traumatic realities within family life were both denied by some family members and/or rendered signs of mental illness of a specific family member (usually the one who had been traumatised). 'Invalidation' in the Laingian sense means both undermining the reality of a situation and turning the person into an 'invalid' (Laing, 1971 [1961]: 144–148; 1976 [1969]: 61–68). In rendering a traumatised person's reality and personhood invalid, the family is able to sustain both the family and the 'family'. Movements of invalidation are sustained through modal collusion. Modal collusion is where allegiances are reciprocally formed (intersubjectively incorporated within modes of existing) to maintain the stability of a family/'family' system and find ways of both partially covering and recognising the reality of the family relations and traumatic encounters with reality contained within the system (Laing, 1972 [1959]: 97–105; 1976 [1969]: 92–111).

In addition to invalidation and collusion, family members can enact 'mystification[s] of experience' (Laing, 1976 [1969]: 86; see also 1985 [1965]). Mystification is the purposeful intersubjective 'misdefinition' of the reality of a situation through 'befuddl[ing], cloud[ing], obscur[ing], mask[ing] whatever is going on, whether this experience, action, or process, or whatever is the issue' (Laing, 1976 [1969]: 29, 86; see also 1990 [1967]: 25). At the extremity, mystification involves the active inducement of a mystified mode of existence, where the person is highly confused and disorientated about their experiences, memories and actions (following Laing, 1985 [1965]). We can see how the disillusionment (disorientation) involved in traumatic confrontations with reality can be heightened through the family, inducing further modal spinning through the enactment of mystification.

Through mystification, family members are able to work on the traumatised person's sense of reality, using verbal and non-verbal invalidations to co-construct denials and augmentations of the confrontations that have been experienced. The label of mental illness enables increased permissiveness among family members to locate the reality-denial or reality-augmentation within the dysfunction of an individual, rather than within the systemic intersubjective worldviews of family members (in relation to the family/'family'). Expressions asserting reality, autonomy and personhood by the traumatised person are frequently met with escalating enactments of discipline and punishment by family members. This is especially the case where the traumatised person attempts to confront the family/'family' with the reality of their situation, and trauma that has occurred within a family system (following Laing, 1971 [1961]: 54; 1976 [1969]: 13).

In the face of reality-denial and reality-augmentation, the traumatised person[8] is confronted with an existential dilemma about whether they can create modes of existing that expand beyond the horizons of those of the immediate family/'family' (building on Laing, 1972 [1959]): 54). Extending on from Laing, the queering potential of traumatic confrontations can (through disillusionment) leave us turning from one horizon to another. For Laing, the existential turns are typified by a dilemma over whether or not one can maintain the integrity of the 'family' or 'destroy' it through generative modal movements. The three turns Laing identified are whether (a) we must sacrifice ourselves (and our reality) to the 'family'; (b) the 'family' will destroy us (and our reality); or (c) we can destroy the 'family' without destroying ourselves (and our reality) (following Laing, 1976 [1969]: 13, see also 85–91).

Laing and Esterson (1974 [1964]) extend Gregory Bateson et al.'s (1978 [1956]) formulation of the *double-bind* to describe how people diagnosed with schizophrenia are systematically positioned in the face of familial reality-denial and reality-augmentation to either (a) choose to concede their reality and maintain the role the family/'family' demands of them, or (b) lose their sense of reality and become 'mad' for the family. I would extend Laing and Esterson's descriptions by drawing attention to specific reoccurring modal responses that I have witnessed both in my clinical work and in conversations with people about their experiences of interpersonal trauma. The first is the mobilisation of what I term *convenient truths*. Convenient truths are truth claims made by people who are attempting to retain their personhood when confronted by invalidation or mystification by other members of the family. Convenient truths are explanatory mechanisms to communicate a simultaneous compliance and rejection of the family's attempts at reality-augmentation.

These truth statements include a person agentically enacting an invalidation (a diagnosed label of post-traumatic stress disorder (PTSD), conduct disorder, autism or attention deficit hyperactivity disorder (ADHD), for example) to explicitly name and confront the family with the reality of situation, without it having to be fully addressed or incorporated by the family system. In turn, the family system increases its tolerance for the person's expressions of reality, without having to acknowledge that the intersubjective position emerges from the traumatised person's need to stay more proximate to the experienced reality. I have seen the use of physical and chemical restraint to silence and regulate the amount of reality confrontation that a human system (or a person within it) can tolerate. The augmented displacement of reality (into the convenient truth of the traumatised person's *madness*) is used as the basis for systemic intervention and control. As such, this represents a mode of existing to survive within confined and constructed human systems. Similar convenient truths operate in situations where the reality-augmentation is located in the traumatised person's pain (*sadness*) or modal expressions (*badness*).

Some model movements result in the traumatised person losing their sense of reality and experiencing themselves, others and the world around them as unreal and irreal (following Laing, 1972 [1959]: 26–28, 47, 52, 69, 77, 85, 145; 1990 [1967]: 18, 26–27). Laing (1972 [1959]: 80) poignantly notes that if the person continues to experience themselves and their world as unreal or irreal, they come to feel 'persecuted by reality itself. The world as it is, and the people as they are, are the dangers' – that is, the denial and augmentation of reality come as a greater threat to them than confronting the traumatic reality of their experience. Extending this analysis, Laing (1990 [1967]: 95) concludes that 'without

exception the experience and behaviour that gets labelled schizophrenic is a special strategy that a person invents in order to live in an unliveable situation'. For
this reason, Laing's advice to existential psychotherapists is to avoid colliding with
the either the 'illusionment or disillusionment' of a family's reality-denying and
reality-augmenting, but rather to focus on articulating the underlying threats
perceived by the family/'family' in confronting the reality of a situation (Laing,
1971 [1961]: 123).

The existential psychotherapists and social workers Jim Lantz and Jacquelyn
Gyamerah [Meshelemiah] take a different stance on how implicated the psychotherapist should be in challenging a family system's reality-denying and
reality-augmenting defences. From a Franklian logotherapeutic perspective, they
characterise the reality of traumatic situations as posing an existential threat to a
family system, and the networked intersubjective meaning-making permeating it.
Lantz and Meshelemiah (2002: 243–255) define trauma, in the family context, as
any situation or experience that disrupts a family system's dimensions of existence
of, *in* and *for* the world. These three existential dimensions of the family build on
the ideas of Frankl (1986 [1946], 1988, 2004 [1959]).

The family system *must* relate to the bio-physical facticity of existence. As
embodied beings *of the world*, they must consume water and food, and attend to
their acute and chronic ill health. Existing *in the world*, family members have some
level of freedom and choice over their proactive and reactive choices. Members of
a family system *can* use their intentionality and limited freedom to choose the ways
in which they agentically respond to a situation or experience within the family
or wider world. Existing *for* the world, family members *find meaning and purpose* in
taking care of each other, other people in their community and the wider environment in which they live.

Lantz and Meshelemiah describe the ways in which family systems defend
themselves against the recognition of traumatic confrontations with reality.
These defences include specific intersubjective relational patterns of 'covering',
'clouding' or 'repressing' the pain and terror that have been experienced by one
or more of the family members (Lantz & Meshelemiah, 2002: 246–247; see also
Lantz & Lantz, 1991: 63). Echoing the observations of Laing, and Stolorow and
Atwood, defensive patterns are precipitated by the family's inability to tolerate the
emotional pain of traumatic confrontations (within or beyond the family), and
thus family members seek to distance themselves from it.

Paradoxically, the attempts to defend the family system from the awareness
of traumatic confrontations (and the intolerability of the pain associated with
them) result in fundamental disruptions in the family's existence *of*, *in* and *for* the
world. The existential disruption occurs from the turning away (re-illusionment)
of the family system from the traumatic reality. For Jim Lantz and Jan Lantz
(1992: 305–306), the disruption emerges from a familial unknowing that our
potential for new meanings and deeper familial intimacy *emerges out of the traumatic
confrontation with the reality of a situation and the associated pain and terror arising from it*.
This is an important description, and the turn towards reality-denial and reality-
augmentation can be understood as both a family system, and the traumatised

person(s), actively (consciously or non-consciously) avoiding the expansive meanings, modal movements and horizons of experiencing that can emerge out of familial disillusionment.

Lantz's existential family trauma therapy (EFTT) aims to directly address the familial patterns of defence against the reality of traumatic experiences. This is achieved through the participatory co-creation of four interweaving phases of psychotherapeutic intervention: *holding up*, *telling*, *mastering* and *honouring* (see Lantz, 1993: 78–85; Lantz & Gregoire, 2000: 23–28, for application to combat trauma; see also Lantz, 2004 for a broader overview). First, the psychotherapist empathetically *holds up* the reality of the traumatic experience, so that it can be acknowledged, recognised, remembered and re-experienced by the family system. Lantz and Lantz (1991: 63; see also Lantz, 1991: 135–136) refer to this as the beginning of a process of 'existential reflection', which opens up the family members' confrontations with traumatic reality. Holding up the reality of the traumatic experience keeps the reality of the situation in view during the psychotherapeutic encounter(s). In doing this, the family is able to find its own ways of first approaching and confronting the reality of the situation, and the pain and terror related to it (Lantz & Meshelemiah, 2002: 247–248; for applications with individual clients see Lantz & Lantz, 1992: 301–304). While the movement described by Lantz and colleagues is a holding up, in practice the psychotherapeutic response bears a striking resemblance to Stolorow and Atwood's notion of *indwelling*, and deep intersubjective meetings to face together the reality of traumatic situations.

The EFTT practice of *telling*, builds on holding up, by explicitly naming the familial defences being used in the present moment to avoid awareness, recognition, pain or terror associated with the confrontation with reality. Through an increasing iteration of psychotherapeutic confrontations, the reality-denials and reality-augmentations are explicitly named by client(s) and psychotherapist. The psychotherapist, in Lantz's formulation of telling, is a queering spectre. As Bugental (1965: 84–85) notes:

> The therapist plays a unique role which is probably also tied in with the shaman […] the therapist is the one who names […] We need to recognise how potent this tool of naming names can be. The therapist is one who is seen as being unafraid to say the unsayable.

The naming brings the reality of the confrontation into the present moment of the psychotherapeutic relationship, and enables the client(s) and therapist to explore and address these defences as they arise (Lantz & Meshelemiah, 2002: 249).[9] Throughout the holding up and telling phases of EFTT, there is significant intersubjective testing of the psychotherapeutic ability to tolerate both the confrontation with reality and the intense feelings of pain and terror that will ensue (following Lantz & Lantz, 1991: 67–68; see also Lantz, 1991: 137–138).

Through the phases of holding up, and telling, the psychotherapist and client(s) can move to focus on *mastering* confrontation(s) with reality. Mastering means the active incorporation of traumatic experience through the experimentation with new modes of relationality within the family system (building on Lantz & Meshelemiah, 2002: 249). In the movement from holding up, through telling, to mastering, the existential concern moves from addressing disruptions in the *of* the world domain, to the *in* the world domain of the family. In experimenting with new agentic modes of (what I would term) disillusioned relationality, the family system opens up intersubjective space for greater expression of freedom, assertiveness, independence and intimacy (following ibid.; see also Lantz & Lantz, 1991, 69–70).

Finally, the family and EFTT psychotherapist can turn to *honouring* the family's confrontation with reality. This involves identifying, exploring and making meaning out of the traumatic experience (Lantz & Meshelemiah, 2002: 250; see also Lantz & Lantz, 1991: 70). The purposeful meaning-making is used as a psychotherapeutic process to transform the pain and terror of traumatic confrontations with reality into healing modes of existence, and increasingly expansive horizons of family experiencing and relational intimacy. As Lantz and Lantz (1991: 64) suggest, it is the meaning potentiality that is repressed through the family's and the person's defence against reality (see also Lantz, 1991: 133–134). Thus, in the EFTT phase of honouring, there is both a recovery of lost meanings and a generative incorporation and elaboration of new meanings. Lantz and Lantz (1992: 305) extend the honouring to incorporate an intentional celebration of the family's capacity to change – and in my terms to expand their horizons of experiencing and elaborate new modes of existing.

Queering systems and spectral turns

Finally, as both Laing and Lantz (1992) suggest, traumatic experiencing brings us into direct confrontation with the ideas, rules and practices (dominate systemic modes) that govern our human systems. Confronting the foundations of our intersubjective *and contextual reality* can bring about significant disillusionments with the ways our society is structured and governed. As we saw with those who elaborate modes of survivalism and survivorism, agentic and collective change become a purposeful and meaningful way to address the permissibility of interpersonal trauma within a contextual human system. In the Anglo-American context, for example, we are indebted to the courage of second-wave feminists who incorporated their own experiences of domestic violence, child sexual abuse, rape and assault to challenge the dominant legislative, cultural, psychological and institutional ideas, rules and practices that allowed (and at times encouraged) enactments of violence between people.

To exist within, and between, *contextual reality* is to queer it. The queering potential of traumatic confrontations with reality is disclosed in the person being simultaneously exposed to the constructions and illusions of existing systemic modes, and the possibility of new horizons of human systemic experiencing. To see the illusionary and re-illusionary movements of human systems is the ground on which to maintain, elaborate and disrupt them. Decentralising (or de-atomising) the confronting with reality from the traumatised person to the contextual reality, allows us to embrace the dispersement of human existence. Further, it provides an extension to my earlier consideration of Ahmed's (2006a: 39) ethno-phenomenological question of what it is we are witnessing as arriving (to meet our own arrival) in a traumatic confrontation. In the witnessing of our own dis-illusionment (*Ernüchterung* or sobering up) to the illusionary foundation of con-textual reality, though our confrontation with traumatic situations, we become aware of the liminal and spectral shadows moving behind, between and within the encounter.

These spectral shadows disclose the symbiotic nature of our reality, and the haunted intergenerational legacy of the modal movement and change within and between human systems. Being confronted with the polysystemic basis of modal movement and its generative elaboration can result in existential horror and terror. Many of the traumatised people I have worked with or spoken to (and myself included) find it intolerable and incomprehensible to participate in a contextual reality that permits interpersonal trauma. It is through agentic generative partici-pation in (or action against) the structures and rules that govern human systems that survivalists and survivorists find their purpose and meaning. Survivalists and survivorists incorporate the spectral shadows into modes of existing within human systems by bringing the haunting and liminal movements of systemic trauma into public awareness and consciousness.

While some might find solace in modes of existing that oscillate and turn within and between survivalism and survivorism, for others the disillusionment of contextual reality is too overwhelming. For these people, modes of existing that incorporate re-illusionments of their contextual reality allow them to rebuild modal expressions of trust, safety and benevolence (following Janoff-Bulman, 1992). Re-illusionment of contextual reality is an active turning towards responsi-bility, although an alternative modal expression to that elaborated in survivalism and survivorism. Responsibility in re-illusionment is a responsibility to become oneself within contextual contingencies and limitations; whereas, responsibility in disillusionment is a responsibility to expand the contextual horizons in which one can make modal movements that incorporate traumatic confrontations with reality.

Queer and liminal modalities are constantly described by clients using mythical states and beings that exist between and within worlds of experience. Extending Laing further, modes of existing that attempt to create distance between the traumatised person and the human or family system can give rise to existential-intersubjective binds. These include the liminal experience of dispersement of the family/'family'. People can become haunted simultaneously by the prospect of no contact from family members and terrorised by the prospect of being in relational contact. We might describe this experience as a mode of existing as a spectre in the family/'family', living between the imaginal, liminal and intersubjective worlds of the family system.

Contextual mythical, horrific and terror-inducing beings act as symbolic acknowledgements of intergenerational confrontations with the reality of trau-matic experiencing, and our human potential to re-turn to the modal horrors of our spectral shadows (building on my reading of the work of Jack Halberstam, 1995). Clients (and sometimes family members) describe themselves (or their relatives) as strange, weird, odd, alien and a freak within their social world. All these descriptions disclose modal incorporation of the liminality of being between worlds and modes of existing. With this in mind, we might explore the movements related to these social and systemic experiences: movements that are (a) unfamiliar and difficult to explain (*strange*), (b) moved (modally) by non-human intentionality (*weird*), (c) contra to the ordinary (*odd*), (d) seemingly of another (modal) world (*alien*), and (e) unexpected in a given situation (*freakish*). These modal movements are all disillusioned modes of existing that are attempting to incorporate confrontations with our primordial dispersement and our intersubjective interdependence.

When considered as movements, people who have seemingly strange, weird, odd and freakish modes of existing might evoke awe and wonderment and inspire new modes of existence and modal expressions in others. Psychotherapeutically, the queering potential of confrontations with contextual reality allow us to ask important phenomenological questions. Rather than assuming that reality-denial or reality-augmentation emerges from the traumatised person's own elaboration, we might inquire as to what is being generatively held on behalf of a human system by the person who has experienced the traumatic situation.

Notes

1 Laing (1971 [1961]: 82) adds in his description that 'collusion may consist of not recognising that there is an injunction for collusion, and not recognising that the enjoined collusion is not possible. In that one finds oneself not simply in conflict, but in such confusion that one does not know what the confusion is about and does not know that one does not know that one is confused'.

2 I have written about this haunting in relation to Heidegger and my own experience of intergenerational trauma elsewhere (Bush [Boaz], 2020a). For me, the incongruity between his formulation of 'Dasein' and the inauthenticity of his own life remain irreconcilable. In part, I follow Morton's (2018: 48, original emphasis) sentiment that 'de-Nazifying Heidegger actually means *being more Heideggerian than Heidegger*', although for me this means moving beyond his vocabulary and inauthenticity, using (where relevant) the work of others who have built upon, critiqued and expanded his work.

3 This account, for me, evokes a full and rich array of human experiencing, and runs contra to the possibility of an 'emptied-out' self that Laing (1972 [1959]: 83) describes in a possible response to the experience of psychosis.

4 Terror management theory (TMT) and anxiety buffer disruption theory (ABDT) would be situated alongside the aforementioned existential theories relating to shattered worldviews. TMT suggests that anxiety emerges from the awareness of one's eventual death or, as they term it, the 'mortality salience', which is primarily inspired by the work of Ernest Becker (2012 [1973]) and Otto Rank (2014 [1929]). For a useful overview of this, readers could consult Burke, Martens and Faucher (2010) and Lewis (2014). In contrast, ABDT is a more recent adaptation of TMT, proposing that trauma symptoms result more specifically from a traumatic disruption of normal death-anxiety-buffering functions that are contained within a person's worldview (see Edmondson et al., 2011; Pyszczynski & Kesebir, 2011).

5 See also Laing (1971 [1961]: 112–117) about the self appearing and disappearing.

6 Freud's suggestion is itself based on an early observation by Jentsch (1995 [1906]).

7 While many of the insights I am drawing on use the model of a Western nuclear family, the sentiments being expressed can equally be applied to any small community or network of belonging – either thrown together by circumstance (i.e. birth or relationship), or chosen through a mode of existing.

8 Those readers questioning the relationship between the phenomena of psychosis that were the primary focus for Laing, and the trauma phenomena explored in this book, should consult Morrison, Frame and Larkin (2003). The authors make a compelling case that psychosis and post-traumatic stress phenomena are part of a spectrum of possible reactions to trauma, and responses to the influences of traumatic life experiences. This sentiment is reflected in a recent special issue of the journal *Schizophrenia Research*, which demonstrates the relationships between childhood and interpersonal trauma and clinically defined symptoms and experiences of psychosis (see Mondelli & Dazzan, 2019). Further, a small-scale study (Read & Mayne, 2017) of young people in New Zealand found that a clinical diagnosis of psychosis was significantly related to the mean number (around three forms) of adversities experienced by their participants in childhood, and more specifically associated with childhood neglect.

9 Direct naming of traumatic reality can be assisted through the use of creative methods, including illustrative, drawn and artistic representations of meanings and dynamics, to make the confrontation tolerable (Lantz & Alford, 1995; Lantz & Lantz, 1991: 69).

Part III

Implications for practice

8 Implications for practice

To take us full circle back to the Introduction of this book, my intention in setting out an existential approach to traumatic experiencing is to tentatively proffer turns and re-turns in our understandings of what is confronted in a traumatic situation and relationship, and the impact this has on the *why, how* and *for whom* we exist. I have described how our modes of existence are confronted by the reality of a traumatic situation, and how this movement leads to forms of disillusionment and re-illusionment. In delving into the reality of traumatic confrontations within this inquiry, I hope to generatively move my own personal and clinical explorations, and support others who are seeking to approach interpersonal trauma existentially.

Existentialism and existential psychiatry, psychology and psychotherapy incorporate a broad international field of research, theory and practice. Those readers seeking empirical and descriptive overviews of the most commonly used contemporary existential-therapeutic methods and practices within the field might want to consult Correia and colleagues (2017), van Deurzen and Adams (2016), Cooper (2017), van Deurzen and Arnold-Baker (2018) and van Deurzen and colleagues (2019). The title of this book is meant somewhat paradoxically. This book is both *an* (just one) existential approach to interpersonal *and* a weaving description of *many* existential approaches to interpersonal trauma. If you have got this far in the book and failed to notice that throughout I have described the clinical practice of many existentialisms and modalities, it might be worth weaving your way back through the text, re-turning again to the chapters that resonated the most with the movements you make, or aspire to explore, in your own clinical work or mode of existing.

My modal existentialism is merely an elaborative synthesis of the many forms of existentialism I practice in my clinical work, and an incorporation of existential features and insights I have (re)(dis)covered from other traditions. As such, this final chapter does not contain a detailed service specification, treatment model or protocol for practice – this is not a practice handbook or manual. Rather, in what follows I set out the features and qualities of an existential approach to interpersonal trauma, and within this describe what the reader may encounter in the exploration of confrontations with reality and modes of experiencing.

DOI: 10.4324/9781003181675-12

Modal expansion and horizons of human experiencing

Baldwin (2017 [1963]: 75) writes that we cannot 'give' towards another way of existing, without risking ourselves. By this, I take him to mean that elaborating new modes of existing involves committing to risking our illusioned and re-illusioned modes. Baldwin (ibid.) continues that rather than 'giving', most people

> guard and keep; they suppose that it is themselves and what they identify with themselves that they are guarding and keeping, whereas what they are actually guarding and keeping is their system of reality and what they assume themselves to be.

Baldwin's words astutely describe *modal singularity*, a turning away from the generative potential of modality and an epistemic reduction of the person, and their world, to one mode of existing. Modal singularities arise from *constricted horizons* of human experiencing and illusioned modes of existing. This is another way of thinking about the traumatic fixing of ideas as described by Janet (1901: 199–200).

Those readers who are familiar with existentialism will know that the philosophical, psychiatric, psychological and psychotherapeutic field is filled with the theoretical and descriptive use of the term *horizons*: from the phenomenology of Husserl (2012 [1931]), to Heidegger's descriptions of Dasein (2010 [1953]), to the existential-hermeneutics of Hans-Georg Gadamer (2013 [1975]). In existentialism, horizons tend to describe the context of all possible existence, including an ever-extending plurality of reference points, grounds and directions for movements. We might build on Merleau-Ponty (2012 [1945]) and Stolorow's (2007) use of horizons to further describe the breadth and depth of possibility in our modes of existing, and the extent to which we can turn and re-turn in an elaborative opening up and closing down of intersubjective and intercorporeal modal movements.

Traumatic confrontations with reality queer the dominant existential ideas about the horizons of human experiencing and modes of existence. As Morton (2019: 93) astutely notes, the real world is

> precisely [...] this tattered, perforated patchwork quilt that doesn't quite start and stop with a definite horizon – temporal as well as spatial horizons are equally full of holes and blurry [...] Our human world is shared with all kinds of other tattered, broken [human and non-human] worlds.

So-called post-traumatic phenomena are full of descriptions of blurry and incomplete horizons of experiencing. One need only re-read the agentic refractions in the aforementioned case of Nathan. The reference to holes and tattered, broken and blurry worlds here is not meant as a negation or denigration of a traumatised person's personhood. Nor should it be taken as me saying that any new mode of existing that emerges from traumatic experiencing is in some way broken or damaged. Rather, it is an acknowledgement that horizons are not linear nor static, and that our movements of constriction and expansion are filled with liminality, spectrality and the primordial dispersement of our existence. Horizons move, we move within them, and through our movements and (re-)turns we generatively elaborate new modes of existing and horizons of experiencing.

Becker (2012 [1973]: 74) rhetorically asks, 'Why does a [person] accept to live a trivial life?' To which he answers, 'Because of the danger of a full horizon of experience, of course.' Confronting the totality and potentiality of our expansive horizons through traumatic experiencing – and their queer qualities and movements (and primordial dispersements) – is existentially horrific to us, and terrorises and haunts our subsequent modes of existing. Modal singularity is an understandable attempt to incorporate the confrontation of reality by closing in the horizons of human experiencing. The movement of turning in, curling up, bracing is to elaborate creative ways of modal movement and expression that deny, avoid and augment our human potentiality for expansion and (dis)covery of new modes of existing. Modal singularity leads to an existential terror of encountering modes of living that elude us, or that exist beyond the narrow horizons that we have created for ourselves. The terror of meeting other people who have realised these terrifying modes of existing leads us to defend, avoid, attack and dismiss their human potentiality, and our own capacity for modal movement. Building on the reflections of Becker (ibid.: 86) further, the mode of existing we have built up to deny, conceal or augment the existential horror and terror of reality, are exactly the modes of existence we need to confront, dissolve and move from, in order to escape our self-imposed limitations on the horizons of experiencing.

In contrast, through our traumatic confrontation of reality, we might turn, weave, twist and spin. In doing so, we expose the unfamiliar and unknown *horizonal potentialities* of human experiencing. Through embracing our own queer movements, and those of the emerging horizon, we face the ambiguity, liminality, uncertainty and unknowing of modal movements. Through unknowing, we (dis)cover and elaborate new modes of existing, and ethics towards ourselves, the other and the world around us. We might call these movements *modal plurality*. Expansion emerges from the courage to face the reality of traumatic situations, and is what emerges from turning beyond the known horizons of modal existence.

Expansion involves queer movements, as the more effortfully we pursue modal change, paradoxically the more we shake and twist within the tensions of our known modes of existing (building on Bush [Boaz], 2019; Levinas, 2001 [1947]). The challenge is not one of forcible effort, but rather a radical openness to unknowing. When we are open to unknown movements emerging within and beyond our horizons, new modes of experiencing generatively appear and make themselves known to us. So modal movement is less about the intentionality of horizons, and more about our openness to experiment with new modes of existing on unknown horizons of experience. Expansion queerly involves movements of ease and tension, and thus modal singularity and constriction have a place in enabling us to find oscillating and vibrating moments within, and between, horizons and modes of existence (modal plurality). New modes of existing can be unformulated and seemingly inarticulable, and many of my clients have described encountering and sensing new modal possibilities (including contra-modal possibilities) and expressions as they expand their horizons in their everyday lives.

On the (re)covery, (dis)covery and (re)(dis)covery of modes of existing

The majority of early and contemporary psychotraumatology has *recovery, resilience, restoration* and *returns* as its primary focus, that is, recovery from post-traumatic stress phenomena, the building of resilience against further adversity and traumatisation in the future, and the restoring or returning to psycho-social functioning, family life and/or an existing way of life. The prefix *(re)* in the terms used to describe the focus of treatments, interventions and practices is disclosive. I ask myself what it is that is being (re)covered, concealed, bounced back, brought back into shape or a previous situation (c.f. Herman, 2015 [1992]; Masten, 2014; Rutter, 1999; Ungar, Ghazinou & Richteret, 2013; van der Kolk, 2014). In early psychotraumatology, it would be the psychic wound that is being (re)covered, and yet in the broader field of medical traumatology, wounds are not re-solved by covering, but rather by attending to the wound, working with the healing flesh and incorporating the wound into the corporeality of the person.

From a modal perspective, (re)covery as a psychotherapeutic intention (of the client or practitioner) works primarily with re-turns, which are movements of re-illusionment through the traumatic confrontation of reality. Re-illusionment involves the generative incorporation of confrontations with reality into modes of existing within known horizons of human experiencing. In contrast, (dis) covery is the psychotherapeutic intention (of the client or practitioner), focusing on turning. Turning works with disillusionment and generatively incorporates confrontation with reality into new modes of existing within emergent horizons of human experiencing. *(Re)* and *(dis)* are modal tensions in the re-covering/discovering of reality through a traumatic confrontation. Between re-illusionment and disillusionment, there are more queer and liminal modal movements. These I have referred to as (re)(dis)covery. (Re)(dis)covery is the modal experimentation within and between known and unknown horizons of human experiencing, to generatively elaborate modes of existing. (Re)(dis)covery is a form of synthesis, which (for me at least) enables people to honour the modes that enabled them to survive traumatic experiences and situations, and the emergent modes of becoming through movement.

When a person approaches us for any orientation of trauma psychotherapy, we are meeting someone who has already survived or is surviving a confrontation with reality. Their movement towards us is an agentic commitment to action, and already incorporates turns (disillusionments) and re-turns (re-illusionments). Ethically, any practitioner seeking to apply a modal existentialism should be prepared to turn and re-turn with their client, finding ways of incorporating confrontations with traumatic reality in ways that resonate with the client. That said, the psychotherapist can remind the client of our horizonal and modal plurality and potentiality, and through (re)(dis)covery encourage them to experiment with unknown modes of existing and ways of relating to themselves and others.

Finally, I am influenced by the existential writings of Martin Buber (1958 [1949], 1996 [1923]), Levinas (2016 [1961], Stolorow (2007) and de Beauvoir (2015 [1948]) on the fundamental relatedness of our intercorporeal existence, and a resulting ethic that is implied in our relation with the other(s). Expansive horizons allow us to encounter and experiment with more possibilities in modes of experiencing that can bring growth, connection, safety, joy and excitement from our modal movements (be it within the constrictions, or between the expansions). For me, Levinas (2016 [1961]: 45–47, 52, 61, 101), in particular, directs our thinking towards a radical ethic towards the other, and even those who have done us harm. His approach denotes a form of radical humanism and an ethic of expansion that recognises the queer intercorporeality and complementarity of interpersonal trauma, and the foundations of our ongoing intersubjective human relatedness.

From this perspective, therapeutic empathy for ourselves, and for the traumatising other, is insufficient. We can *feel into* (the etymological route of empathy (*Einfühlung*)) the intercorporeality of traumatic experiencing to understand it. However, it does not necessarily provide the turning movements leading to more expansive (re)(dis) covery of horizonal and modal plurality and potentiality. Stolorow and Atwood (2019c: 116–117) note the inadequacy of merely feeling into in their own formulation of *indwelling*. Explorations of expanded horizons allow us to incorporate the confrontations and harms of interpersonal trauma by generatively *(re)(dis)turning* the interpersonal confrontation into the reality of our human existence. This generative (re)(dis)turning allows for the possibility of ethical communication between people. (Re)(dis)turning does not negate the uses and possible needs for epistemological devices – for example, of human forgiveness (Miller, 2009), compassion, care (Heidegger, 2010 [1953]), love (Binswanger, 1942), kindness – but rather allows us to synthesise them into ethical modal movements. The ethical concern is not one of re-storation with the traumatising other(s). Rather, it is how we will embrace expansive modes of existence, which seek to confront the realities of our intercorporeality and incorporate this into horizonal and modal plurality. Further, (re)(dis)turning implies an ethic of promoting human healing, growth and liberation. My suggestion here is that expanded horizons constitute an ethic that is akin to a constant answering of our primordial call to philosophise, and in doing so contributes to the healing of ourselves, others and the world in the face of reality (and human systems of reality-denial and reality-augmentation).

Features and qualities of an existential approach

The central features of my existential approach to interpersonal trauma are modes of existence (and modal movements) and traumatic confrontations with reality. As such, the core practice considerations offered below relate to these elements. The linearity of many psychotraumatological models gives a false sense of vertical-directional movement – moving from a starting position of traumatisation to an end of post-traumatic re-covery or growth. Lantz attempts to address this within his own meaning-focused, existential family trauma therapy (*holding up, telling, mastering* and *honouring*), by noting that phasic models, in practice, interweave, overlap, spiral and are cyclical (following Lantz, 1993, 2004). If there was a phasic component to my own existential model, it would be (a) establishing and expanding horizonal communication, (b) enquiring into traumatic confrontations with reality, (c) examining past and present modes of existing and (d) expanding and experimenting with new modal movements and modes of existing.

For the practical application of my approach, I have stripped my discussion back to the core considerations. In the previous chapter, I set out more nuanced existential and psychotherapeutically technical descriptions of how to understand and work with modes of disillusionment and re-illusionment in traumatic confrontations with reality. The rationale for only giving the core features and qualities in what follows, is to allow for generative incorporation and synthesis of my approach within and between other existing modalities (both existential and non-existential). Generative movements and modal expansion are a core premise of my own description, and thus I would celebrate pluralistic and elaborative syntheses of these descriptions into existing schools of psychological and psychotheraputic practice (following Cooper, 2015).

Communication on the horizon

In order to work with traumatic confrontations with reality, the client and psychotherapist need to establish a foundational safety, trust and tolerance to examine their (past, present and emergent) modes of existing and the disillusioned and re-illusioned turns incorporated within them. The establishment and maintenance of safety, trust and tolerance require a *radical equalisation* of power within the psychotheraputic relationship between client(s) and psychotherapist. I call this radical equalisation *communication on the horizon*. Communication on the horizon has been described elsewhere in the existential-humanistic field as *I–Thou dialogue* (Buber, 1996 [1923]), *co-presence* (by Laing; see Nuttall, 2019 for overview), and *relational depth* (Mearns & Cooper, 2018).

Communication on the horizon demands radical modal movements of acceptance, openness, honesty and presence in the psychotheraputic relationship, and in each relational moment. The intention is to establish relational mutuality and reciprocity, which both the psychotherapist and the client(s) take responsibility for maintaining and deepening. This allows for psychotheraputic intimacy to emerge, and the ground for sharing in turns and re-turns in modal incorporation and elaboration. In the existential language of Stolorow and Atwood (2019c), the psychotheraputic intimacy required would be the previously explored mode of *indwelling*. Stolorow (2007, 2011c) would add a modal quality of kinship-in-the-same-darkness, and Schütz (1967 [1932]) might draw our attention to the sensing of synchronicity experienced in establishing the *we-relationship* of the Umwelt.

Within service and private-based settings, the psychotheraputic relationship is more usually initiated and established on a vertical plane. Many clients come to psychotherapy with a fixative or curative attitude echoing the dominant discourse, frameworks and practices in psychotraumatology, and the contexts in which they live. Fixative and curative relationships require verticalisation. While a client might initially seem satisfied with a position that is subject to the will of the practitioner, over time this is problematic as it removes the communicative and experiential ground required for modal experimentation and movements. Verticalised psycho-therapeutic relationships involve moments of going up and down: fighting, tossing, grappling, wrestling, combating, struggling against and conceding our own modal movements, and those of the other. Alfred Adler (2013 [1928]) described this modal entwinement as a dynamic between superiority and inferiority, and Sartre (2003 [1943]: 383–452) as oscillating 'masochistic' and 'sadist' attitudes.

Eger (2018: 10) reflects that in reality 'there is no hierarchy [verticalisation] of suffering, and comparisons are misleading and meaningless'. And so, when psychotherapeutic relationships are founded on a vertical plane, communication becomes conflictual and intolerable – *and from the intolerable, intolerance springs forth*, that is, intersubjective intolerance co-created by the psychotherapist and client(s) for each other's interweaving modes of existing, and the modal dynamic they are enacting, and participating in. The client(s) and psychotherapist alike become too proximate and too distant from each other to tolerate the confrontation of each other, let alone the traumatic confrontation(s) of reality. Some psychotherapists then revert to a more verticalised and professionalised mode of existing, expressing directional enactments and attempting to induce an unethical docility in the modality and modal movements of the client. To borrow a turn of phrase from Becker (2012 [1973]: 186), we might understand verticalisation as a 'problem of too much narrowness toward the world or too much openness'; a turn away from relation depth at every moment. Communication on the vertical results in intersubjective overwhelm, where simultaneously there is a clashing (narrowness) co-confrontation of reality *and* a leaping or jumping away (openness) from the confrontation. This dynamic then manifests as a modal movement of denial of the suffering (or even existence) of the other (moving on top), or conceding to the suffering (or existence) of the other (elaborating on the Sartrean dynamic, see Sartre, 2003 [1943]).

Committing to communication on the horizon, and taking responsibility to stay equal, is where intersubjective equality emerges from and thus the ground and potential for modal dialogue and experimentation. Schütz and the mentalisation theorists, in different ways, draw our attention to the importance of honestly and explicitly disclosing our intentionality within the psychotherapeutic relationship. This is especially important given the confusion, distress and incomprehensi-bility of intentionality that can arise from the confronted reality in interpersonal trauma. Turning on the horizonal means naming explicitly what we are experi-encing intercorporeally when we encounter our clients, and inviting and encour-aging them to do the same. As psychologists and psychotherapists, communication on the horizon is to turn and re-turn alongside the client. This involves a radical appreciation and valuing of the insights that our clients bring about human exist-ence, honouring the modal change they have explored in their lives and their agentic potential to move, and move us, and to be moved by what we co-create together.

As Morton (2019) reminds us, communication on the horizon is primordially infused with a spectral patchwork of voids, absences and mis-turns. As such, both the client(s) and psychotherapist will encounter the unfamiliar and unknown *horizonal potentialities* of human experiencing through dialogue. This will especially be the case in moments where the client or psychotherapist experiences their intercorporeal modal expressions and movements as invalid, mystified, incomprehensible, liminal, irreal, unreal, surreal or ab-real. Ambiguous communications and miscommunications require close and honest intersubjective attending to unknowing, and attunement to the existential horror, terror, fright and liberation that might emerge in encountering the communicative uncertainty and expansive potentiality.

Communicative ambiguity and miscommunication are important psychotherapeutic opportunities to (re)(dis)turn towards each other and expand the horizons of human experiencing. Further, they provide the ground to reflect on the modal movements (of the psychotherapist and client(s)) that generated specific modal responses. Communication on the horizon requires the agentic participation of a psychotherapist whom a client can push against, whose mode of existing and modal expression can be experienced as really there. The phenomena of turning with and turning from each other, at moments of ambiguous or miscommunication, can be opened up through inquiry and disclosure of our perceptive and imaginal experiences of the other. This also builds intersubjective competence, and a shared language for describing the specific dynamics of modes of existing. In my own personal and clinical practice, the use of movement and/or metaphors of movements can be especially powerful in co-creating referents for modal turns, re-turns and (re)(dis)turning. Communication on the horizon is aided through a reciprocal attitude of enduring curiosity; even (and especially) in moments when a modal expression evokes a movement away from the other, in attempts to re-turn to a verticalised mode of relating, and/or where we encounter the liminal and spectral dimensions of traumatic experiencing. With clients, I have found it useful to elaborate and agree how we will name and indicate if we feel we have turned away from each other, and the movements we might explore to coming back to dialogue.

The commitment of the psychotherapist is to demystify themselves and psychotherapy within the intersubjective field. We can do this in the immediacy of communication on the horizon by inviting the client(s) to clarify their experiences, to critically reflect on the modal consequences of our co-created dialogue, and to radically celebrate the client's agentic movements and expressions within the intersubjective field. In this way, the communication is generatively elaborated and deepened. Co-commitment and responsibility for relational mutuality require professional humility on behalf of the psychologist or psychotherapist. The psychologist or psychotherapist in this mode of relating is open to noticing the ways in which their modal moments and responses might have disrupted communication on the horizon.[1] To be radically co-creative does not mean the psychotherapist loses all sense of professional ethics and boundaries. Disclosure within and between horizonal communication does not require the flooding of the client's movements with statements of fact or data about one's life. Rather, disclosure is the honest and mutual presence and generative movement of the psychotherapist in the psychotherapeutic relationship, turning, re-turning and (re)(dis)turning alongside the client. The purpose of disclosing is to establish and explore synchronicity, intentionality and the possibility of intersubjective meeting that recognises, names, holds and celebrates differences in modal movements and modes of experiencing.

Inquiring into traumatic confrontations with reality

Communication on the horizon provides the intersubjective ground for dialogue on, and explorations of, traumatic experiences. By way of re-emphasis: a client who meets us, has already been disillusioned by the traumatic confrontation with reality and incorporated this (disillusionment or re-illusionment) into their modes of existence. Carl Rogers, the founder of person-centred psychotherapy, asks us to imagine what might happen if we move from a 'grudging tolerance' of another person's worldview to a 'full acceptance' of the person and their right to have a worldview. He speculates that this could open us up to being more willing to explore the person's reality, rather than 'shutting out' their realities as being 'absurd or dangerous or heretical or stupid' (Rogers, 1995 [1980]: 105).

While I come to a different perspective on the individualised nature of reality, Rogers (ibid., 2004 [1961]) asks important questions about how we phenomenologically inquire about traumatic confrontations with reality within and between communication on the horizon.

Within existential psychiatry, psychology and psychotherapy, we can phenomenologically inquire about the person's experience of their world, the embodied sense of self and relationships with others (for more detailed methodological description, see van Deurzen & Adams, 2016; Spinelli, 2005). Through dialogue we open up the client's descriptions (verbal and non-verbal) of reality, and the modal movements they make through their confrontation(s) with traumatic situations and relationships. I use phenomenological *inquiry* to signal the mode of horizonal communication, which is more deliberately expansive. For me, inquiry seeks to open up our modes of existence and confrontations with reality. The intention of the inquiry is to retain an awareness of the commonalities and difference between our modes of existence and those of the other person, and the co-created movements resulting from the communication within, and between us. In contrast, enquiry in this formulation is an act of questioning that one might experience from a friend, family member, colleague or acquaintance. Engagement in enquiry involves the conscious and non-conscious intent of simultaneously opening up and closing down the modality of the person(s). We have all experienced the seemingly engaged and empathetic questioning of a friend, family member, or acquaintance, which over the course of the conversation turns out to be an explicit closing down of our modal expression; perhaps because the other person finds it intolerable to be confronted with our different modal movements.

Dominant contemporary dimensional frameworks within existential psychology and psychotherapy include Längle's (motivational) confrontations with fundamental structures of existence (c.f. Längle, 2020), and Spinelli's four interrelational *I-focused*, *you-focused*, *we-focused* and *they-focused* realms and how we descriptively experience these in our encounters with ourselves, others and the world around us (c.f. Spinelli, 2005: 148–149). Frankl (1986 [1946]: 177) describes his own four worlds of inquiry: physical, psychic, social or contextual, and what he describes as 'as a mode of existence', which incorporates our values, meanings, purpose and way we live our lives. All of these are compatible with a phenomenological inquiry of people's movements in confronting the reality of traumatic experiencing.

One of the increasingly prominent dimensional models is van Deurzen's four worlds (van Deurzen, 2010: 129–168; see also 2012; van Deurzen & Adams, 2016; van Deurzen & Arnold-Baker, 2018). Building on the work of Binswanger (c.f. 1958, 1963), van Deurzen describes four interrelated dimensions of existence: physical (*Umwelt*), our being with nature; social (*Mitwelt*), being with others; personal (*Eigenwelt*), being with oneself; and spiritual (*Überwelt*), being with values and meaning. She draws our attention to the expansive horizon of human experiencing that could be accessed by the client through an embracing of all four interweaving worlds.

van Deurzen suggests we might open up new perspectives, understandings, values and meanings by exploring and encouraging clients to describe their experiences through the other existential dimensions (see Bush [Boaz], 2020b, for an illustrative application of the four worlds to descriptive accounts of the early COVID-19 lockdown in the United Kingdom). Within the phenomenological description of existential dimensions, van Deurzen demonstrates how focusing on polarity, paradox and seeming inconsistency in descriptions can enable clients to find new ways of existing, relating to others and the world around them (following van Deurzen, 2010: 138). Given the modal movements of disillusionment and re-illusionment in the traumatic confrontation with reality, van Deurzen's four-worlds model provides a framework for a descriptive and thematic exploration of the modal expression and elements of modes of existing that have emerged for the client.

More recently, existential psychotherapists have demonstrated the limitations of more Westernised and individualised dimensional frameworks for clients who come from, and live in, more collaborative and collectivist cultures (see Spinelli, 2015: 21–22, for a brief inclusion of the South African concept of *ubuntu*; see also for useful contemporary discussion: Eliastam, 2015; Müller, Eliastam & Trahar, 2020). For example, Paul Murray Wilson and Stephen William Appel (2013) provide an important contribution to this conversation in describing how the Māori model of well-being (*Whare Tapa Wha*), can be used as an alternative dimensional framework. *Whare Tapa Wha* as a four-worlds framework includes the existential domains of *tinana*, or our capacity for bodily (physical) health, growth and development; *taha whanau*, or our capacity for belonging, caring and sharing, and our interdependence and reciprocity of extended human relationships and family;

taha hinengaro, or our capacity to *think-feel* (thoughts and emotions arise from the same source in Māori understandings), express and communicate this to ourselves and others; and *taha wairua*, or our capacity for ecological and spiritual connection and communion.

Using *Whare Tapa Wha* as a four-worlds model is inherently more systemic, in that the client is always located within the health and well-being of the wider family, and collectively our *mauri* (life force). However, rather than focusing on the freedom and individuation of the person, *Whare Tapa Wha* reminds us to ask what the individual person is disclosing about the collective reality of our existence when they are confronted with traumatic situations and relationships. Further, its foundational basis in collectivist culture turns our inquiry towards the intercorporeality and generative elaboration of our modal movements within the contextuality of our lived existence. The Māori *Whare Tapa Wha* intersubjectively and spatio-temporally incorporates our ancestors, living relatives and future descendants (*Taha Whanau*), and our communions with tribal lands and cultural practices (*Taha Wairua*). This interweaving contextuality enables more active engagement and recognition with the historical realities and enactments of cultural traumas (including colonisation, institutional racism and enforced sterilisation) that frame contemporary enactments and experiences of interpersonal trauma (see also Pihama et al., 2017). In many ways, the form of phenomenological inquiry advocated for within *communication on the horizon* lends itself more readily to the Māori ideals for psychotherapeutic practice emerging from *Whare Tapa Wha*. These are described by Wilson and Appel (2013: 138–139, 144) as an expansive and intersubjective mode of phenomenological inquiry, which seeks to practise caring (*manaakitanga*), encouragement (*whakamanawa*), and reciprocity (*whanaungatanga*) across the existential dimensions.

My own modal existentialist framework proposes phenomenological inquiry across the dimensions of personal reality, intersubjective reality, contextual reality and dispersed existence. Modal existentialism is premised on the notion of our primordial dispersed intercorporeality and generatively agentic participation in modal movement. The existential focus is on turns/re-turns/(re)(dis)turns and disillusionments/re-illusionments/(re)(dis)illusionments within, and between, our modes of existing and horizons of human experiencing. I equally seek to open up the queerer experiential and imaginal descriptions within and between the four dimensions of existence. These spectral and liminal descriptions emerge out of our traumatic confrontation(s) with reality, and include experiences of our queer realities, irrealities, unrealities, surrealities and ab-realities.

My own offering here is a synthesis of both individualised and collectivised dimensional frameworks for phenomenological inquiry. As such, it is compatible with, and can be used alongside, existing dimensional frameworks used within existential and non-existential orientations. Further, my proposal is that practitioners find new ways of synthesising the modal existentialist approach within their existing training, orientation or modality, and the ethical and professional frameworks governing these practices. Paradoxically, even curative and fixative psychologies and psychotherapies can have their place in a synthesised model.

Curative and fixative models can intersubjectively demonstrate to the client movements that open up to them across a more expanded (even if still constricted) horizon of experience, and can enact the potentiality of modal movement.

The advocation of this synthesising approach emerges from long discussions I have had with two of my own existential supervisors, and insightful psychiatrists, psychologists and psychotherapists outside of the tradition of existentialism. There are modes of phenomenological inquiry and modal expression that exist beyond any given psychologist's or psychotherapist's horizon of human experiencing. Knowing the potentiality of more expansive horizons is an important tool in maintaining communication on the horizon. It enables practitioners to reflect on their intersubjective turns and re-turns with clients across the horizon. There will be moments where the client feels they want to explore new modes of existing or the expansive horizon beyond the particular psychotherapeutic relationship that has been established. Other moments will arise where the psychologist or psychotherapist understands that the horizon, mode of existing or modal expressions are beyond their known and experiential reality. This can be addressed within and between communication on the horizon. The wise and honest practitioner will recognise the value of plurality in modalities in the psychiatric, psychological and psychotherapeutic professions, and when the time comes will explore with the client where their new turn, re-turn or (re)(dis)turn might take them (building on Cooper, 2015). Recognition of modal limitations is a fundamental aspect of confronting the reality of traumatic experiences, as it discloses the generative foundations of intersubjective modal movement and elaboration.

Finally, phenomenological inquiry into traumatic confrontations with reality is not a linear process. Even within modal singularity, the client actively re-illusions themselves and constricts the horizons of human experiencing in order to deny, avoid or augment the turning, re-turning and (re)(dis)turning movements of our primordial modality. Phenomenological inquiry manifests in circular and spiralling movements, oscillating in distance and proximity to the confronted reality and incorporations into modes of existence. The reality of a traumatic situation is difficult to approach because our generative elaborations within and between modes of existence already incorporate our turns and re-turns, disorientations and re-orientations, and disillusionments and re-illusionment.

Psychotherapeutic confrontations with reality, within communication on the horizon, have their own ground and pacing (building on Lantz & Lantz, 1991: 64–65; 1992: 299–300). The ground and the pacing of inquiring about traumatic confrontations is co-created consensually between the psychotherapist and client. With some clients I use the metaphor of walking through a forest and describe the proximity to known and unknown confrontations, employing imagery suitable for this imaginal location. Other clients have used metaphors of bodies of water, mountains, rooms, boxes, digestion, elemental states, colours and tastes to describe their pacing and oscillations between distance and proximity to traumatic confrontations with reality. Clients sometimes experience this as an incomprehensible *Stravaig*, and other times a spiritual exploration into the unknown. Other clients use communication on the horizon to disclose the existence and awareness of traumatic confrontations of modal responses they find (for example) frightening or shaming, and to signal that they are not yet ready to turn to inquire about, or examine, them. Co-creating the pacing of confrontations is a vital quality in opening up the (re)(dis)covery of modes of existing.

Encouragement in the confrontation of reality

The Chinese existential psychologist Xuefu Wang (2011, 2016) describes the existential attitude of *Zhi Mian* (直面). Initially coined by the writer Xun Lu (2009), *Zhi Mian* means 'directly facing' reality. Reflecting on Xun's writings, Wang draws out a specific form of courage required to face the reality of existence. This courage is not described as physical courage, but rather a daring courage to 'face life directly as it is […] and to look unflinchingly at one's circumstance' (Xun quoted in Wang, 2016: 9). As Wang notes, this form of courage has some equivalency to the *courage to be* described by Paul Tillich (2000 [1952]). Psychotherapeutically, we can extend Wang's framing to see *Zhi Mian* as being an encouragement of *both* confrontation with the reality of existence and our modes of existing (movements) within it – and thus is a mode of (re)(dis)covery.

Zhi Mian-existential psychotherapy, according to Wang (2011, 2016), is focused more explicitly on exploring reality, and courageously facing the confrontation with reality as we find it. Extending the propositions of Wang (2016: 11–12), life choices and modal movements emerge from the awareness of the reality of a situation, and remain disillusioned and (re)(dis)illusioned in the face of this awareness. In Western psychotraumatology, what we call psychiatric or psychological symptoms are seen in *Zhi Mian* psychotherapy as lived expressions of our experience of reality and/or our avoidance of the reality of our existence, and active participation within it (Wang, 2011: 242–243). Wang (2016: 12–14) demonstrates how alluring the movement towards re-illusionment is, and the ways in which the psychotherapist can enable the client to rediscover the wisdom contained within the reality of their experience.

Wang recognises in *Zhi Mian* that our modal propensity is to re-turn towards re-illusionment. This is because incorporating the disillusionary and queer potentialities of *Zhi Mian* into our modal movement is 'extremely difficult' (ibid.: 10). To stay with our disillusionment, our traumatic confrontation with reality, and to (re)(dis)cover new horizons and modes of existing, *Zhi Mian* psychotherapy cultivates the balancing of two existential and modal movements. These two existential movements are characterised by Wang as the *hero-rebel* and the *gentle warrior*. The hero-rebel movements cultivate resistance against 'forces and powers that obstruct and damage' our disillusioned modes of existing, in order that we might 'defy a thousand pointing fingers' (ibid.). The hero-rebel is a defiant mode of existence, seeking to incorporate the traumatic confrontation with reality into modal movements and expressions. The modal incorporation is through defiance or contra-positioning to intersubjective and systemic pressures to re-illusion oneself.

Utilising Xun's image of an iron house, Wang (2019) describes the (reality-denying and reality-augmenting) human systems and the self-illusioned modes of existing which seem to provide meaning, but that, however, are sheltering people from the reality of their existence. While a shelter from reality might seem comforting to people, it prevents existential growth and modal expansion. The hero-rebel movements seek to noisily wake up those in the iron house, encouraging them to become disillusioned and face reality alongside us in a generative turn. In response, Wang sees three forms of modal response: (a) being the person outside the iron house shouting; (b) being inside, waking to the shouting and being eager for action and movement; and (c) sleeping through the shouting, not wishing to wake up from our sleep. I would add a fourth response (d) of having re-illusioned oneself to experience oneself as the iron house or instruments of noise in the hero-rebel's hands. The choice, according to Wang, is between (a) surviving reality by turning and re-turning away from it and (b) really existing by (re)(dis)covering new modes that incorporate the disillusionment of the reality of traumatic experiencing. Both modes are meaningful, although the mode of *Zhi Mian* describes the latter (re)(dis)turns towards reality, and modes of existing that can tolerate uncertainty, curiosity and unknowing.

The second fundamental existential movement, balancing that of the hero-rebel, is of the gentle warrior (ibid.: 10–11). The gentle warrior is a mode of existence through service to reality, and the other. This can best be understood as serving the self and others through leading exposures and confrontations with reality through movements of love, kindness and tenderness. Echoing the psychotraumatology of Winnicott (1991 [1964]: 69–74), the gentle warrior turns towards reality by offering others gentle and attuned protections, mediations and confrontations with reality. Both the modes of the hero-rebel and the gentle warrior are required, as the struggle to confront the reality of our situation involves attending to our own re-illusioned and disillusioned modes of existing within the limitations and conditions of our life (Wang, 2011: 244).

Following Wang (ibid.: 243), I would suggest that when we experience the existential liminality of our traumatic confrontations with reality, existential horror and terror draw us to turn back to re-illusionment. Extending Wang's description, in the face of existential horror and terror,

> We would rather believe in an illusion and never see that it is a fantasy [re-illusionment] by ourselves. We run, run and run, even dare not to take a pause or to turn back for a glimpse of what we are escaping from. We lack the courage to do so.
>
> (Wang, 2016: 12; see also 2011: 243)

This echoes Becker's (2012 [1973]) observations that giving up our illusions about reality gives way to terror – although I would propose this terror is about our primordial dispersement, with death being a modal expression of this. Building on Becker (ibid.: 189), our existential horror and existential terror give rise to a *reality/illusion paradox*. Traumatic experiencing goes to the heart of this paradox, in that the confrontation with reality is a simultaneous confrontation with the unbearable state of reality/unreality. As such, the shaking, shocking and trembling movements of traumatic experiencing are the spectral and intercorporeal quake of our exposure to the reality/illusion paradox.

Described allegorically through the movements of a tiger, Wang (2016) proposes that we can build our courage to face traumatic reality by cautiously experimenting with modes of (re)(dis)covery. These modes enable us to both recognise the reality that has been faced and retain our modal movement in proximity to it. Further, Wang re-emphasises that in confronting the reality of a traumatic situation or relationship, we are also simultaneously inquiring into our modal movements and modes of existing in the face of it. The traumatic confrontation and our modal movement are inseparable. All phenomenological inquiry must recognise that when we open up a traumatic reality, we open up the person who was, and still is, moving within the traumatic confrontation(s). Contra to some schools of psychotraumatology, the person we encounter in the psychotherapeutic relation-ship is a person primordially and generatively in the midst of modal movement, no matter how subtle or still-like they appear to be.

On awe and wonderment

Examining our past and present modes of existing and experimenting with new modal movements can be excruciating. Previously, I described the traumatic iden-tities that can arise from modal disillusionment and re-illusionment, and the states of existential guilt, regret, shame and humiliation we can experience in relation to our own movements. To confront reality is to confront our own modes of existing. In finding the courage to examine the traumatic reality we have confronted, we must also find the *Zhi Mian* to face our own modal movements of incorporation. The potential for re-traumatisation emerges from movements of (re)(dis)covery, despite their expansive horizons. When we move into new elaborative modes of existing, there are the spectral remnants of another modal expression and enact-ment haunting us. Further, new modes can result in people verticalising against older modes of existing, attacking, defending and experiencing existential shame and humiliation over the agentic movements they previously have made to survive traumatic situations or relationships, and the people they were becoming.

The existential mode of the gentle warrior can be instrumental in co-creating the psychotherapeutic and intersubjective space required to experiment with existing and new modal movements. Within my own practice, I co-create with the client a *modal perspective-taking*, which aims to find constructive, contextual and tender dialogue between the modal movements of a person's past, present and imagined future (this could be seen as akin to parts-work in internal family systems therapy, c.f. Schwartz, 2021; Schwartz & Sweezy, 2020; see also Lantz, 2004: 171–172, on the treatment dynamic in the *fullness of time*). The aim is to find value and meaning in the confrontation with reality, and to understand what insight modes of existence and modal expressions might offer the client about the turns they want to experiment with in the present and the future. I also use Längle's method of *personal existential analysis* (PEA) to co-explore the value (even if it is experienced as paradoxical by the client) of former modes of existing. Längle

(2003b, 2011) distinguishes between three steps in the existential motivation process. Modifying his language use slightly, we could describe these three steps as (a) *recognising* the situational value and meaning of our modal movements and enactments; (b) *harmonising or incorporating* the value, challenge or meaning into new modal experimentations and expressions; and (c) giving oneself *permission* (Längle uses the term 'inner consent') to enact the generative modal elaboration within the psychotherapeutic relationship and in one's life.

Generative modal elaboration can be further encouraged psychotherapeutically through a mutual ethic and impulsion to philosophise. An existential mode of awe and wonderment enables expansions both in the horizons of human experiencing and modal experimentation (following Schneider, 2008, 2011). Nietzsche (1969 [1883]), Jaspers (2003 [1954]) and Eger (2018: 81–230) all draw on the philosophical idea of a moving child. The existential modal movements of the child are used to denote a modal attitude towards unknowing, awe and wonderment. Traumatic confrontations with reality expose us to the expansive existential horror and terror of our existence, and the potentiality of unknown horizons of human experiencing. Building on Winnicott (1991 [1971]), psychotherapeutic play and experimentation enable the intercorporeal (re)(dis)covery of modes of existing and modal expressions. Lantz (2004: 173) describes the psychotherapeutic moment as *surprise*, when clients (re)(dis)cover their agentic potential to incorporate their traumatic confrontation into modal movements neither they nor the psychotherapist were expecting. Surprise, awe and wonderment provide the basis of hope, joy, celebration and honouring of the client's capacity to generatively elaborate new modes of existing. As Charlie Smith (2020) describes it, 'Hope emerges through the gentle tilt forward into the unknown; embracing our experimentation, our play, our joy, and our explorations.'

Note

1 Different psychotherapeutic modalities and traditions have their own existing ways of describing such intersubjective disruptions, including the mechanisms of defence, transference, countertransference, projection and displacement.

References

Abi-Rached, J. & Rose, N. (2010). 'The birth of the neuromolecular gaze' *History of the Human Sciences* 23(1): 11–26.

Abram, D. (2011). *Becoming animal: an earthly cosmology*. New York: Vintage.

Adams, M. (2019). *An existential approach to human development: philosophical and therapeutic perspectives*. London: Palgrave.

Adler, A. (2013 [1928]). *Understanding human nature*. Hove: Routledge.

Ahmed, S. (2004). *The cultural politics of emotion*. Edinburgh: Edinburgh University Press.

Ahmed, S. (2006a). *Queer phenomenology*. London: Duke University Press.

Ahmed, S. (2006b). 'Orientations: toward a queer phenomenology' *GLQ: Journal of Lesbian and Gay Studies* 12(4): 543–574.

Alisic, E., Zalta, A. K., van Wesel, F., Larsen, S. E., Hafstad, G. S., Hassanpour, K. & Smid, G. E. (2014). 'Rates of post-traumatic stress disorder in trauma-exposed children and adolescents: meta-analysis' *British Journal of Psychiatry* 204(5): 335–340.

Allen, D. J. & Oleson, T. (1999). 'Shame and internalized homophobia in gay men' *Journal of Homosexuality* 37(3): 33–43.

Allen, J. G. (2001). *Traumatic relationships and serious mental disorders*. Chichester: Wiley.

Allen, J. G. (2005). *Coping with trauma: hope through understanding* (2nd ed.). Washington, DC: American Psychiatric Publishing.

Allen, J. G. (2013). *Mentalizing in the development and treatment of attachment trauma*. Oxon: Routledge.

Allen, J. G., Fonagy, P. & Bateman, A. (2008). *Mentalizing in clinical practice*. Arlington, VA: American Psychiatric Publishing.

Amemiya, A., Fujiwara, T., Shirai, K., Kondo, K., Oksanen, T., Pentti, J. & Vahtera, J. (2019). 'Association between adverse childhood experiences and adult diseases in older adults: a comparative cross-sectional study in Japan and Finland' *BMJ Open* 9: e024609.

American Psychiatric Association (APA) (2013). *Diagnostic and statistical manual of mental disorders* (5th ed. – *DSM-5*). Washington, DC: American Psychiatric Publishing.

Andersen, T., Lahav, Y., Ellegaard, H. & Manniche, C. (2017). 'A randomized controlled trial of brief somatic experiencing for chronic low back pain and comorbid post-traumatic stress disorder symptoms' *European Journal of Psychotraumatology* 308(1): 1331108.

Anton, B. S. (2010). 'Proceedings of the American Psychological Association for the legislative year 2009: minutes of the annual meeting of the Council of Representatives and minutes of the meetings of the Board of Directors' *American Psychologist* 65: 385–475.

Archer, M. S. (1995). *Realist social theory: the morphogenetic approach*. Cambridge, UK: Cambridge University Press.

Arnault, D. S. & O'Halloran, S. (2015). 'Biodynamic psychotherapy for trauma recovery: a pilot study' *International Body Psychotherapy Journal* 14(1): 20–35.

Arnold, L. & Pinkston, A. (2014). 'Other-being: traumatic stress and dissociation in existential therapy' *International Journal of Existential Psychology & Psychotherapy* 5(1): 96–104.

Ascher, L. M. (1981). 'Employing paradoxical intention in the treatment of agoraphobia' *Behaviour Research & Therapy* 19(6): 533–542.

Ascher, L. M. (1989). *Therapeutic paradox*. New York: Guilford Press.

Ascher, L. M. & Schotte, D. E. (1999). 'Paradoxical intention and recursive anxiety' *Journal of Behavior Therapy & Experimental Psychiatry* 30(2): 71–79.

Austin, S. (2016). 'Working with chronic and relentless self-hatred, self-harm and existential shame: a clinical study and reflections' *Journal of Analytical Psychology* 61(1): 24–43.

Balchin, R., Barry, V., Bazan, A., Blechner, M. J., Clarici, A., Flores Mosri, D., Fotopoulou, A(K)., Goergen, M. S., Kessler, R., Matthis, I., Fernando, J., Zúñiga, M., Northoff, G., Olds, D., Oppenheim, L., Reismann-Lagrèze, D., Tsakiris, M., Watt, D., Yeates, G. & Zellner, M. (2019). 'Reflections on 20 years of neuropsychoanalysis' *Neuropsychoanalysis* 21(2): 89–123.

Baldwin, J. (2017 [1955]). *Notes of a native son*. London: Penguin.

Baldwin, J. (2017 [1963]). *The fire next time*. London: Penguin.

Baldwin, J. R., Reuben, A., Newbury, J. B. & Danese, A. (2019). 'Agreement between prospective and retrospective measures of childhood victimization: a systematic review and meta-analysis' *JAMA Psychiatry* 76(6): 584–593.

Balint, M. (1969). 'Trauma and object relationship' *International Journal of Psychoanalysis* 50(4): 429–435.

Balint, M. (2015 [1968]). *The basic fault: therapeutic aspects of regression*. Oxon: Routledge.

Baron-Cohen, S. (2017). 'Neurodiversity – a revolutionary concept for autism and psychiatry' *Journal of Child Psychology & Psychiatry* 58(6): 744–747.

Bateson, G., Jackson, D. D., Haley, J. & Weakland, J. (1978 [1956]). 'Towards a theory of schizophrenia' in M. M. Berger (ed.) *Beyond the double bind: communication and family systems, theories, and techniques with schizophrenics*. New York: Brunner/Mazel, pp. 3–28.

Beck, A. T. (1963). 'Thinking and depression I: idiosyncratic content and cognitive distortions' *Archives of General Psychiatry* 9(4): 324–333.

Beck, A. T. (1964). 'Thinking and depression II: theory and therapy' *Archives of General Psychiatry* 10(6): 561–571.

Becker, E. (2012 [1973]). *The denial of death*. London: Souvenir Press.

Bellis, M. A., Ashtoni, K., Hughes, K., Fordii, K., Bishopi, J. & Paranjothyi, S. (2015). *Welsh adverse childhood experiences (ACE) study: adverse childhood experiences and their impact on health-harming behaviours in the Welsh adult population*. Cardiff: Public Health Wales NHS Trust.

Bellis, M. A., Hughes, K., Leckenby, N., Hardcastle, K. A., Perkins, C. & Lowey, H. (2015). 'Measuring mortality and the burden of adult disease associated with adverse childhood experiences in England: a national survey' *Journal of Public Health* 37(3): 445–454.

Bellis, M. A., Hughes, K., Leckenby, N., Jones, L., Baban, A., Kachaeva, M., Povilaitis, R., Pudule, I., Qirjako, G., Ulukol, B., Ralevah, M. & Terzici, N. (2014). 'Adverse childhood experiences and associations with health-harming behaviours in young adults: surveys in eight eastern European countries' *Bulletin of the World Health Organization* 92(9): 641–655.

Berceli, D. (2005). *Trauma releasing exercises: a revolutionary new method for stress and trauma recovery*. Scotts Valley, CA: CreateSpace Independent Publishing.

Berceli, D. (2008). *The revolutionary trauma release process: transcend your toughest times*. Vancouver: Namaste Publishing.

Berceli, D. (2015). *Shake it off naturally: reduce stress, anxiety, and tension with [TRE]*. Scotts Valley, CA: CreateSpace Independent Publishing.

Bergson, H. (1889 [1927]). *Essai sur les données immédiates de la conscience*. Paris: Presses Universitaires de France.

Bergson, H. (1941). *L'évolution Créatrice*. Paris: Presses Universitaires de France.

Berlin, L. J., Appleyard, K. & Dodge, K. A. (2011). 'Intergenerational continuity in child maltreatment: mediating mechanisms and implications for prevention' *Child Development* 82(1): 162–176.

Bethell, C. D., Carle, A., Hudziak, J., Gombojav, N. Powers, K., Wade, R. & Braveman, P. (2017). 'Methods to assess adverse childhood experiences of children and families: toward approaches to promote child well-being in policy and practice' *Academic Pediatrics* 17(7 Suppl): S51–S69.

Bettelheim, B. (1979). *Surviving and other essays*. New York: Knopf.

Bezoa, B. & Maggib, S. (2015). 'Living in "survival mode": intergenerational transmission of trauma from the Holodomor genocide of 1932–1933 in Ukraine' *Social Science & Medicine* 134: 87–94.

Binswanger, L. (1942). *Grundformen und Erkenntnis Menschlichen Daseins*. Munich: Ernst Reinhardt.

Binswanger, L. (1958 [1946]). 'The existential analysis school of thought' in R. May, 'Contributions of existential psychotherapy' in R. May, E. Angel & H. F. Ellenberger (eds and trans.) *Existence: a new dimension in psychiatry and psychology*. New York: Basic Books, pp. 191–213.

Binswanger, L. (1958). 'The case of Ellen West' W. M. Mandel & J. Lyons (trans.) in R. May, E. Angel & H. F. Ellenberger (eds) *Existence: a new dimension in psychiatry and psychology*. New York: Simon & Schuster, pp. 237–364.

Binswanger, L. (1963). *Being in the world: selected papers of Ludwig Binswanger*. J. Needleman (trans.). New York: Basic Books.

Binswanger, L. (1986 [1930]). 'Dream and existence' J. Needleman (trans.) in M. Foucault & L. Binswanger. *Dream and existence* (Studies in Existential Psychology & Psychiatry). K. Hoeller (ed.). Seattle, WA: Review of Existential Psychology and Psychiatry, pp. 79–106.

Bion, W. R. (2004 [1962]). *Learning from experience*. Lanham, MD: Rowman & Littlefield.

Boals, A. (2018). 'Trauma in the eye of the beholder: objective and subjective definitions of trauma' *Journal of Psychotherapy Integration* 28(1): 77 89.

Boss, M. (1963). *Psychoanalysis and Daseinsanalysis*. New York: Basic Books.

Bourdieu, P. (2003 [1979]). *Distinction: a social critique of the judgement of taste*. R. Nice (trans.). London: Routledge.

Bowers, M. E. & Yehuda, R. (2016). 'Intergenerational transmission of stress in humans' *Neuropsychopharmacology* 41: 232–244.

Bowlby, J. (1955). 'The growth of independence in the young child' *Royal Society of Health* 76(9): 587–591.

Bowlby, J. (1973). *Attachment and loss: separation, anxiety and anger* (vol. II). London: Hogarth Press and the Institute of Psychoanalysis.

Bowlby, J. (1979). *The making & breaking of affectional bonds*. London: Tavistock Publications.

Bowlby, J. (1982 [1969]). *Attachment and loss: attachment* (vol. I, 2nd ed.). New York: Basic Books.

Bowlby, J. (2005 [1988]). *A secure base*. Oxon: Routledge.

Bowlby, J. (2020 [1933–1983]). *Trauma and loss: key texts from the John Bowlby archive*. R. Duschinsky & K. White (eds). London: Routledge.

Bowlby, J., Miller, E. & Winnicott, D. W. (1939). 'Evacuation of small children' *British Medical Journal* 2: 1202–1203.

Boyd, J. (2007). 'The rhythm method' *Body Movement and Dance in Psychotherapy* 2(1): 57–67.

Bremness, A. & Polzin, W. (2014). 'Developmental trauma disorder: a missed opportunity in DSM V' *Journal of the Canadian Academy of Child and Adolescent Psychiatry* 23(2): 142–145.

Brennan, R., Bush [Boaz], M. & Trickey, D. with Levene, C. & Watson, J. (2019). *Adversity & trauma-informed practice: a short guide for professionals working on the frontline.* London: YoungMinds, Anna Freud National Centre for Children and Families, and Body & Soul.

Breuer, J. & Freud, S. (1982 [1908]). *Studies on hysteria (Studien über Hysterie)* (2nd ed.). J. Strachey (ed. and trans.). New York: Basic Books.

Briquet, P. (1859). *Traité Clinique et Thérapeutique de L'Hystérie.* Paris: J.-B. Bailliére & Fils.

Brom, D., Stokar, Y., Lawi, C., Nuriel-Porat, V., Ziv, Y., Lerner, K. & Ross, G. (2017). 'Somatic experiencing for posttraumatic stress disorder: a randomized controlled outcome study' *Journal of Traumatic Stress* 30(3): 304–312.

Brown, D. W., Anda, R. F., Tiemeier, H., Felitti, V. J., Edwards, V. J., Croft, J. B., Giles, W. H. (2009). 'Adverse childhood experiences and the risk of premature mortality' *American Journal of Preventive Medicine* 37(5): 389–396.

Brown, L. S. (2004). 'Feminist paradigms of trauma treatment' *Psychotherapy: Theory, Research, Practice, Training* 41(4): 464–471.

Brownmiller, S. (1975). *Against our will: men, women and rape.* New York: Simon & Schuster.

Brunner, J. (1991). 'Psychiatry, psychoanalysis, and politics during the First World War' *Journal of the History of the Behavioral Sciences* 27(4): 352–365.

Buber, M. (1958 [1949]). *Paths in utopia.* R. F. C. Hull (trans.). Boston, MA: Beacon Press.

Buber, M. (1996 [1923]). *I and thou.* W. Kaufmann (trans.). New York: Touchstone.

The Buddhist Society (2020). *Fundamental teachings.* www.thebuddhistsociety.org/page/fundamental-teachings.

Bugental, J. F. T. (1965). *The search for authenticity: an existential-analytic approach to psychotherapy.* New York: Holt, Rinehart & Winston.

Burgermeister, D. (2007). 'Childhood adversity: a review of measurement instruments' *Journal of Nursing Measurement* 15(3): 163–176.

Burgess, A. W. (1985). *Rape and sexual assault: a research handbook.* London: Garland.

Burgess, A. W. & Holmstrom, L. (1974). 'Rape trauma syndrome' *American Journal of Psychiatry* 131(9): 981–986.

Burke, B. L., Martens, A. & Faucher, E. H. (2010). 'Two decades of terror management theory: a meta-analysis of mortality salience research' *Personality and Social Psychology Review* 14(2): 155–195.

Bush [Boaz], M. (2018a). 'Between fantasy and finitude: re-appraising Kierkegaard's philosophy of despair with a contemporary existential-psychotherapeutic attitude of (de) spero' *Existential Analysis* 29(1): 123–134.

Bush [Boaz], M. (2018b). 'Childhood adversity and trauma' in M. Bush [Boaz] (ed.) *Addressing adversity: prioritising adversity and trauma-informed care for children and young people in England.* London: YoungMinds/Health Education England, pp. 26–55.

Bush [Boaz], M. (2018c). 'On the phenomenon of Enttäuschung: a rejoinder to Roy Schafer's psychoanalytic formulation of "disappointment" and "disappointedness"' *Existential Analysis* 29(2): 189–197.

Bush [Boaz], M. (2019). 'Action in the present: towards the application of Levinasian approaches to fatigue in cognitive-behavioural environments' *Existential Analysis* 30(2): 248–259.

Bush [Boaz], M. (2020a). 'Haunted by Heidegger' *Hermeneutic Circular* (April): 6–8.

Bush [Boaz], M. (2020b). 'Paradox, polarity and the pandemic: making sense of the existential impacts of COVID-19 on people's lives' *Existential Analysis* 31(2): 225–236.

Bush [Boaz], M. (2020c). 'Refractions in time: a Minkowskian understanding of being dislocated in time.' *Existential Analysis* 31(1): 133–141.

Butler, J. (2011 [1993]). *Bodies that matter: on the discursive limits of sex*. Oxon: Routledge.

Calhoun, L. G. & Tedeschi, R. G. (2013). *Post-traumatic growth in clinical practice*. London: Routledge.

Camus, A. (2005 [1942]). *The myth of Sisyphus*. J. O'Brien (trans.). London: Penguin.

Cannon, W. B. (1963 [1932]). *Wisdom of the body: how the human body reacts to disturbance and dancer and maintains the stability essential to life* (rev. ed.). New York: W. W. Norton.

Carroll, R. (2002). 'Biodynamic massage in psychotherapy: re-integrating, re-owning and re-associating though the body' in T. Staunton (ed.) *Body psychotherapy*. London: Routledge, pp. 78–100.

Castro-Vale, I., Severo, M., Carvalho, D. & Mota-Cardoso, R. (2019). 'Intergenerational transmission of war-related trauma assessed 40 years after exposure' *Annals of General Psychiatry* 18: 14.

Cesario, J., Johnson, D. J. & Eisthen, H. L. (2020). 'Your brain is not an onion with a tiny reptile inside' *Current Directions in Psychological Science* 9(3): 255–260.

Chandan, J. D., Thomas, T., Gokhale, K. M., Bandyopadhyay, S., Taylor, J. & Nirantharakumar, K. (2019). 'The burden of mental ill health associated with childhood maltreatment in the UK, using the Health Improvement Network database: a population-based retrospective cohort study' *Lancet Psychiatry* 6(11): 926–934.

Charcot, J. M. (1873). *Leçons sur les maladies du système nerveux, faites a la Salpêtrière*. Paris: Place De L'école-De-Medicine (accessed on the digital archive.org).

Children Act [2004]. www.legislation.gov.uk/ukpga/2004/31/section/58.

Cohen, J. A., Deblinger, E. & Mannarino, A. P. (2018). 'Trauma-focused cognitive behavioral therapy for children and families' *Psychotherapy Research* 28(1): 47–57.

Cohen, J. A. & Mannarino, A. P. (2015). 'Trauma-focused cognitive behavior therapy for traumatized children and families' *Child and Adolescent Psychiatric Clinics of North America* 24(3): 557–570.

Cohen, J. A., Mannarino, A. P. & Deblinger, E. (2017). *Treating trauma and traumatic grief in children and adolescents* (2nd ed.). New York: Guilford Press.

Cohen, J. A., Mannarino, A. P. & Murray, L. K. (2011). 'Trauma-focused CBT for youth who experience ongoing traumas' *Child Abuse & Neglect* 35(8): 637–646.

Cohen, S. (2002 [1972]). *Folk devils and moral panics: the creation of mods and rockers* (3rd ed.). New York: Routledge.

Cohn, H W. (1997). *Existential thought and therapeutic practice: an introduction to existential psychotherapy*. London: SAGE.

Conway, C., Raposa, E. B., Hammen, C. & Brennan, P. A. (2018). 'Transdiagnostic pathways from early social stress to psychopathology: a 20-year prospective study' *Journal of Child Psychology and Psychiatry* 59(8): 855–862.

Cooper, M. (2015). *Existential psychotherapy and counselling: contributions to a pluralistic practice*. London: SAGE.

Cooper, M. (2017). *Existential therapies* (2nd ed.). London: SAGE.

Copeland, W. E., Keeler, G., Angold, A. & Costello E. J. (2007). 'Traumatic events and post-traumatic stress in childhood' *Archives of General Psychiatry* 64(5): 577–584.

Correia, E. A., Cooper, M., Berdondini, L. & Correia, K. (2017). 'Characteristic practices of existential psychotherapy: a worldwide survey of practitioners' perspectives' *The Humanistic Psychologist* 45(3): 217–237.

Correia, E. A., Cooper, M., Berdondini, L. & Correia, K. (2018). 'Existential psychotherapies: similarities and differences among the main branches' *Journal of Humanistic Psychology* 58(2): 119–143.

Corrie, S. & Milton, M. (2000). 'The relationship between existential-phenomenological and cognitive-behaviour therapies' *Journal of Psychotherapy & Health* 3(1): 7–24.

Craig, A. D. (2003). 'Interoception: the sense of the physiological condition of the body' *Current Opinion in Neurobiology* 13(4): 500–505.

Craig, A. D. (2015). *How do you feel? An interoceptive moment with your neurobiological self.* Princeton, NJ: Princeton University Press.

Cramer, H., Anheyer, D., Saha, F. J. & Dobos, G. (2018). 'Yoga for post-traumatic stress disorder: a systematic review and meta-analysis' *BMC Psychiatry* 18: 72.

Cristobal, K. A. (2018). 'Power of touch: working with survivors of sexual abuse within dance/movement therapy' *American Journal of Dance Therapy* 40(1): 68–86.

Crittenden, P. M. & Ainsworth, M. D. S. (1989). 'Child maltreatment and attachment theory' in D. Cicchetti & D. Carlson (eds) *Childhood maltreatment: theory and research on the causes and consequences of child abuse and neglect.* Cambridge, UK: Cambridge University Press, pp. 432–463.

Cromby, J. & Standen, P. (1999). 'Taking ourselves seriously' in D. Nightingale & J. Cromby (eds) *Social constructionist psychology: a critical analysis of theory and practice.* Buckingham: Open University Press, pp. 141–155.

Cronholm, F. P., Forke, C. M., Wade, R., Bair-Merritt, M. H., Davis, M., Harkins-Schwarz, M., Pachter, L. M. & Fein, J. A. (2015). 'Adverse childhood experiences: expanding the concept of adversity' *American Journal of Preventive Medicine* 49(3): 354–361.

Dalgleish, T., Black, M., Johnston, D. & Bevan, A. (2020). 'Transdiagnostic approaches to mental health problems: current status and future directions' *Journal of Consulting and Clinical Psychology* 88(3): 179–195.

Danese, A. & Widom, C. S. (2020). 'Objective and subjective experiences of child maltreatment and their relationships with psychopathology' *Nature Human Behaviour* 4(8): 811–818.

Dashorst, P., Mooren, T. M., Kleber, R. J. de Jong, P. J. & Huntjens, R. J. C. (2019). 'Intergenerational consequences of the Holocaust on offspring mental health: a systematic review of associated factors and mechanism' *European Journal of Psychotraumatology* 10(1): 1654065.

Davis, A. Y. (2019 [1981]). *Women, race & class.* London: Penguin.

de Beauvoir, S. (2015 [1948]). *The ethics of ambiguity.* New York: Philosophical Library.

de Roos, M. S. & Jones, D. N. (2020). 'Self-affirmation and false allegations: the effects on responses to disclosures of sexual victimization' *Journal of Interpersonal Violence*: 1–24. doi:10.1177/0886260520980387.

Debanné, M. & Nolte, T. (2019). 'Contemporary neuroscientific research' in A. W. Bateman & P. Fonagy (eds) *Handbook of mentalizing in mental health practice* (2nd ed.). Washington, DC: American Psychiatric Association, pp. 21–36.

Dennett, D. C. (1991). *Consciousness explained.* London: Little, Brown & Company.

Di Cesare, D. (2018). *Heidegger and the Jews: the black notebooks.* M. Baca (trans.). Cambridge, UK: Polity Press.

Domestic Abuse Bill [2020]. https://services.parliament.uk/Bills/2019-21/domesticabuse/documents.html.

Douglas, M. (1986). *Risk acceptability according to the social sciences.* London: Routledge.

Douglas, M. & Wildavsky, A. (1982). *Risk and culture.* Oxford: Blackwell.

Downs, A. (2012). *The velvet rage: overcoming the pain of growing up gay in a straight man's world* (revised and updated 2nd ed.). Boston, MA: Da Capo Press.

Dowset, G. W. (2009). 'The "gay plague" revisited: AIDS and its enduring moral panic' in G. Herdt (ed.) *Moral panics, sex panics: fear and the fight over sexual rights.* London: New York University Press, pp. 130–156.

Drescher, J. (2009). 'Queer diagnoses: parallels and contrasts in the history of homosexuality, gender variance, and the Diagnostic and Statistical Manual' *Archives of Sexual Behavior* 39(2): 427–460.

Duke, L. A., Allen, D. N., Rozee, P. D. & Bommaritto, M. (2008). 'The sensitivity and specificity of flashbacks and nightmares to trauma' *Journal of Anxiety Disorders* 22(2): 319–327.

Dunleavy, K. & Kubo Slowik, A. (2012). 'Emergence of delayed post-traumatic stress disorder symptoms related to sexual trauma: patient-centered and trauma-cognizant management by physical therapists' *Physical Therapy* 92(2): 339–351.

Dworkin, A. (1974). *Woman hating.* New York: Plume.

Dworkin, A. (1993 [1989]). 'What battery really is' in A. Dworkin. *Letters from a war zone.* New York: Lawrence Hill Books, pp. 329–334.

Early Intervention Foundation (2020). *Adverse childhood experiences: what we know, what we don't know, and what should happen next.* London: EFI.

Edmondson, D., Chaudoir, S. R. Mills, M. A., Park, C. L., Holub, J. & Bartkowiak, J. M. (2011). 'From shattered assumptions to weakened worldviews: trauma symptoms signal anxiety buffer disruption' *Journal of Loss & Trauma* 16(4): 358–385.

Edwards, D. J. A. (1990). 'Cognitive-behavioral and existential-phenomenological approaches to therapy: complementary or conflicting paradigms? *Journal of Cognitive Psychotherapy* 4(2): 105–120.

Eger, E. (2018). *The choice: even in hell hope can flower.* London: Rider.

Ehlers, A. & Clark, D. M. (2000). 'A cognitive model of post-traumatic stress disorder' *Behaviour Research & Therapy* 38(4): 319–345.

Ehrenreich-May, J. & Chu, B. C. (2014). 'Overview of transdiagnostic mechanisms and treatments for youth psychopathology' in J. Ehrenreich-May & B. Chu (eds) *Transdiagnostic treatments for children and adolescents: principles and practice.* New York: Guilford Press, pp. 3–14.

Eliastam, J. L. B. (2015). 'Exploring ubuntu discourse in South Africa: loss, liminality and hope' *Verbum et Ecclesia* 36(2): 1–8.

Ellenberger, H. F. (1970). *The discovery of the unconscious: the history and evolution of dynamic psychiatry.* New York: Basic Books.

Ellis, A. (1957). 'Rational psychotherapy and individual psychology' *Journal of Individual Psychology* 13(1): 38–44.

Ellis, A. (1963). *Rational-emotive psychotherapy.* New York: Institute for Rational-Emotive Therapy.

Emerson, D. (2015). *Trauma-sensitive yoga in therapy: bringing the body into treatment.* London: W. W. Norton.

Emerson, D. & Hopper, E. (2011). *Overcoming trauma through yoga: reclaiming your body.* Berkeley, CA: North Atlantic Books.

Engel, G. (1977). 'The need for a new medical model: a challenge for biomedicine' *Science* 196(4286): 129–136.

Esterson, A. (2001). 'The mythologizing of psychoanalytic history: deception and self-deception in Freud's accounts of the seduction theory episode' *History of Psychiatry* 12(47): 329–352.

European Court of Human Rights (ECHR). [1997]. Case of *A. v. The United Kingdom* (100/1997/884/1096).

Evans, J. S. (2008). 'Dual-processing accounts of reasoning, judgment, and social cognition' *Annual Review of Psychology* 59: 255–278.

Faimberg, H. (2007). 'A plea for a broader concept of *Nachträglichkeit*' *Psychoanalytic Quarterly* 76: 1221–1240.

Fairbairn, W. R. D. (1994 [1943a]). 'The repression and the return of bad objects (with special reference to the "war neuroses")' in W. R. D, Fairbairn *Psychoanalytic studies of the personality*. London: Routledge, pp. 59–81.

Fairbairn, W. R. D. (1994 [1943b]). 'The war neuroses – their nature and significance' in W. R. D. Fairbairn *Psychoanalytic studies of the personality*. London: Routledge, pp. 256–288.

Fairbairn, W. R. D. (1994 [1944]). 'Endopsychic structure considered in terms of object-relationships' in W. R. D. Fairbairn *Psychoanalytic studies of the personality*. London: Routledge, pp. 82–136.

Fairbairn, W. R. D. (1994 [1951]). 'A synopsis of the development of the author's views regarding the structure of the personality' in W. R. D. Fairbairn *Psychoanalytic studies of the personality*. London: Routledge, pp. 162–182.

Fanon, F. (2004 [1961]). *The wretched of the earth*. R. Philcox (trans.). New York: Grove Press.

Fanon, F. (2008 [1952]). *Black skin, white masks*. R. Philcox (trans.). New York: Grove Press.

Farin, I. & Malpas, J. (2018). *Reading Heidegger's black notebooks 1931–1941*. Cambridge, MA: MIT Press.

Feldman Barrett, L. (2006). 'Solving the emotion paradox: categorization and the experience of emotion' *Personality and Social Psychology Review* 10(1): 20–46.

Feldman Barrett, L. (2009). 'The future of psychology: connecting mind to brain' *Perspectives on Psychological Science* 4(4): 326–339.

Feldman Barrett, L. (2017a). *How emotions are made: the secret life of the brain*. London: Macmillan.

Feldman Barrett, L. (2017b). 'The theory of constructed emotion: an active inference account of interoception and categorization' *Social Cognitive & Affective Neuroscience* 12(1): 1–23.

Feldman Barrett, L. (2021). *Seven and a half lessons about the brain*. London: Picador.

Felitti, V. J., Anda, R. F., Nordenberg, D., Williamson, D. F., Spitz, A. M., Edwards, V., Koss, M. P. & Marks, J. S. (1998). 'Relationship of childhood abuse and household dysfunction to many of the leading causes of death in adults: the adverse childhood experiences (ACE) study' *American Journal of Preventative Medicine* 14(4): 245–258.

Ferenczi, S. (1926 [1916/1917]). 'Two types of war neuroses' in J. Rickman (ed.), J. I. Suttie, (trans.) *Further contributions to the theory and technique of psycho-analysis*. New York: Boni & Liverlight, pp. 124–141.

Ferenczi, S. (1949 [1932]). 'Confusion of the tongues between the adults and the child (the language of tenderness and of passion). Balint, M. (trans.). *International Journal of Psychoanalysis* 30(4): 225–230.

Ferenczi, S. (1988 [1932]). *The clinical diary of Sandor Ferenczi*. J. Dupont (ed.), M. Balint & N. Z. Jackson (trans.). Cambridge, MA: Harvard University Press.

Ferenczi, S., Abraham, K. A., Simmel, E. & Jones, E. (1921 [1919]). *Psychoanalysis and the war neuroses*. London: International Psychoanalytic Press.

Fitzgerald, E., Given, M., Gough, M., Kelso, L, Mcilwaine, V. & Miskelly, C. (2017). *The transgenerational impact of 'the troubles' in Northern Ireland*. Belfast: Queen's University Belfast. www.qub.ac.uk/schools/psy/files/Filetoupload,784073,en.pdf.

Foa, E. B. (2011). 'Prolonged exposure therapy: past, present, and future' *Depression & Anxiety* 28(12): 1043–1047.

Foa, E. B., Chrestman, K. & Gilboa-Schechtman, E. (2009). *Prolonged exposure therapy for adolescents with PTSD: emotional processing of traumatic experiences (therapist's guide).* Oxford: Oxford University Press.

Fonagy, P. (2001). *Attachment theory and psychoanalysis.* London: Karnac Books.

Fonagy, P. & Allison, E. (2014). 'The role of mentalizing and epistemic trust in the therapeutic relationship' *Psychotherapy* 51(3): 372–380.

Fonagy, P. & Bateman, A. W. (2016). 'Adversity, attachment, and mentalizing' *Comprehensive Psychiatry* 64: 59–66.

Fonagy, P. & Bateman, A. W. (2019). 'Introduction' in A. W. Bateman & P. Fonagy (eds) *Handbook of mentalizing in mental health practice* (2nd ed.). Washington, DC: American Psychiatric Association, pp. 3–20.

Foucault, M. (1979). *Discipline & punish: the birth of the prison.* A. Sheridan (trans.). London: Penguin.

Foucault, M. (1983). 'The subject and power' in H. Dreyfus & P. Rabinow (eds) *Michel Foucault: beyond structuralism and hermeneutics* (2nd ed.). Chicago: University of Chicago Press, pp. 208–223.

Foucault, M. (1990 [1984]). *The history of sexuality: the care of the self.* R. Hurley (trans.). London: Penguin.

Foucault, M. (1998 [1976]). *The history of sexuality: the will to knowledge.* R. Hurley (trans.). London: Penguin.

Foucault, M. (2000 [1970]). 'The discourse of language' A. Sheridan & R. Sawyer (trans.) in L. Burke, T. Crowley & A. Girvin (eds) *The Routledge language and cultural theory reader.* London: Routledge, pp. 231–240.

Foucault, M. (2002 [1969]). *The archaeology of knowledge.* A. M. Sheridan Smith (trans.). Oxon: Routledge.

Foucault, M. (2003 [1963]). *The birth of the clinic.* A. M. Sheridan (trans.). Oxon: Routledge.

Foucault, M. (2003 [1999]). *Abnormal: lectures at the Collège de France 1974–1975.* G. Burchell (trans.). New York: Picador.

Foucault, M. (2009 [1961]). *History of madness.* J. Murphy & J. Khalfa (trans.), J. Khalfa (ed.). Oxon: Routledge.

Foucault, M. (2010 [2004]). *The birth of biopolitics: lectures at the Collège de France 1978–1979.* G. Burchell (trans.). New York: Palgrave Macmillan.

Frances, A. (2013). *Saving normal: an insider's revolt against out-of-control psychiatric diagnosis, DSM-5, big pharma, and the medicalization of ordinary life.* New York: William Morrow.

Frankel, J. (2004). 'Identification with the aggressor and the "normal traumas": clinical implications' *International Forum of Psychoanalysis* 13(1/2): 78–83.

Frankl, V. E. (1960). 'Paradoxical intention: a logotherapeutic technique' *American Journal of Psychotherapy* 14(3): 520–535.

Frankl, V. E. (1967). *Psychotherapy and existentialism: selected papers on Logotherapy.* London: Pelican.

Frankl, V. E. (1975). 'Paradoxical intention and dereflection' *Psychotherapy: Theory, Research & Practice* 12(3): 226–237.

Frankl, V. E. (1986 [1946]). *The doctor and the soul: from psychotherapy to logotherapy* (3rd ed., revised and expanded). R. Winston & C. Winston (trans.). New York: Vintage Books.

Frankl, V. E. (1988). *The will to meaning: foundations and applications of logotherapy* (expanded ed.). New York: Plume.

Frankl, V. E. (2004 [1959]). *Man's search for meaning.* London: Rider.

Frankl, V. E. (2020 [1946]). *Yes to life: in spite of everything.* J. Young (trans.). London: Penguin.

Freud, A. (1967). 'Comments on trauma' in S. S. Furst (ed.) *Psychic trauma.* New York: Basic Books, pp. 235–245.

Freud, A. (2018 [1936]). *The ego and the mechanisms of defence*. Oxon: Routledge.

Freud, S. (1909). *Selected papers on hysteria and other psychoneuroses*. A. Brill (trans.). New York: Journal of Nervous and Mental Disease Pub. Co.

Freud, S. (1931 [1899]). *The interpretation of dreams*. A. A. Brill. (trans.). London: Allen & Unwin.

Freud, S. (1940). *Moses and monotheism* (2nd ed.) K. Jones (trans.). London: Hogarth Press/ Institute of Psychoanalysis.

Freud, S. (1953 [1914/18]). 'From the history of an infantile neurosis' in J. Strachey (trans.) *Standard edition of the complete psychological works of Sigmund Freud* (vol. 17). London: Hogarth Press.

Freud, S. (1955 [1919]). 'The "uncanny"' in *The standard edition of the complete psychological works of Sigmund Freud. Vol. XVII (1917–1919): an infantile neurosis and other works*. J. Strachey (ed. and trans.). London: Hogarth Press and the Institute of Psychoanalysis.

Freud, S. (1963 [1940]). *An outline of psychoanalysis*. J. Strachey (trans.). New York: W. W. Norton.

Freud, S. (1966 [1895]). 'Project for a scientific psychology' in J. Strachey (trans.) *Standard edition of the complete psychological works of Sigmund Freud* (vol. 1). London: Hogarth Press.

Freud, S. (2012 [1920]). 'Eighteenth lecture: traumatic fixation – the unconscious' in G. Stanley Hall (trans.) *A general introduction to psychoanalysis*. Hertfordshire: Wordsworth, pp. 231–242.

Freyd, J. (1994). 'Betrayal trauma: traumatic amnesia as an adaptive response to childhood abuse' *Ethics & Behavior* 4(4): 307–329.

Freyd, J. (1996). *Betrayal trauma: the logic of forgetting childhood abuse*. Cambridge, MA: Harvard University Press.

Frith, C. D. & Frith, U. (2006). 'The neural basis of mentalizing' *Neuron* 50(4): 531–534.

Fuchs, T. (2013). 'Temporality and psychopathology' *Phenomenology and the Cognitive Sciences* 12(1): 75–104.

Fuchs, T. & De Jaegher, H (2009). 'Enactive intersubjectivity: participatory sense-making and mutual incorporation' *Phenomenology and the Cognitive Sciences* 8(4): 465–486.

Fuchs, T. & Koch, S. C. (2014). 'Embodied affectivity: on moving and being moved' *Frontiers in Psychology* 5(408). doi:10.3389/fpsyg.2014.00508.

Gabaya, R., Hameiribc, B., Rubel-Lifschitz, T. & Nadlera, A. (2020). 'The tendency for interpersonal victimhood: the personality construct and its consequences' *Personality & Individual Differences* 165: 110134.

Gadamer, H.-G. (2013 [1975]). *Truth and method*. J. Weinsheimer & D. G. Marshall (trans.). London: Bloomsbury.

Garfinkel, H. (1967). *Studies in ethnomethodology*. Englewood Cliffs, NJ: Prentice-Hall.

Gil, E. & Dias, T. (2014). 'The integration of drama therapy and play therapy in attachment work with traumatised children' in C. A. Malchoiodi & D. A. Crenshaw (eds) *Creative arts and play therapy for attachment problems*. London: Guilford Press.

Gilbert, P. (2013). *The compassionate mind* (rev. ed.). London: Constable.

Goffman, E. (1963). *Behaviour in public places: notes on the social organization of gatherings*. New York: Free Press.

Goffman, E. (1967). *Interaction ritual: essays on face-to-face behaviour*. New York: Anchor Books.

Goffman, E. (1968 [1961]). *Asylums: essays on the social situation of mental patients and other inmates*. London: Pelican.

Goffman, E. (1986 [1974]). *Frame analysis: an essay on the organization of experience*. Boston, MA: Northeastern University Press.

Goffman, E. (1990 [1959]). *The presentation of the self in everyday life*. London: Penguin.

Goffman, E. (1990 [1963]). *Stigma: notes on the management of spoiled identity*. London: Penguin.

Gray, A. E. L. (2017). 'Polyvagal-informed dance/movement therapy for trauma: a global perspective' *American Journal of Dance Therapy* 39(1): 43–46.

Greenberg, D. M., Baron-Cohen, S., Rosenberg, N., Fonagy, P. & Rentfrow, P. J. (2018). 'Elevated empathy in adults following childhood trauma' *PLoS ONE* 13(10): e0203886.

Hacking, I. (1991). 'The making and moulding of child abuse' *Critical Inquiry* 17: 253–288.

Hacking, I. (1992). 'World-making by kind-making: child abuse for example' in M. Douglas & D. Hull (eds) *How classification works: Nelson Goodman among the social sciences*. Edinburgh: Edinburgh University Press, pp. 180–237.

Hacking, I. (1995). *Rewriting the soul: multiple personality and the science of memory*. Princeton, NJ: Princeton University.

Hacking, I. (1998). *Mad travellers: reflections on the reality of transient mental illness*. Charlottesville, VA: University of Virginia Press.

Hacking, I. (1999). *The social construction of what?* London: Harvard University Press.

Hacking, I. (2007). 'Kinds of people: moving targets' *Proceedings of the British Academy* 151: 285–318.

Hacking, I. (2009). 'Autistic autobiography' *Philosophical Transactions of the Royal Society* 364: 1467–1473.

Halberstam, J. (1995). *Skin shows: gothic horror and the technology of monsters*. London: Duke University Press.

Hambrick, E. P., Brawner, T. W. & Perry, B. D. (2019). 'Timing of early-life stress and the development of brain-related capacities' *Frontiers in Behavioural Neuroscience* 13. doi.org/10.3389/fnbeh.2019.00183.

Harvey, M. R. (1996). 'An ecological view of psychological trauma and trauma recovery' *Journal of Traumatic Stress* 9(1): 3–23.

Hebb, D. O. (1949). *The organization of behavior: a neuropsychological theory*. London: Chapman & Hall.

Heidegger, M. (2001). *Zollikon seminars: protocols-conversations-letters*. M. Boss (ed.), R. Askay & F. Mayr (trans.). Evanston, IL: Northwestern University Press.

Heidegger, M. (2010 [1953]). *Being and time*. J. Stambaugh (trans.). Albany, NY: State University of New York Press.

Heidegger, M. (2016 [2014]). *Ponderings II–VI: black notebooks 1931–1938* (Studies in Continental Thought). R. Rojcewicz (trans.). Bloomington, IN: Indiana University Press.

Heidegger, M. (2017a [2014]). *Ponderings VII–XI: black notebooks 1938–1939* (Studies in Continental Thought). R. Rojcewicz (trans.). Bloomington, IN: Indiana University Press.

Heidegger, M. (2017b [2014]). *Ponderings XII–XV: black notebooks 1939–1941* (Studies in Continental Thought). R. Rojcewicz (trans.). Bloomington, IN: Indiana University Press.

Heidenreich, T., Noyon, A., Worrell, M. & Menzies, R. (2021). 'Existential approaches and cognitive behavior therapy: challenges and potential' *International Journal of Cognitive Therapy* 14: 209–234.

Heim, G. & Bühler, K.-E. (2006). 'Psychological trauma and fixed ideas in Pierre Janet's conception of dissociative disorders' *American Journal of Psychotherapy* 60(2): 111–129.

Herman, J. L. (1985). 'Father–daughter incest' in A. W. Burgess (ed.) *Rape and sexual assault: a research handbook*. London: Garland Publishing, pp. 83–96.

Herman, J. L. (1992). 'Complex PTSD: A syndrome in survivors of prolonged and repeated trauma' *Journal of Traumatic Stress* 5(3): 377–391.

Herman, J. L. (1998). 'Recovery from psychological trauma' *Psychiatry and Clinical Neurosciences* 52(1): 98–103.

Herman, J. L. (2015 [1992]). *Trauma and recovery: the aftermath of violence – from domestic abuse to political terror*. New York: Basic Books.

Herman, J. L. with Hirschman, J. (1981). *Father–daughter incest*. Cambridge, MA: Harvard University Press.

Hesse, E. & Main, M. (2000). 'Disorganized infant, child, and adult attachment: collapse in behavioral and attentional strategies' *Journal of the American Psychoanalytic Association* 48(4): 1097–1127.

Hesse, E. & Main, M. (2006). 'Frightened, threatening, and dissociative parental behavior in low-risk samples: description, discussion, and interpretations' *Development & Psychopathology* 18(2): 309–343.

Hodges, A. (2014 [1983]). *Alan Turing: the enigma*. London: Penguin.

Holzhey-Kunz, A. (2014). *Daseinsanalysis*. London: Free Association Books.

Holzhey-Kunz, A. (2016). 'Why the distinction between ontic and ontological trauma matters for existential therapists' *Existential Analysis* 27(1): 16–27.

hooks, b. (2015 [1981]). *Ain't I a woman: black women and feminism*. London: Routledge.

hooks, b. (2015 [1984]). *Feminist theory: from margin to centre*. Oxon: Routledge.

Hoppena, T. H. & Chalder, T. (2018). 'Childhood adversity as a transdiagnostic risk factor for affective disorders in adulthood: a systematic review focusing on biopsychosocial moderating and mediating variables' *Clinical Psychology Review* 65: 81–151,

Horowitz, M. J. (1976). *Stress response syndromes*. New York: Jason Aronson.

Horowitz, M. J. (1986). 'Stress-response syndromes: a review of posttraumatic and adjustment disorders' *Hospital & Community Psychiatry* 37(3): 241–249.

Horowitz, M. J. (1993). 'Stress-response syndromes: a review of posttraumatic stress and adjustment disorders' in J. P. Wilson & B. Raphael (eds) *International handbook of traumatic stress syndromes*. New York: Plenum Press, pp. 49–60.

Horwitz, A. & Wakefield, J. (2007). *The loss of sadness: how psychiatry transformed normal sorrow into depressive disorder*. New York: Oxford University Press.

Horwitz, A. V. (2018). *PTSD: a short history*. Lanham, MD: Johns Hopkins University Press.

Hughes, D., Golding, K. S. & Hudson, J. (2019). *Healing relational trauma with attachment-focused interventions*. London: W. W. Norton.

Hughes, K., Lowey, H., Quigg, Z. & Bellis, M. A. (2016). 'Relationships between adverse child- hood experiences and adult mental well-being: results from an English national household survey' *BMC Public Health* 16: 222.

Hulette, A. C., Kaehler, L. A. & Freyd, J. J. (2011). 'Intergenerational associations between trauma and dissociation' *Journal of Family Violence* 26: 217–225.

Husserl, E. (2012 [1931]). *Ideas: general introduction to pure phenomenology*. W. R. Boyce Gibson (trans.). London: Routledge.

Iacovou, S. & Paidoussis-Mitchell, C. (2017). 'The impact of active service on the intimate relationships of British Royal Naval Veterans of the Falklands War' *Existential Analysis* 28(2): 385–405.

Illich, I. (1976). *Limits to medicine: medical nemesis – the expropriation of health*. London: Marion Boyars.

Independent Inquiry into Child Sexual Abuse (IICSA) (2018). *Interim report of the independent inquiry into child sexual abuse*. London: HM Stationery Office.

Independent Inquiry into Child Sexual Abuse (IICSA) (2020a). *The Anglican Church: investigation report*. London: HM Stationery Office.

Independent Inquiry into Child Sexual Abuse (IICSA) (2020b). *The Roman Catholic Church: investigation report*. London: HM Stationery Office.

Independent Inquiry into Child Sexual Abuse (IICSA) (2020c). *Safeguarding children from sexual abuse in residential schools.* London: HM Stationery Office.

Insel, T. R. & Young, L. J. (2001). 'The neurobiology of attachment' *Nature Reviews (Neuroscience)* 2: 129–136.

Irigaray, L. (1992 [1982]). *Elemental passions.* J. Collie & J. Still (trans.). London: Athlone Press.

Jacobsen, B. (2006). 'The life crisis in an existential perspective: can trauma and crisis be seen as an aid in personal development?' *Existential Analysis* 17(1): 39–53.

Jacobsen, B. (2007). *Invitation to existential psychology: a psychology for the unique human being and its applications in therapy.* Hoboken, NJ: John Wiley & Sons.

Janet, P. (1901). *The mental state of hystericals: a study of mental stigmata and mental accidents.* C. Rollin Corson (trans.). London: G. P. Putnam's & Sons.

Janet, P. (1911). *L'état Mental Des Hystériques (deuxième edition).* Paris: Ancienne Librairie Germer Bailliere et Felix Alcan.

Janoff-Bulman, R. (1989). 'The benefits of illusions, the threat of disillusionment and the limits of inaccuracy' *Journal of Social and Clinical Psychology* 8(2): 158–176.

Janoff-Bulman, R. (1992). *Shattered assumptions: towards a new psychology of trauma.* Oxford: Free Press.

Janoff-Bulman, R. & Berg, M. (2013 [1998]). 'Disillusionment and the creation of value: from traumatic losses to existential gains' in J. H. Harvey (ed.) *Perspectives on loss: a sourcebook.* New York: Routledge, pp. 35–47.

Jaspers, K. (1948). *Philosophie.* Berlin: Springer-Verlag.

Jaspers, K. (1956). *Philosophie.* Berlin: Springer-Verlag.

Jaspers, K. (1995 [1971]). *Philosophy of existence.* R. F. Grabay (trans.). Philadelphia, PA: University of Pennsylvania Press.

Jaspers, K. (2003 [1954]). *Way to wisdom: an introduction to philosophy* (2nd ed.). New Haven, CT: Yale University Press.

Jentsch, E. (1995 [1906]). 'On the psychology of the uncanny' R. Sellars (trans.). *Angelaki* 2(1): 7–16.

Kandel, E. R. (1998). 'A new intellectual framework for psychiatry' *American Journal of Psychiatry* 155(4): 457–469.

Kandel, E. R. (2006). *In search of memory: the emergence of a new science of mind.* New York: W. W. Norton.

Kandel, E. R. (2013). 'The new science of mind and the future of knowledge' *Neuron* 80(3): 546–560.

Kardiner, A. (1941). *The traumatic neurosis of war.* Menasha, WI: George Banta Publishing.

Kaufman, G. & Raphael, L. (1996). *Coming out of shame: transforming gay and lesbian lives.* London: Doubleday.

Kaufman, J. & Zigler, E. (1987). 'Do abused children become abusive parents?' *American Journal of Orthopsychiatry* 57(2): 186–192.

Kelly-Irving, M., Lepage, B., Dedieu, D., Bartley, M., Blane, D., Grosclaude, P., Lang, T., Delpierre, C. (2013). 'Adverse childhood experiences and premature all-cause mortality' *European Journal of Epidemiology* 28(9): 721–734.

Kierkegaard, S. (2008 [1849]). *The sickness unto death [Sygdommen til Døden].* A. Hannay (trans.). London: Penguin.

King, P. & Steiner, R. (1991). *The Freud–Klein Controversies 1941–45* (New Library of Psychoanalysis). London: Routledge/Institute of Psychoanalysis.

Kitzinger, K. (1996). 'The Freudian coverup: a reappraisal' *Feminism & Psychology* 6(2): 251–259.

Klein, M. (1997 [1975]). *Envy and gratitude and other works 1946–1963.* London: Vintage.

Klein, M. (1998 [1975]). *Love, guilt and reparation and other works 1921–1945.* London: Vintage.

Kohut, H. (1971). *The analysis of the self: a systematic approach to the psychoanalytic treatment of narcissistic personality disorders.* New York: International Universities Press.

Kohut, H. (1984). *How does analysis cure?* A. Goldberg with P. Stepansky (eds). Chicago: University of Chicago Press.

Køster, A. (2017). 'Mentalization, embodiment, and narrative: critical comments on the social ontology of mentalization theory' *Theory & Psychology* 27(3): 1–19.

Krippner, S. & Pitchford, D. B. (2018). 'Humanistic and existential approaches in the treatment of PTSD' in R. House, D. Kalisch & J. Maidman (eds) *Humanistic psychology: current trends and future prospects.* Oxon: Routledge, pp. 174–185.

Krippner, S., Pitchford, D. B. & Davies, J. (2012). *Post-traumatic stress disorder (biographies of disease).* Santa Barbara, CA: Greenwood.

Lacan, J. (1991 [1975]). *Freud's papers on technique: 1953–54 (The seminars of Jacques Lacan Book 1).* J.-A. Miller (ed.), J. Forrester (trans.). London: W. W. Norton.

Lacan, J. (2001 [1966]). *Écrits: a selection.* A. Sheridan (trans.). Oxon: Routledge.

Laing, R. D. (1971 [1961]). *Self and others.* London: Pelican.

Laing, R. D. (1972 [1959]). *The divided self: an existential in sanity and madness.* London: Pelican.

Laing, R. D. (1976 [1969]). *The politics of the family and other essays.* London: Pelican.

Laing, R. D. (1985 [1965]). 'Mystification, confusion & conflict' in I. Boszormenyi-Nagy & J. L. Framo (eds) *Intensive family therapy: theoretical and practical aspects.* New York: Brunner/Mazel, pp. 343–363.

Laing, R. D. (1990 [1967]). *The politics of experiences and the bird of paradise.* London: Penguin.

Laing, R. D. & Esterson, A. (1974 [1964]). *Sanity, madness and the family.* London: Pelican.

Lakoff, G. & Johnson, M. (2003 [1980]). *Metaphors we live by.* London: University of Chicago Press.

Landolt, M. A., Schnyder, U., Maier, T., Schoenbucher, V. & Mohler-Kuo, M. (2013). 'Trauma exposure and posttraumatic stress disorder in adolescents: a national survey in Switzerland' *Journal of Trauma Stress* 26(2): 209–216.

Längle, A. (1993). 'Ein Gespräch zur Selbstfindung anhand der Personalen Existenzanalyse' *Bulletin der Gesellschaft für Logotherapie und Existentzanalyse* 10(2): 3–11.

Längle, A. (2003a). 'The art of involving the person: fundamental existential motivations as the structure of the motivational process' *European Psychotherapy* 4(1): 25–36.

Längle, A. (2003b). 'The method of "personal existential analysis"' *European Psychotherapy* 4(1): 37–53.

Längle, A. (2005). 'Persönlichkeitsstörungen und Traumagenese: Existenzanalyse traumabedingter Persönlichkeitsstörungen' *Existenzanalyse* 22(2): 4–18.

Längle, A. (2007). 'Trauma und Existenz' *Psychotherapie Forum* 15: 109–116.

Längle, A. (2008). 'Suffering – an existential challenge: understanding, dealing and coping with suffering from an existential-analytic perspective' in G. von Kirchbach (trans.) *International Journal of Existential Psychology & Psychotherapy* 2(1): 1–10.

Längle, A. (2011). 'The existential fundamental motivations structuring the motivational process' in D. A. Leontiev (ed.) *Psychology of emotions, motivations and actions: motivation, consciousness and self-regulation.* New York: Nova, pp. 27–42.

Längle, A. (2020). *Existenzanalyse Und Logotherapie.* Stuttgart: Kohlhammer.

Lanius, R. A. (2015). 'Trauma-related dissociation and altered states of consciousness: a call for clinical, treatment, and neuroscience research' *European Journal of Psychotraumatology* 6(1): 27905.

Lanius, R. A., Vermetten, E., Loewenstein, R. J., Brand, B., Schmahl, C., Bremner, J. D. & Spiegel, D. (2010). 'Emotion modulation in PTSD: clinical and neurobiological evidence for a dissociative subtype' *American Journal of Psychiatry* 167(6): 640–647.

Lantz, J. (1991). 'Franklian treatment with Vietnam veteran couples' *Journal of Religion & Health* 30(2): 131–138.

Lantz, J. (1993). *Existential family therapy: using the concepts of Viktor Frankl.* Northvale, NJ: Jason Aronson.

Lantz, J. (2004). 'World view concepts in existential family therapy' *Contemporary Family Therapy* 26(2): 165–178.

Lantz, J. & Alford, K. (1995). 'Art in existential psychotherapy with couples and families' *Contemporary Family Therapy* 17(3): 331–342.

Lantz, J. & Gregoire, T. (2000). 'Existential psychotherapy with Vietnam veteran couples: a twenty-five-year report' *Contemporary Family Therapy* 22(1): 19–37.

Lantz, J. & Gyamerah [Meshelemiah], J. (2002). 'Existential family trauma therapy' *Contemporary Family Therapy* 24(2): 243–255.

Lantz, J. & Lantz, J. (1991). 'Franklian treatment with the traumatized family' *Journal of Family Psychotherapy* 2(2): 61–73.

Lantz, J. & Lantz, J. (1992). 'Franklian psychotherapy with adults molested as children' *Journal of Religion & Health* 31(4): 297–307.

Laplanche, J. (1999). *Essays on otherness.* Oxon: Routledge.

Latour, B. (2005). *Reassembling the social: an introduction to actor-network-theory.* Oxford: Oxford University Press.

Latour, B. & Woolgar, S. (1979). *Laboratory life: the construction of scientific facts.* London: SAGE.

Lee, N. (2005). *Childhood and human value: development, separation and separability.* Berkshire: Open University Press.

Leuenberger, R. (2008). 'Die EMDR-Methode und ihr Bezug zur ersten Grundmotivation' *Existenzanalyse* 1: 44–53.

Levi, P. (2013 [1958/1963]). *If this is a man/the truce.* S. Woolf (trans.). London: Abacus.

Levin, H. B. & Brown, L. J. (2013). *Growth and turbulence in the container/contained: Bion's continuing legacy.* Sussex: Routledge.

Levinas, E. (2001 [1947]). *Existence and existents.* A. Lingis (trans.). Pittsburgh, PA: Duquesne University Press.

Levinas, E. (2016 [1961]). *Totality and infinity: an essay on exteriority.* A. Lingis. (trans.). Pittsburgh, PA: Duquesne University Press.

Levine, B. & Land, H. M. (2015). 'A meta-synthesis of qualitative findings about dance/movement therapy for individuals with trauma' *Qualitative Health Research* 26(3): 330–344.

Levine, P. A. (2010). *In an unspoken voice: how the body releases trauma and restores goodness.* Berkeley, CA: North Atlantic Books.

Levine, P. A. with Frederick, A. (1997). *Waking the tiger: healing trauma.* Berkeley, CA: North Atlantic Books.

Lewey, J. H., Smith, C. L., Burcham, B., Saunders, N. L., Elfallal, D. & O'Toole, S. K. (2018). 'Comparing the effectiveness of EMDR and TF-CBT for children and adolescents: a meta-analysis' *Journal of Child & Adolescent Trauma* 11: 457–472.

Lewis, A. M. (2014). 'Terror management theory applied clinically: implications for existential-integrative psychotherapy' *Death Studies* 38(6): 412–417.

Lewis, S. L., Arseneault, L., Caspi, A., Fisher, H. L., Matthews, T., Moffitt, T. E., Odgers, C. L., Stahl, D., Teng, J. Y. & Danese, A. (2019). 'The epidemiology of trauma and post-traumatic stress disorder in a representative cohort of young people in England and Wales' *Lancet Psychiatry* 6(3): 247–256.

Leys, R. (2000). *Trauma: a genealogy*. London: University of Chicago Press.

Likierman, M. (1995). 'The debate between Anna Freud and Melanie Klein: an historical survey' *Journal of Child Psychotherapy* 21(3): 313–325.

Lindquist, K. A., Wager, T. D., Kober, H., Bliss-Moreau, E. & Feldman Barrett, L. (2012). 'The brain basis of emotion: a meta-analytic review' *Behavioral and Brain Sciences* 35(3): 121–143.

Loparic, Z. (2002). 'Winnicott's paradigm outlined' *Revista Latinoamericana de Psicopatologia Fundamental* 5(1): 61–98.

Lucas, M. (2004 [1959]). 'Existential regret: a crossroads of existential anxiety and existential guilt'. *Journal of Humanistic Psychology* 44(1): 58–70.

Lucero, I. (2018). 'Written in the body? Healing the epigenetic molecular wounds of complex trauma through empathy and kindness' *Journal of Child & Adolescent Trauma* 11(4): 443–455.

Lupton, D. (1993). 'Risk as moral danger: the social and political functions of risk discourse in public health' *International Journal of Health Services* 23(3): 425–435.

Lupton, D. (2004). 'Foucault and the medicalisation critique' in G. Scambler (ed.) *Medical sociology: major themes in health and social welfare. Vol. 1: the nature of medical sociology.* London: Routledge, pp. 245–258.

Lupton, D. (2013a). *Risk* (2nd ed.). New York: Routledge.

Lupton, D. (2013b). 'Risk and emotion: towards an alternative theoretical perspective' *Health, Risk & Society* 15(8): 634–647.

Lupton, D. (2016). *The quantified self: a sociology of self-tracking*. Cambridge, UK: Polity Press.

Luyten, P. & Fonagy, P. (2015). 'The neurobiology of mentalizing' *Personality Disorders* 6(4): 366–379.

Luyten, P. & Fonagy, P. (2019). 'Mentalizing and trauma' in A. W. Bateman & P. Fonagy (eds) *Handbook of mentalizing in mental health practice* (2nd ed.). Washington, DC: American Psychiatric Association, pp. 79–102.

Luyten, P., Malcorps, S., Fonagy, P. & Ensink, K. (2019). 'Assessment of mentalizing' in A. W. Bateman & P. Fonagy (eds) *Handbook of mentalizing in mental health practice* (2nd ed.). Washington, DC: American Psychiatric Association, pp. 37–62.

Lyons-Ruth, K. & Block, D. (1996). The disturbed caregiving system: relations among childhood trauma, maternal caregiving, and infant affect and attachment' *Infant Mental Health Journal* 17(3): 257–275.

Lyons-Ruth, K. & Spielman, E. (2004). 'Disorganized infant attachment strategies and helpless-fearful profiles of parenting: integrating attachment research with clinical intervention' *Infant Mental Health Journal* 25(4): 318–335.

Mackey, T. F., Hacker, S. S., Weissfeld, L. A., Ambrose, N. C., Fisher, M. G. & Zobel, D. L. (1991). 'Comparative effects of sexual assault on sexual functioning of child sexual abuse survivors and others' *Issues in Mental Health Nursing* 12(1): 89–112.

MacLean, P. D. (1990). *The triune brain in evolution: role in paleocerebral functions*. New York: Plenum.

Macquarrie, J. (1972). *Existentialism*. London: Penguin.

Maercker A., Brewin, C. R., Bryant, R. A., Cloitre, M., van Ommeren, M., Jones, L. M., Humayan, A., Kagee, A., Llosa, A. E., Rousseau, C., Somasundaram, D. J., Souza, R., Suzuki, Y., Weissbecker, I. & Wessely, S. C. (2013). 'Diagnosis and classification of disorders specifically associated with stress: proposals for ICD-11' *World Psychiatry* 12(3): 198–206.

Mai, F. M. & Merskey, H. (1981). 'Briquet's concept of hysteria: an historical perspective' *Canadian Journal of Psychiatry* 26(1): 57–63.

Main, M. & Hesse, E. (1990). 'Parents' unresolved traumatic experiences are related to infant disorganized attachment status: us frightened and/or frightening parental behavior the linking mechanism?' in M. Greenberg, D. Cicchetti & E. M. Cummings (eds) *Attachment in the preschool years: theory, research and intervention*. Chicago: University of Chicago Press, pp. 161–184.

Main, M. & Solomon, J. (1990). 'Procedures for identifying infants as disorganized/disoriented during the Ainsworth strange situation' in M. Greenberg, D. Cicchetti & E. M. Cummings (eds) *Attachment in the preschool years: theory, research and intervention*. Chicago: University of Chicago Press, pp. 121–160.

Marcel, G. (1949). *Being and having*. K. Farrer (trans.). Glasgow: Glasgow University Press.

Marcel, G. (1950). *The mystery of being: reflection and mystery*. G. S. Fraser (trans.). London: Harvill Press.

Marcel, G. (1952 [1927]). *Metaphysical journal*. B. Wall (trans.). Chicago, IL: Henry Regnery.

Marlock, G. & Weiss, H. with Young, C. & Soth, M. (2015). *The handbook of body psychotherapy & somatic psychology*. Berkeley, CA: North Atlantic Books.

Masson, J. M. (1984). *The assault on truth: Freud's suppression of the seduction theory*. New York: Farrar, Strauss & Giroux.

Masten, A. S. (2014). *Ordinary magic: resilience in development*. London: Guilford Press.

Maté, G. (2019 [2003]). *When the body says no: the cost of hidden stress*. London: Vermillion.

Matto, M., McNiel, D. E. & Binder, R. L. (2021). 'A systematic approach to the detection of false PTSD' *Journal of the American Academy of Psychiatry and the Law Online* 49(2): 325–334.

Maxfield, M. G. & Widom, C. S. (1996). 'The cycle of violence: revisited six years later' *Archives of Pediatric and Adolescent Medicine* 150(4): 390–395.

May, R. (1953). *Man's search for himself*. London: W. W. Norton.

May, R. (1958). 'Contributions of existential psychotherapy' in R. May, E. Angel & H. F. Ellenberger (eds) *Existence: a new dimension in psychiatry and psychology*. New York: Basic Books, pp. 37–91.

May, R. (1972). *Power and innocence*. New York: W. W. Norton.

May, R. (1992). *The art of counselling* (rev. ed.). London: Souvenir Press.

May, R. (2015 [1950]). *The meaning of anxiety*. London: W. W. Norton.

McCrory, E. J., Gerin, M. I. & Viding, E. (2017). 'Childhood maltreatment, latent vulnerability and the shift to preventative psychiatry – the contribution of functional brain imaging' *Journal of Child Psychology and Psychiatry* 58(4): 338–357.

McCrory, E. J., Puetz, V. B., Maguire, E. A., Mechelli, A., Palmer, A., Gerin, M. I., Kelly, P. A, Koutoufa, I. & Viding, E. (2017). 'Autobiographical memory: a candidate latent vulnerability mechanism for psychiatric disorder following childhood maltreatment' *British Journal of Psychiatry* 211(4): 216–222.

McCrory, E. J. & Viding, E. (2015). 'The theory of latent vulnerability: reconceptualizing the link between childhood maltreatment and psychiatric disorder' *Development and Psychopathology* 27(2): 493–505.

McLaughlin, K. A., Colich, N. L., Rodman & A. M. Weissman, D. G. (2020). 'Mechanisms linking childhood trauma exposure and psychopathology: a transdiagnostic model of risk and resilience' *BMC Medicine* 18: 96.

McLaughlin, K. A., Koenen, K. C., Hill, E. D., Petukhova, M., Sampson, N. A., Zaslavsky, A. M. & Kessler, R. C. (2013). 'Trauma exposure and posttraumatic stress disorder in a national sample of adolescents' *Journal of the American Academy of Child and Adolescent Psychiatry* 52(8): 815–830.

McNally, R. J. (2005). *Remembering trauma*. London: Belknap Press.

Mearns, D. & Cooper, M. (2018). *Working at relational depth in counselling and psychotherapy* (2nd ed.). London: SAGE.

Merleau-Ponty, M. (1968 [1964]). *The visible and the invisible.* C. Lefort (ed.), A. Lingis. (trans.). Evanston, IL: Northwestern University Press.

Merleau-Ponty, M. (2010 [2001]). *Child psychology and pedagogy: the Sorbonne lectures 1949–1952.* T. Welsh (trans.). Evanston, IL: Northwestern University Press.

Merleau-Ponty, M. (2012 [1945]). *Phenomenology of perception* [*Phénoménologie de la Perception*]. D. A. Landes (trans.). London: Routledge.

Mersky, J. P., Janczewski, C. E. & Topitzes, J. (2017). 'Rethinking the measurement of adversity: moving toward second-generation research on adverse childhood experiences' *Child Maltreatment* 22(1): 58–68.

Micale, M. C. (1985). 'The Salpetriere in the age of Charcot: an institutional perspective on medical history in the late nineteenth century' *Journal of Contemporary History* 20(4): 703–731.

Miller, A. (1984 [1981]). *Thou shalt not be aware: society's betrayal of the child.* H. & H. Hannum (trans.). New York: Farrar, Straus & Giroux.

Miller, A. (1990 [1980]). *For your own good: hidden cruelty in child-rearing and the roots of violence.* H. & H. Hannum (trans.). New York: Farrar, Straus & Giroux.

Miller, A. (1990 [1988]). *Banished knowledge: facing childhood injuries.* L. Vennewitz (trans.). London: Doubleday.

Miller, J. A. (2009). 'The trauma of evil and the traumatological conception of forgiveness' *Continental Philosophy Review* 42: 401–419.

Miller, M. (2018). *The true 'drama of a gifted child': the phantom Alice Miller – the real person.* B. Rogers & R. Peterson (trans.). n.p.: Martin Miller.

Minkowski, E. (1958). 'Findings in a case of schizophrenic depression'. B. Bliss (trans.) in R. May, E. Angel & H. F. Ellenberger (eds) *Existence: a new dimension in psychiatry and psychology.* New York: Simon & Schuster, pp. 127–138.

Minkowski, E. (1970 [1933]). *Lived time: phenomenological and psychopathological studies.* Mitzel, N. (trans.). Evanston, IL: Northwestern University Press.

Minton, K., Ogden, P. & Pain, C. (2006). *Trauma and the body: a sensorimotor approach to psychotherapy.* London: W. W. Norton.

Mirea, D. & Hickes, M. (2011). 'Cognitive behavioural therapy and existential phenomenological psychotherapy: rival paradigms or fertile ground for therapeutic synthesis?' *Existential Analysis* 23(1): 15–31.

Mitchell, A. J. & Trawny, P. (2017). *Heidegger's black notebooks: responses to anti-Semitism.* New York: Columbia University Press.

Mondelli, V. & Dazzan, P. (2019). 'Childhood trauma and psychosis: moving the field forward' *Schizophrenia Research* 205: 1–3.

Morina, N., Koerssena, R. & Polletc, T. V. (2016). 'Interventions for children and adolescents with posttraumatic stress disorder: A meta-analysis of comparative outcome studies' *Clinical Psychology Review* 47: 41–54.

Morrison, A. P., Frame, L. & Larkin, W. (2003). 'Relationships between trauma and psychosis: a review and integration' *British Journal of Clinical Psychology* 42: 331–353.

Morton, T. (2018). *Being ecological.* London: Pelican.

Morton, T. (2019). *Humankind: solidarity with nonhuman people.* London: Verso.

Mudrik, L. & Maoz, U. (2015). '"Me & my brain": exposing neuroscience's closet dualism' *Journal of Cognitive Neuroscience* 27(2): 211–221.

Müller, J., Eliastam, J. & Trahar, S. (2020). *Unfolding narratives of ubuntu in southern Africa.* Oxford: Routledge.

National Collaborating Centre for Mental Health (NCCMH) (2019). *The improving access to psychological therapies manual*. London: NHS England.

National Institute for Health and Care Excellence (NICE). (2018). *NICE guideline [NG116]: Post-traumatic stress disorder*. Manchester: NICE.

National Institute for the Clinical Application of Behavioral Medicine. (2019). *How trauma can affect your window of tolerance* (infographic). www.nicabm.com/trauma-how-to-help-your-clients-understand-their-window-of-tolerance.

National Society for the Prevention of Cruelty to Children (NSPCC). (2020). *The impact of the coronavirus pandemic on child welfare: sexual abuse*. https://learning.nspcc.org.uk/media/2280/impact-of-coronavirus-pandemic-on-child-welfare-sexual-abuse.pdf.

Newbury, J., Arseneault, L., Moffitt, T. E., Caspi, A., Danese, A., Baldwin, J. R. & Fisher, H. (2018). 'Measuring childhood maltreatment to predict early-adult psychopathology: comparison of prospective informant-reports and retrospective self-reports' *Journal of Psychiatric Research* 96: 57–64.

NHS England, NHS Scotland, Scottish Government, ACC, BABCP, BACP, BPC, BPS, COSRT, GLADD, NCS, Pace, Pink Therapy, RCGP, RCPsych, Relate, UKCP (2015). *Memorandum of understanding on conversion therapy in the UK*. www.psychotherapy.org.uk/wp-content/uploads/2016/09/Memorandum-of-understanding-on-conversion-therapy.pdf.

Nicki, A. (2001). 'The abused mind: feminist theory, psychiatric disability, and trauma' *Hypatia* 16(4): 80–104.

Nicki, A. (2016). 'Borderline personality disorder, discrimination, and survivors of chronic childhood trauma' *International Journal of Feminist Approaches to Bioethics* 9(1): 218–245.

Nietzsche, F. (1914). *The will to power (book I and II): an attempted transvaluation of all values*. O. Levy (ed.), A. M. Ludovici (trans.). Edinburgh: T. N. Foulis.

Nietzsche, F. (1969 [1883]). *Thus spake Zarathustra*. R. J. Hollingdale (trans.). London: Penguin.

Norcross, J. C. (1987). 'A rational and empirical analysis of existential psychotherapy' *Journal of Humanistic Psychology* 27(1): 41–68.

Northoff, G. (2011). *Neuropsychoanalysis in practice: brain, self and objects*. Oxford: Oxford University Press.

Nuttall, M. D, (2019). 'Co-presence and the transpersonal field according to R. D. Laing: pointing towards holism' *Journal of Transpersonal Psychology* 51(2): 225–241.

Oei, T. I., Verhoeven, W. M. A., Westenberg, H. G. M., Zwart, F. M. & Van Ree, J. M. (1990). 'Anhedonia, suicide ideation and Dexamethasone non-suppression in depressed patients' *Journal of Psychiatric Research* 24(1): 25–35.

Office of National Statistics (ONS) (2020). *Domestic abuse during the coronavirus (COVID-19) pandemic, England and Wales: November 2020*. www.ons.gov.uk/peoplepopulationand community/crimeandjustice/articles/domesticabuseduringthecoronaviruscovid19pandemi cenglandandwales/november2020.

Ogden, P. (2015). 'Proximity, defence and boundaries with children and care-givers: a Sensorimotor psychotherapy perspective' *Children Australia* 40(2): 139–146.

Ogden, P. & Fisher, J. (2015). *Sensorimotor psychotherapy: interventions for trauma and attachment*. New York: W. W. Norton.

Ogden, P. & Minton, K. (2000). 'Sensorimotor psychotherapy: one method for processing traumatic memory' *Traumatology* 6(3): 149–173.

Paidoussis-Mitchell, C. (2012). 'Traumatic bereavement: a phenomenological study' *Existential Analysis* 23(1): 32–45.

Pat-Horenczyk, R., Zamir, O., Yochman, A., Schiff, M., Brickman, S., Lerner, M. & Brom, D. (2020). 'Long-term impact of maternal posttraumatic symptoms on children's regulatory functioning: a four-year follow-up study'. *Psychological Trauma: Theory, Research, Practice, and Policy* 12(2): 131–137.

Pears, K. C. & Capaldi, D. M. (2001). 'Intergenerational transmission of abuse: a two-generational prospective study of an at-risk sample' *Child Abuse & Neglect* 25(11): 1439–1461.

Perry, B. D. (2009). 'Examining child maltreatment through a neurodevelopmental lens: clinical applications of the neurosequential model of therapeutics' *Journal of Loss and Trauma* 14(4): 240–255.

Perry, B. D., Pollard, R. A., Blakley, T. L. Baker, W. L. & Vigilante, D. (1995). 'Childhood trauma, the neurobiology of adaptation, and "use-dependent" development of the brain: How "states" become "traits"' *Infant Mental Health Journal* 16(4): 271–291.

Perry, B. D. with Szalavitz, M. (2011). *Born for love: why empathy is essential and endangered* (rev. ed.). New York: HarperCollins.

Perry, B. D. with Szalavitz, M. (2017). *The boy who was raised as a dog and other stories from a child psychiatrist's notebook* (3rd ed.). New York: Basic Books.

Pesso, A. (1972). *Experience in action: a psychomotor psychology*. New York: New York University Press.

Pierce, L. (2014). 'The integrative power of dance/movement therapy: implications for the treatment of dissociation and developmental trauma' *The Arts in Psychotherapy* 41(1): 7–15.

Pihama, L. Tuhiwai Smith, L., Evans-Campbell, T., Kohu-Morgan, H., Cameron, N., Mataki, T., Te Nana, R., Skipper, H. & Southey, K. (2017). 'Investigating Māori approaches to trauma informed care' *Journal of Indigenous Wellbeing* 2(3): 18–31.

Pinel, P. H. (1806). *A treatise on insanity* [*Traité Médico-Philosophique Sur L'aliénation Mentale*], D. D. Davis (trans.). Sheffield: W. Todd.

Pitchford, D. B. (2009). 'The existentialism of Rollo May: an influence on trauma treatment' *Journal of Humanistic Psychology* 49(4): 441–461.

Policing and Crime Act [2017]. www.legislation.gov.uk/ukpga/2017/3/part/9/chapter/1/crossheading/pardons-for-certain-abolished-offences-etc/2017-05-02.

Porges, S. W. (2003). 'Social engagement and attachment: a phylogenetic perspective' *Annals of the New York Academy of Sciences* 1008: 31–47.

Porges, S. W. (2009). 'The polyvagal theory: new insights into adaptive reactions of the autonomic nervous system' *Cleveland Clinic Journal of Medicine* 76(2): 86–90.

Porges, S. W. (2011). *The polyvagal theory: neurophysiological foundations of emotions, attachment, communication, and self-regulation*. London: W. W. Norton.

Porter, R. (1985). 'Under the influence: mesmerism in England' *History Today* 35(9): 22–29.

Public Health Wales (2018). *Working to achieve a healthier future for Wales: long-term strategy 2018–30*. Cardiff: Public Health Wales.

Putnam, F. W. (1989). 'Pierre Janet and modern views of dissociation' *Journal of Traumatic Stress* 2(4): 413–429.

Pyszczynski, T. & Kesebir, P. (2011). 'Anxiety buffer disruption theory: a terror management account of post-traumatic stress disorder' *Anxiety, Stress, & Coping* 24(1): 3–26.

Quigg, Z., Wallis, S. & Butler, N. (2018). *Routine enquiry about adverse childhood experiences: implementation pack pilot evaluation (final report)*. Liverpool: LHMU Public Health Institute.

R v R [1991] UKHL 12.

R v R [1991] 3 WLR 767.

Rachman, S. (2015). 'The evolution of behaviour therapy and cognitive behaviour therapy' *Behaviour Research and Therapy* 64: 1–8.

Rank, O. (1936). *Will therapy: an analysis of the therapeutic process in terms of relationship*. New York: A. A. Knopf.

Rank, O. (2014 [1929]). *The trauma of birth*. Oxfordshire: Routledge.

Ratcliffe, M., Ruddell, M. & Smith, B. (2014). 'What is a "sense of foreshortened future?": a phenomenological study of trauma, trust, and time' *Frontiers in Psychology* 5(1026). doi:10.3389/fpsyg.2014.01026.

Read, J. & Mayne, R. (2017). 'Understanding the long-term effects of childhood adversities: beyond diagnosis and abuse' *Journal of Child & Adolescent Trauma* 10: 289–297.

Rellini, A. H. & Meston, C. M. (2011). 'Sexual self-schemas, sexual dysfunction, and the sexual responses of women with a history of childhood sexual abuse' *Archives of Sexual Behavior* 40(2): 351–362.

Renner, L. M. & Slack, K. S. (2006). 'Intimate partner violence and child maltreatment: understanding intra-and intergenerational connections' *Child Abuse & Neglect* 30(6): 599–617.

Reuben, A., Moffitt, T. E., Caspi, A., Belsky, D. W., Harrington, H., Schroeder, F., Hogan, S., Ramrakha, S., Poulton, R. & Danese, A. (2016). 'Lest we forget: comparing retrospective and prospective assessments of adverse childhood experiences in the prediction of adult health' *Journal of Child Psychology and Psychiatry* 57(10): 1103–1112.

Rogers, C. R. (1995 [1980]). *A way of being*. New York: Houghton Mifflin.

Rogers, C. R. (2004 [1961]). *On becoming a person: a therapist's view of psychotherapy*. London: Constable.

Rose, N. & Abi-Rached, J. (2013). *Neuro: the new brain science and the management of the mind*. Oxford: Princeton University Press.

Roth, M., Neuner, F. & Elbert, T. (2014). 'Transgenerational consequences of PTSD: risk factors for the mental health of children whose mothers have been exposed to the Rwandan genocide' *International Journal of Mental Health Systems* 8(12).

Rothschild, B. (2000). *The body remembers: the psychophysiology of trauma and trauma treatment*. London: W. W. Norton.

Rush, F. (1996 [1977]). 'The Freudian coverup' *Feminism & Psychology* 6(2): 261–276.

Rutter, M. (1999). 'Resilience concepts and findings: implications for family therapy' *Journal of Family Therapy* 21(2): 119–144.

Sagan, C. (1977). *The dragons of Eden: speculations on the evolution of human intelligence*. New York: Random House.

Salter Ainsworth, M. D., Blehar, M. C., Waters, E. & Wall, S. (2014 [1978]). *Patterns of attachment: a psychological study of the strange situation*. London: Psychology Press.

Sandel, M. (2012). *What money can't buy: the moral limits of markets*. London: Penguin.

Sarfati, G.-E. (2016). 'Meaning and trauma: from psychosocial recovery to existential affirmation. A note on V. Frankl's contribution to the treatment of psychological trauma' in A. Batthyány (ed.) *Logotherapy and existential analysis: proceedings of the Viktor Frankl Institute, Vienna* (vol. 1). Basel, Switzerland: Springer, pp. 237–243.

Sartre, J.-P. (2003 [1943]). *Being and nothingness: an essay on phenomenological ontology* (2nd ed.). H. E. Barnes (trans.). London: Routledge.

Sartre, J.-P. (2007 [1946]). *Existentialism is a humanism [L'Existentialisme est un humanisme]*. C. Macomber. (trans.). London: Yale University Press.

Scaer, R. (2014). *The body bears the burden: trauma, dissociation, and disease*. London: Routledge.

Scalzo, C. (2010). *Therapy with children: an existential perspective*. London: Karnac Books.

Scambler, G. (1989). *Epilepsy*. London: Tavistock.

Scambler, G. & Hopkins, A. (1986). 'Being epileptic: coming to terms with illness' *Sociology of Health & Illness* 8(1): 26–43.

Schauer, M., Neuner, F. & Elbert, T. (2011). *Narrative exposure therapy: a short-term treatment for traumatic stress disorders (second revised and expanded edition)*. Göttingen: Hogrefe.

Schierholz, A., Krüger, A., Barenbrügge, J. & Ehring, T. (2016). 'What mediates the link between childhood trauma and depression? The role of emotion dysregulation, attachment, and attributional style' *European Journal of Psychotraumatology* 7: 32652.

Schmid, M., Petermann, F. & Fegert, J. M. (2013). 'Developmental trauma disorder: pros and cons of including formal criteria in the psychiatric diagnostic systems' *BMC Psychiatry* 13(3). www.ncbi.nlm.nih.gov/pmc/articles/PMC3541245/pdf/1471-244X-13-3.pdf.

Schneider, K. J. (2008). 'From segregation to integration' in K. J. Schneider (ed.) *Existential-integrative psychotherapy: guideposts to the core of practice*. Oxon: Routledge, pp. 15–22.

Schneider, K. J. (2011). 'Awakening to an awe-based psychology' *The Humanistic Psychologist* 39(3): 247–252.

Schnyder, U., Ehlers, A., Elbert, T., Foa, E. B., Gersons, B P. R. Resick, P. A., Shapiro, F. & Cloitre, M. (2015). 'Psychotherapies for PTSD: what do they have in common?' *European Journal of Psychotraumatology* 6: 28186.

Schopenhauer, A. (2004 [1850]). *On the suffering of the world*. London: Penguin.

Schütz, A. (1967 [1932]. *The phenomenology of the social world*. G. Walsh & F. Lehnert (trans.). Evanston, IL: Northwestern University Press.

Schütz, A. & Luckmann, T. (1973). *The structures of the life-world* (vol. 1). R. M. Zaner & H. T. Engelhardt (trans.). Evanston, IL: Northwestern University Press.

Schütz, A. & Luckmann, T. (1989 [1983]). *The structures of the life-World* (vol. 2). R. M. Zaner & D. J. Parent (trans.). Evanston, IL: Northwestern University Press.

Schwartz, C. (2016). *In the mind fields: exploring the new science of neuropsychoanalysis*. London: Vintage.

Schwartz, R. C. (2021). *No bad parts: healing trauma and restoring wholeness with the internal family systems model*. Boulder, CO: SoundsTrue.

Schwartz, R. C. & Sweezy, M. (2020). *Internal family systems therapy* (2nd ed.). New York: Guilford Press.

Science and Technology Committee (2018). *Evidence-based early years Intervention (inquiry report)*. London: House of Commons.

Scottish Government (2017). *A nation with ambition: the government's programme for Scotland 2017–18*. Edinburgh: Scottish Government.

Seligman, S. (2016). 'Disorders of temporality and the subjective experience of time: unresponsive objects and the vacuity of the future' *Psychoanalytic Dialogues* 26(2): 110–128.

Sexual Offences Act [2003]. www.legislation.gov.uk/ukpga/2003/42/contents.

Shah, P. E., Fonagy, P. & Strathearn, L. (2010). 'Is attachment transmitted across generations? The plot thickens' *Clinical Child Psychology and Psychiatry* 15(3): 329–345.

Shapiro, F. (2018). *Eye-movement desensitization and reprocessing (EMDR) therapy: basic principles, protocols, and procedures* (3rd ed.). London: Guilford Press.

Sharpe Lohrasbe, R. & Ogden, P. (2017). 'Somatic resources: sensorimotor psychotherapy approach to stabilising arousal in child and family treatment' *Australian and New Zealand Journal of Family Therapy* 38: 573–581.

Shaw, C. & Proctor, G. (2005). 'Women at the margins: a critique of the diagnosis of borderline personality disorder' *Feminism & Psychology* 15(4): 483–490.

Sherin, J. E. & Nemeroff, C. (2011). 'Post-traumatic stress disorder: the neurobiological impact of psychological trauma' *Dialogues in Clinical Neuroscience* 13(3): 263–278.

Sidebotham, P., Golding, J. & ALSPAC Study Team – Avon Longitudinal Study of Parents and Children (2001). 'Child maltreatment in the "children of the nineties": a longitudinal study of parental risk factors' *Child Abuse & Neglect* 25(9): 1177–1200.

Siegel, D. J. (2006). 'An interpersonal neurobiology approach to psychotherapy' *Psychiatric Annals* 36(4): 248–256.

Siegel, D. J. (2020). *The developing mind: how relationships and the brain interact to shape who we are* (3rd ed.). New York: Guilford Press.

Siegel, D. J. & Solomon, M. (2003). *Healing trauma: attachment, mind, body and brain*. London: W. W. Norton.

Siegel, E. H., Sands, M. K., van den Noortgate, W., Condon, P., Chang, Y., Dy, J., Quigley, K. S. & Feldman Barrett, L. (2018). Emotion fingerprints or emotion populations: a meta-analytic investigation of autonomic features of emotion categories' *Psychological Bulletin* 144(4): 343–393.

Silberman, S. (2015). *NeuroTribes: the legacy of autism and how to think smarter about people who think differently*. London: Allen & Unwin.

Simon, W. (2009). 'Mourning the person one could have become: the existential transition for the psychotherapy clients experienced by abuse or neglect' *Aggression and Violent Behavior* 14: 423–432.

Smith, C. (2020). Personal correspondence with the author.

Smith, C. U. M. (2010). 'The triune brain in antiquity: Plato, Aristotle, Erasistratus' *Journal of the History of the Neurosciences* 19(1): 1–14.

Smith, D. (2014). 'The diminished resistance to medicalization in psychiatry: psychoanalysis meets the medical model of mental illness' *Society and Mental Health* 4(2): 75–91.

Smith, E. (1998). *Touch in psychotherapy: theory, research and practice*. New York: Guilford Press.

Solinski, S. (2020a). 'Recovered memories of child sexual abuse: forgetting to remember and remembering to forget. Part 1: a perennial controversy' *Frontiers in the Psychotherapy of Trauma and Dissociation* 4(1): 17–27.

Solinski, S. (2020b). 'Recovered memories of child sexual abuse: forgetting to remember and remembering to forget. Part 2: the nature of memory and ordinary forgetting' *Frontiers in the Psychotherapy of Trauma and Dissociation* 4(1): 28–61.

Solinski, S. (2020c). 'Recovered memories of child sexual abuse: forgetting to remember and remembering to forget. Part 3: the role of disassociation in extraordinary forgetting' *Frontiers in the Psychotherapy of Trauma and Dissociation* 4(1): 62–92.

Solms, M. (2004). 'Freud returns' *Scientific American* 290(5): 82–88.

Song, S. J., Tol, W. & de Jong, J. (2014). 'Indero: intergenerational trauma and resilience between Burundian former child soldiers and their children' *Family Process* 53(2): 239–251.

Spinelli, E. (2005). *The interpreted world: an introduction to phenomenological psychology* (2nd ed.). London: SAGE.

Spinelli, E. (2015). *Practising existential therapy: the relational world* (2nd ed.). London: SAGE.

Stanek, D. (2015). 'Bridging past and present: embodied intergenerational trauma and the implications for dance/movement therapy' *Body, Movement and Dance in Psychotherapy* 10(2): 94–105.

Steenkamp, J. O. (2012). 'Introducing SHIPB as a psychotherapeutic model to access the body memory of traumatised clients: depathologising expressions of trauma' *South African Journal of Psychology*, 42(2): 202–213.

Steiner, C. M. (1990). *Scripts people live: transactional analysis of life scripts* (2nd ed.). New York: Grove Press.

Stern, D. B. (2003). *Unformulated experience: from dissociation to imagination in psychoanalysis*. Mahwah, NJ: Analytic Press.

Stern, D. B. (2010). *Partners in thought: working with unformulated experience, dissociation, and enactment*. Hove: Routledge.

Stern, D. B. (2017). 'Unformulated experience, dissociation, and *Nachträglichkeit*' *Journal of Analytical Psychology* 62(4): 501–525.

Stern, D. B. (2019). *The infinity of the unsaid: unformulated experience, language, and the nonverbal.* Oxon: Routledge.

Stolorow, R. D. (2003). 'Trauma and temporality' *Psychoanalytic Psychology* 20(1): 158–161.

Stolorow, R. D. (2007). *Trauma and human existence: autobiographical, psychoanalytic, and philosophical reflections.* Oxon: Analytic Press.

Stolorow, R. D. (2011a). 'Portkeys, eternal recurrence, and the phenomenology of traumatic temporality' *International Journal of Psychoanalytic Self Psychology* 6(3): 433–436.

Stolorow, R. D. (2011b). 'Toward greater authenticity: from shame to existential guilt, anxiety, and grief' *International Journal of Psychoanalytic Self Psychology* 6(2): 285–287.

Stolorow, R. D. (2011c). *World, affectivity, trauma: Heidegger and post-Cartesian psychoanalysis.* London: Routledge.

Stolorow, R. D. (2019a). 'Emotional disturbance, trauma and authenticity: a phenomenological-contextualist perspective' in R. D. Stolorow & G. E. Atwood *The power of phenomenology: psychoanalytic and philosophical perspectives.* Oxon: Routledge, pp. 71–84.

Stolorow, R. D. (2019b). 'Phenomenology and metaphysical realism' in R. D. Stolorow & G. E. Atwood *The power of phenomenology: psychoanalytic and philosophical perspectives.* Oxon: Routledge, pp. 97–104.

Stolorow, R. D. & Atwood, G. E. (2002 [1992]). *Contexts of being: the intersubjective foundations of psychological life.* London: Routledge.

Stolorow, R. D. & Atwood, G. E. (2019a). 'Experiencing selfhood is not "a self"' in R. D. Stolorow & G. E. Atwood *The power of phenomenology: psychoanalytic and philosophical perspectives.* Oxon: Routledge, pp. 91–96.

Stolorow, R. D. & Atwood, G. E. (2019b). 'The phenomenology of language and the metaphysicalizing of the real' in R. D. Stolorow & G. E. Atwood *The power of phenomenology: psychoanalytic and philosophical perspectives.* Oxon: Routledge, pp. 85–90.

Stolorow, R. D. & Atwood, G. E. (2019c). 'Walking the tightrope of emotional dwelling' in R. D. Stolorow & G. E. Atwood *The power of phenomenology: psychoanalytic and philosophical perspectives.* Oxon: Routledge, pp. 113–118.

Stolorow, R. D., Atwood, G. & Orange, D. (2002). *Worlds of experience: interweaving philosophical and clinical dimensions in psychoanalysis.* New York: Basic Books.

Tanaka, S. (2013). 'The notion of intercorporeality and its psychology' *Bulletin of Liberal Arts Education Center, Tokai University* 33: 101–109.

Tanaka, S. (2015). 'Intercorporeality as a theory of social cognition' *Theory & Psychology* 25(4): 455–472.

Tasca, C., Rapetti, M., Carta, M. G. & Fadda, B. (2012). 'Women and hysteria in the history of mental health' *Clinical Practice & Epidemiology in Mental Health* 8: 110–119.

Tedeschi, R. G. & Calhoun, L. G. (2004). 'Posttraumatic growth: conceptual foundations and empirical evidence' *Psychological Inquiry* 15(1): 1–18.

Teicher, M. H. & Samson, J. A. (2013). 'Childhood maltreatment and psychopathology: a case for ecophenotypic variants as clinically and neurobiologically distinct subtypes' *American Journal of Psychiatry* 70(10): 1114–1133.

Thomä, H. & Cheshire, N. (1991). 'Freud's *Nachträglichkeit* and Strachey's "deferred action": trauma, constructions and the direction of causality' *International Review of Psycho-Analysis* 18: 407–427.

Thornberry, T. P., Knight, K. E. & Lovegrove, P. J. (2012). 'Does maltreatment beget maltreatment? A systematic review of the intergenerational literature' *Trauma, Violence, & Abuse* 13(3): 135–152.

Tillich, P. (2000 [1952]). *The courage to be* (2nd ed.). New Haven, CT: Yale University Press.

Tord, P. & Bräuninger, I. (2015). 'Grounding: theoretical application and practice in dance movement therapy' *The Arts in Psychotherapy* 43(1): 16–22.

Totten, N. (2015). *Embodied relating: the ground of psychotherapy*. Oxon: Karnac Books.

Tulloch, J. & Lupton, D. (2003). *Risk and everyday life*. London: SAGE.

Ungar, M., Ghazinour, M. & Richter, J. (2013). 'Annual research review: what is resilience within the social ecology of human development?' *Journal of Family Therapy* 54(4): 348–366.

United Nations High Commissioner for Refugees (UNHCR) (2012). *The Buddhist core values and perspective for protection challenges: faith and protection*. Geneva, Switzerland: UNHCR.

Vachon, M., Bessette, P. C. & Goyette, C. (2016). 'Growing from an invisible wound: a humanistic-existential approach to PTSD' in G. El-Baalbaki & C. Fortin (eds) *A multidimensional approach to post-traumatic stress disorder: from theory to practice*. London: IntechOpen, pp. 179–203.

van der Hart, O. & Horst, R. (1989). 'The dissociation theory of Pierre Janet' *Journal of Traumatic Stress* 2(4): 397–412.

van der Hart, O., van Dijke, A., van Son, M. & Steele, K. (2001). 'Somatoform dissociation in traumatized World War I combat soldiers: a neglected clinical heritage' *Journal of Trauma & Dissociation* 1(4): 33–66.

van der Kolk, B. A. (1989). 'The compulsion to repeat the trauma: re-enactment, revictimization, and masochism' *Psychiatric Clinics of North America* 12(2): 389–411.

van der Kolk, B. (2005). 'Developmental trauma disorder: toward a rational diagnosis for children with complex trauma histories' *Psychiatric Annals* 35(5): 401–408. www.traumacenter.org/products/Developmental_Trauma_Disorder.pdf.

van der Kolk, B. (2006). 'Clinical implications of neuroscience research in PTSD' *Annals of the New York Academy of Sciences* 1071: 277–293.

van der Kolk, B. (2014). *The body keeps score: mind, brain and body in the transformation of trauma*. London: Penguin.

van der Kolk, B. A. & van der Hart, O. (1989). 'Pierre Janet and the breakdown of adaptation in psychological trauma' *American Journal of Psychiatry* 146(12): 1530–1540.

van der Kolk, B. A., Brown, P. & van der Hart, O. (1989). 'Pierre Janet on post-traumatic stress' *Journal of Traumatic Stress* 2(4): 365–378.

van der Kolk, B. A., Weiseath, L. & van der Hart, O. (1996). 'History of trauma in psychiatry' in B. A. van der Kolk, A. C. McFarlane & L. Weisaeth (eds) *Traumatic stress: the effects of overwhelming experience on mind, body and society*. London: Guilford Press, pp. 47–75.

van Deurzen, E. (2010). *Everyday mysteries: a handbook of existential psychotherapy* (2nd ed.). Sussex: Routledge.

van Deurzen, E. (2012). *Existential counselling & psychotherapy in practice* (3rd ed.). London: SAGE.

van Deurzen, E. & Adams, M. (2016). *Skills in existential counselling & psychotherapy* (2nd ed.). London: SAGE.

van Deurzen, E. & Arnold-Baker, C. (2018). *Existential therapy: distinctive features*. Oxon: Routledge.

van Deurzen, E., Craig, E., Längle, A., Schneider, K. J., Tantam, D., du Plock, S. (2019). *The Wiley world handbook of existential psychotherapy*. Chichester: Wiley Blackwell.

van IJzendoorn, M. H., Bakermans-Kranenburg, M. J. & Sagi-Schwartz, A. (2003). 'Are children of Holocaust survivors less well-adapted? A meta-analytic investigation of secondary traumatization' *Journal of Traumatic Stress* 16: 459–469.

Varese, F., Smeets, F., Drukker, M., Lieverse, R., Lataster, T., Viechtbauer, W., Read, J., van Os, J. & Bentall, R. P. (2012). 'Childhood adversities increase the risk of psychosis: a meta-analysis of patient-control, prospective- and cross-sectional cohort studies' *Schizophrenia Bulletin* 38(4): 661–671.

Vogt, R. (2018). 'Trauma severity: parallels between SPIM 30 and polyvagal theory' in S. W. Porges & D. Dana (eds) *Clinical applications of the polyvagal theory: the emergence of Polyvagal-informed therapies*. London: W. W. Norton, pp. 285–302.

Vos, J. (2018). *Meaning in life: an evidence-based handbook for practitioners*. London: Palgrave Macmillan.

Wang, X. (2011). 'Zhi Mian and existential psychology' *The Humanistic Psychologist* 39(3): 240–246.

Wang, X. (2016). 'Zhi Mian: approaching healing/therapy through facing reality: a Chinese approach to existential thinking and practice (lecture from World Congress for Existential Therapy 2015) *Existential Analysis* 27(1): 4–15.

Wang, X. (2019). 'The symbol of the iron house: from survivalism to existentialism' in L. Hoffman, M. Yang, M. Mansilla, J. Dias, M. Moats & T. Claypool (eds) *Existential psychology East–West*. Colorado Springs, CO: University Professors Press, pp. 3–16.

Waters, E., Merrick, S. Treboux, D. Crowell, J. & Albersheim, L. (2000). 'Attachment security in infancy and early adulthood: a twenty-year longitudinal study' *Child Development* 71(3): 684–689.

Weiser, D. A. (2017). 'Confronting myths about sexual assault: a feminist analysis of the false report literature' *Family Relations* 66(1): 46–60.

Weissman, D. G., Bitran, D., Bryant Miller, A, Schaefer, J. D., Sheridan, M. A. & McLaughlin, K. A. (2019). 'Difficulties with emotion regulation as a transdiagnostic mechanism linking child maltreatment with the emergence of psychopathology' *Development and Psychopathology* 31(3): 899–915.

Widom, C. S. (1989a). 'The cycle of violence' *Science* 244(4901): 160–166.

Widom, C. S. (1989b). 'Does violence beget violence: a critical examination of the literature?' *Psychological Bulletin* 106(1): 3–28.

Widom, C. S. (1999). 'Post-traumatic stress disorder in abused and neglected children grown up' *American Journal of Psychiatry* 156(8): 1223–1229.

Widom, C. S., Czaja, S. & DuMont, K. A. (2015). 'Intergenerational transmission of child abuse and neglect: real or detection bias?' *Science* 347(6229): 1480–1485.

Widom, C. S. & Osborn, M. (2021). 'The cycle of violence: abused and neglected girls to adult female offenders' *Feminist Criminology* 16(3): 266–285.

Wilde, O. (1907 [1897]). *De Profundis: the writings of Oscar Wilde*. H. Zick (trans.). London: A. R. Keller.

Wilson, P. M. & Appel, S. W. (2013). 'Existential counselling and psychotherapy and Māori clients' *Asia Pacific Journal of Counselling and Psychotherapy* 4(2): 137–146.

Winnicott, D. W. (1953). 'Transitional objects and transitional phenomena: a study of the first not-me possession' *International Journal of Psychoanalysis* 34(2): 89–97.

Winnicott, D. W. (1974). 'Fear of breakdown' *International Review of Psycho-Analysis* 1(1–2): 103–107.

Winnicott, D. W. (1991 [1964]). *The child, the family, and the outside world*. London: Penguin.

Winnicott, D. W. (1991 [1971]). *Playing and reality*. London: Routledge.

Winnicott, D. W. (2006 [1965]). *The family and individual development*. London: Routledge.

Winnicott, D. W. (2018a [1965]). 'The concept of trauma in relation to the development of the individual within the family' in C. Winnicott, R. Shepherd & M. Davis (eds) *Psychoanalytic explorations*. London: Routledge, pp. 130–148.

Winnicott, D. W. (2018b [1965]). *The maturational processes and the facilitating environment: studies in the theory of emotional development*. Oxon: Routledge.

World Health Organisation (2018). *Adverse childhood experiences international questionnaire (ACE-IQ)*. Geneva, Switzerland: WHO.

World Health Organization (2019). *The international classification of diseases (proposed ICD-11)*. https://icd.who.int/browse11/l-m/en#/http%3a%2f%2fid.who.int%2ficd%2fentity%2f585833559.

Xun, L. (2009). *The real story of Ah-Q and other tales of China: the complete fiction of Lu Xun*. J. Lovell (trans.). London: Penguin.

Yalom, I. D. (1980). *Existential psychotherapy*. New York: Basic Books.

Yalom, I. D. (2011 [2008]). *Staring at the sun: overcoming the dread of death*. London: Piatkus.

Yalom, I. D. & Leszcz, M. (2005). *Theory and practice of group psychotherapy* (5th ed.). New York: Basic Books.

Yalom, I. D. & Yalom, M. (2021). *A matter of death and life: love, loss and what matters in the end*. London: Piatkus.

Yehuda, R. & Bierer, L. M. (2008). 'Transgenerational transmission of cortisol and PTSD risk' *Progress in Brain Research* 167: 121–135.

Yehuda, R., Daskalakis, N. P., Bierer, L. M., Bader, H. N., Klengel, T., Holsboer, F. & Binder, E. B. (2016). 'Holocaust exposure induced intergenerational effects on FKBP5 methylation' *Biological Psychiatry* 80(5): 372–380.

Yehuda, R., Lehrner, A. & Bierer, L. M. (2018). 'The public reception of putative epigenetic mechanisms in the transgenerational effects of trauma' *Environmental Epigenetics* 4(2): 1–7.

Young, A. (1995). *The harmony of illusions: inventing post-traumatic stress disorder*. Princeton, NJ: Princeton University Press.

Youssef, N. A., Lockwood, L., Su, S., Hao, G. & Rutten, B. P. F. (2018). 'The effects of trauma, with or without PTSD, on the transgenerational DNA methylation alterations in human offsprings' *Brain Sciences* 8(5): 83.

Zola, I. K. (1982). *Socio-medical inquiries: recollections, reflections and reconsiderations*. Philadelphia, PA: Temple University Press.

Zuravin, S., McMillen, C., DePanfilis, D & Risley-Curtiss, C. (1991). 'The intergenerational cycle of child maltreatment: continuity versus discontinuity' *Journal of Interpersonal Violence* 11: 315–334.

Zyromski, B., Dollarhide, C. T., Aras, Y., Geiger, S., Oehrtman, J. P. & Clarke, H. (2018). 'Beyond complex trauma: an existential view of adverse childhood experiences' *Journal of Humanistic Counselling* 57(3): 156–172.

Index

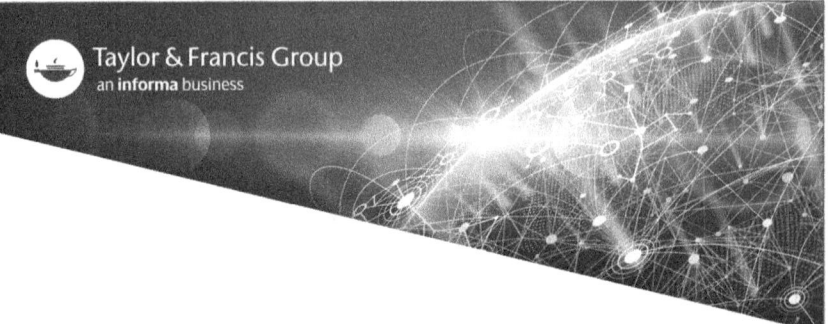
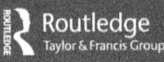
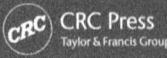